Case Studies in Urology

Case Studies in Urology

Editor: Bellamy Burton

AMERICAN
MEDICAL PUBLISHERS
www.americanmedicalpublishers.com

AMERICAN
MEDICAL PUBLISHERS
www.americanmedicalpublishers.com

Cataloging-in-Publication Data

Case studies in urology / edited by Bellamy Burton.
p. cm.
Includes bibliographical references and index.
ISBN 979-8-88740-618-3
1. Urology. 2. Genitourinary organs--Diseases. 3. Urinary organs--Diseases.
4. Evidence-based medicine. I. Burton, Bellamy.
RC871 .E85 2023
616.6--dc23

American Medical Publishers,
41 Flatbush Avenue,
1st Floor, New York,
NY 11217, USA

ISBN 979-8-88740-618-3 (Hardback)

Contents

Preface ... XI

Chapter 1 **Locally Recurrent Leiomyoma of the Bladder Refractory to Visually Complete Transurethral Resection: An Indication for Cystoprostatectomy** ... 1
Katharina Mitchell, John Barnard and Adam Luchey

Chapter 2 **A Rare Case of Isolated Ureteral Diaphragmatic Herniation: Case Report and Review of Literature** ... 4
Nassib Abou Heidar, Hussein Elsemesmani, Ahmad Elamine and Mustafa Natout

Chapter 3 **The Association of Renal Agenesis and Ipsilateral Seminal Vesicle Cyst: Zinner Syndrome Case Report** ... 8
Mishal AlArifi, Magdi Al-Gahwary and Mohamed Gomha

Chapter 4 **Subcutaneous Dorsal Penile Vein Thrombosis or Penile Mondor's Disease: A Case Report and Literature Review** ... 11
Adama Ouattara, Abdoul Karim Paré, Aristide F. Kaboré, Clotaire Yaméogo, Gnimdou Botcho, Désiré Ky, Abdoul Aziz Ouédraogo, Amidou Bako, Rigobert Kiba, Zakari Nikiéma and Timothée Kambou

Chapter 5 **Penile Fracture: Delayed Presentation, Primary Urethral Repair and Satisfactory Outcome** ... 14
Bashir Yunusa, Kalamon Wullie, Soeghen E. Willie, Solomane Konneh, Swaliho Sherriff, Ayun Cassell and Edit Ikpi

Chapter 6 **A Paratesticular Angiolipoma: A Case Report of a Rare Benign Scrotal Mass and Review of Literature** ... 18
Mohamed Ali Nouioui, Tarek Taktak, Seif Mokadem, Faten Gargouri, Houssem Mediouni, Ramzi Khiari and Samir Ghozzi

Chapter 7 **Organ-Sparing Surgery for a Giant Verrucous Carcinoma of the Penile Shaft: A Case Report and Review of the Literature** ... 21
Prodromos Philippou, Christos Kitsios, Maria Miliatou, Christiana Poullou and Pavlos Konstantinou

Chapter 8 **Perinephric Hematoma with Active Arterial Hemorrhage following Extracorporeal Shockwave Lithotripsy** ... 25
Edward Assaf, Rawad Abou Zahr, Elie Ghabi and Imad Ghantous

Chapter 9 **Unusual Mechanisms of Penile Amputation** ... 28
Julian Fazi, David Adkins, Jennifer Knight and Adam Luchey

Chapter 10 **Tumefactive Fat Necrosis with Multinucleate Giant Cell Reaction Mimicking Recurrent Renal Cell Carcinoma following Percutaneous Renal Cryoablation** ... 32
Amanda E. Kahn, Kevin J. Wu and David D. Thiel

Chapter 11 **Plexiform Schwannoma of the Penis: A Rare Subtype of Genital Schwannoma** ... 36
Chrysovalantis Gkekas, Vasileios Kalyvas, Evangelos N. Symeonidis, Apostolos Malioris, Michail Papathanasiou, Nikolaos Kalinderis, Kyriakos Moisidis and Konstantinos Hatzimouratidis

Chapter 12 **Necrotizing Epididymo-Orchitis: A Rare Manifestation of COVID-19** ... 40
Ali Tavoosian, Sana Ahmadi and Seyed Mohammad Kazem Aghamir

Chapter 13 **The Intraoperative use of a Portable Cone-Beam Computed Tomography System for the Diagnosis of Intraperitoneal Bladder Perforation** ... 44
Ankur Choksi, Benjamin Press, Cayce Nawaf, Shannon Longyear, Marc Ferrante and Thomas V. Martin

Chapter 14 **A Mislocated Intrauterine Device Migrating to the Urinary Bladder: An Uncommon Complication Leading to Stone Formation** ... 48
Mohamed Ali Nouioui, Tarek Taktak, Seif Mokadem, Houssem Mediouni, Ramzi Khiari and Samir Ghozzi

Chapter 15 **Septic Shock Immediately following Percutaneous Suprapubic Catheterization** ... 52
Cale E. Leeson, Brianna-Lee Beaudry and Geoffrey R. Wignall

Chapter 16 **Pulmonary Embolism following Percutaneous Nephrolithotomy: An Uncommon and Life-Threatening Complication** ... 55
Spyridon Paparidis, Antonios Katsimantas, Dimitrios Oikonomidis and Nikolaos Ferakis

Chapter 17 **Exceptional Response of Metastatic Chromophobe Renal Cell Carcinoma to Vascular Endothelial Growth Factor (VEGF) Inhibitors: Should Increased VEGF-C Expression be used to Guide Treatment?** ... 59
Jacob W. Bruinius, Karl J. Dykema, Sabrina L. Noyes, Bin Tean Teh and Brian R. Lane

Chapter 18 **Macrocystic Adult Penile Lymphangioma: A Rare Presentation** ... 65
Jaisukh Kalathia, Kaushal Patel and Santosh Agrawal

Chapter 19 **Colon Cancer Metastasis to the Right Testis: Case Report and Review of Literature** ... 68
Mizuki Kasahara, Tomo Shimizu, Hiroshi Aoki, Mizuho Okawa, Fumito Yamabe, Hideyuki Kobayashi, Koichi Nagao, Koichi Nakajima and Yozo Mitsui

Chapter 20 **Doubling of Decipher Biopsy Genomic Score is Related to Disease Reclassification on Subsequent Surveillance Biopsy but not Adverse Features on Radical Prostatectomy** ... 72
Kamyar Ghabili, Nathan Paulson, Jamil S. Syed, Cayce B. Nawaf, Ghazal Khajir, Darryl T. Martin, John Onofrey, Michael S. Leapman, Angelique Levi, Jeffrey C. Weinreb, Peter A. Humphrey and Preston C. Sprenkle

Chapter 21 **Reconstruction of a Scrotum by Combining Two Skin Flaps in a Ball Shape** ... 76
Kazuya Kashiyama, Motoi Nakano, Akihito Higashi, Shoko Ashizuka, Yuki Moriuchi, Atsuhiko Iwao and Katsumi Tanaka

Chapter 22 **Bladder Leiomyoma with Synchronous Solitary Fibrous Tumor of the Pleura** ... 82
Charalampos Mavridis, George Georgiadis, Eleni D. Lagoudaki, Iordanis Skamagkas, Ioannis Heretis, Anastasios V. Koutsopoulos and Charalampos Mamoulakis

Chapter 23 **Extensive Prostatic Abscess in an Elderly Patient Requiring Multidisciplinary Drainage** 86
John Michael Nesemann, Kathy Huen and Jonathan Bergman

Chapter 24 **Male Perineal Carcinoma: Experience in 4 Cases and Literature Review** 92
Agustín Fraile Poblador, Manuel Hevia Palacios, Manuel Rodríguez Vegas, Alberto Artiles Medina, Enrique Sanz Mayayo, Silvia García Barreras, Guillermo Fernández Conejo, Rafael Rodríguez Patrón, Varona Crespo Constatino, Ana Saiz González and Javier Burgos Revilla

Chapter 25 **Functional Bladder Paraganglioma Treated by Partial Cystectomy** 97
Amine Hermi, Hamza Ichaoui, Aziz Kacem, Houcem Hedhli, Faten Gargouri, Ramzi Khiari and Samir Ghozzi

Chapter 26 **Isolated Fungal Balls in Urinary Bladder Presenting as Acute Retention of Urine** 101
Tariq Hameed, Sudhir Kumar Jain, Faiz Manzar Ansari and Amrita Dua

Chapter 27 **Delayed Presentation of Iliac Vein Injury: A Severe Complication at Retropubic Midurethral Sling Arm Removal** 104
Pansy Uberoi and Forrest Jellison

Chapter 28 **A Rare Case Report of Giant Urinary Bladder Stone Causing Recurrent Dysuria in a Woman** 107
Rojan Adhikari, Hari Prasad Baral, Utsav Bhattarai, Ravi Kiran Gautam, Kiran Jung Kunwar, Dipesh Shrestha and Bijay Mansingh Katwal

Chapter 29 **Ureteral Diaphragmatic Hernia Treated with Ureteral Stenting: A Case Report and Review of the Literature** 110
Tateki Yoshino, Ayako Itakura, Shinnosuke Fujikawa, Tomoyuki Sugitani, Kazuo Kawakami, Emi Ishibashi, Koji Kodama and Shota Oshima

Chapter 30 **Initial Diagnosis and Detection of Very Late Local Recurrence of a Ductal Prostate Cancer due to a Ureteral Stone** 115
Manolis Pratsinis, Charlotte Düwel, Olivia Köhle, Annette Enzler-Tschudy, Hans-Peter Schmid and Patrick Betschart

Chapter 31 **Total Penectomy for Recurrent Chordoma of the Corpus Cavernosum** 119
Lennert Eismann, Sabine Kess, Christian G. Stief and Frank Strittmatter

Chapter 32 **Vulvar Pyogenic Granuloma in Adult Female Population: A Case Report and Review of the Literature** 123
Nastaran Mahmoudnejad, Alireza Zadmehr and Mohammad Hamidi Madani

Chapter 33 **Leptomeningeal Carcinomatosis in Urothelial Carcinoma of the Urinary Bladder: A Report of a Patient with a Fulminant Course Who Died of Cancer after Definitive Therapies** 127
Masayuki Tomioka, Makoto Kawase, Daiki Kato, Manabu Takai, Koji Iinuma, Kengo Horie, Keita Nakane, Natsuko Suzui, Tatsuhiko Miyazaki and Takuya Koie

Chapter 34 **Effectiveness of Steroid Pulse Therapy for Systemic Side Effects after Bacillus Calmette-Guérin Intravesical Instillation Therapy: A Series of Five Cases** 131
Tatsuya Umemoto, Jun Naruse, Yukio Usui, Hidenori Zakoji, Hideshi Miyakita and Akira Miyajima

Chapter 35 **Squamous Cell Carcinoma Developing in a Buccal Mucosa Graft after Urethroplasty: A Report of 2 Cases of Malignant Degeneration** 137
Catti Massimo, Nappo Gerocarni Simona, Tadini Barbara, Cerchia Elisa, Ferrero Luisa, Gambella Alessandro, Pacchioni Donatella, Elisabetta Teruzzi, Marco Falcone, Sedigh Omidreza and Gontero Paolo

Chapter 36 **Clear Cell Adenocarcinoma of the Ureter Similar to Clear Cell Renal Cell Carcinoma Histology** 141
Kazuhiro Watanabe, Go Hasegawa, Yohei Ikeda, Noboru Hara and Tsutomu Nishiyama

Chapter 37 **Leptomeningeal Metastases in a Patient with Castration-Resistant Prostate Cancer** 145
Takuya Koie, Yasuhiro Hashimoto, Yuichiro Suzuki, Yoshiomi Hatayama and Futoshi Kimura

Chapter 38 **Pulsed Electromagnetic Field Therapy as a Complementary Alternative for Chronic Pelvic Pain Management in an Interstitial Cystitis/Bladder Pain Syndrome Patient** 148
Tyler L. Overholt, Christina Ross, Robert J. Evans and Stephen J. Walker

Chapter 39 **New Methods of Reconstruction for Old Challenges: The Use of the Integra Graft in Necrotizing Soft Tissue Infections of the Male Genitalia** 151
Katharina Mitchell, Chad Crigger, Chad Morley, John Barnard and Vidas Dumasius

Chapter 40 **Simultaneous Laparoscopic Surgery for Bladder Diverticulum and Urachal Remnant: A Case Report** 156
Masaki Murata, Kohei Inui, Moto Hasegawa, Yohei Ikeda, Yuki Nakagawa, Noboru Hara and Tsutomu Nishiyama

Chapter 41 **Penile Glans Amputation following Circumcision: A Case Report of a Rare Complication** 160
Salman Soltani, Mahdi Mottaghi, Amir Jafarpisheh and Mahmoud Tavakkoli

Chapter 42 **An Unusual Location for a Nonurachal Bladder Adenocarcinoma** 163
George Khludenev, Akshay Reddy, Sinan Akosman and Michael J. Whalen

Chapter 43 **Use of Cadaveric Pericardial Tissue in the Surgical Treatment of Neurogenic Bladder** 169
Madison Caja, Michaela Lamonde, John Barnard, Stanley Zaslau and Robert E. Shapiro

Chapter 44 **Rare Case of Multiple Perirenal, Extra-Adrenal Myelolipoma: Case Report, Current Management Options and Literature Review** 173
Goran Benko, Andrina Kopjar, Marin Plantak, Danijel Cvetko, Vicko Glunčić and Anita Lukić

Chapter 45 **Use of the T-1470 LiteTouch™ Laser in the En Bloc Resection of an Upper Tract Urothelial Cancer** 177
Ezra Shoen, Benjamin Zollinger, Tripp Gresham, Katayoon M. Rezaei and Michael Whalen

Chapter 46 **Rare Associations with Posterior Urethral Valves** 181
Ahmed Osama Mohamed, Bala Eradi, Anthony Owen and Ashok Rajimwale

Chapter 47 **A Giant Solitary Adrenal Plasmacytoma in a Patient with HIV: A Rare Case Report and Review of the Literature** ... 185
Mehdi Chennoufi, Ibrahim Boukhannous, Mohamed Mokhtari, Anouar El Moudane, Mohamed Irzi, Abdelghani Ouraghi, Issam Jandou, Achraf Miry and Ali Barki

Chapter 48 **Abdominoscrotal Hydrocele: An Uncommon Cause of Abdominoscrotal Cystic Swelling** ... 191
Manish Swarnkar and Pathan Tanveer Khan

Chapter 49 **A Conservative Approach to Inflammatory Myofibroblastic Tumor of the Bladder: A Case Report and Review of Literature** ... 194
Rawad Abou Zahr, Elie Ghabi, Mehdi Idrissi-Kaitouni and Thierry Roumeguere

Chapter 50 **Penile Glans Necrosis following Prostatic Artery Embolization for the Treatment of Benign Prostatic Hyperplasia: A Rare but Serious Complication** ... 198
Eric Chung

Chapter 51 **Brain Complete Response to Cabozantinib prior to Radiation Therapy in Metastatic Renal Cell Carcinoma** ... 201
An Uche, Chad Sila, Tad Tanoura, James Yeh, Neil Bhowmick, Edwin Posadas, Robert Figlin and Jun Gong

Chapter 52 **Pyelolithotomy in a Patient with Complete Coraliform Calcification Induced by a Double-J Ureteral Stent** ... 205
Miguel Bonfitto, Analaura de Oliveira Cury, Victoria Caroline Pagelkopf, Vinicius Ramos Bezerra de Morais and Carlos Abib Cury

Chapter 53 **Normotensive, Oversized Pheochromocytoma in Twin-Pregnancy: Analysis of Therapeutic Challenges in a Rare Case** ... 208
Bora Özveren, Halim Ulugöl and Levent Türkeri

Chapter 54 **Giant Primary Scrotal Lipoma: A Rare Entity with Diagnostic Pitfalls** ... 212
Louis Vignot, Elie Saad, Michael Peyromaure and Nicolas Barry Delongchamps

Chapter 55 **Dorsal Onlay Oral Mucosa Graft Urethroplasty: A Case Report and Review of Literature** ... 215
Kwaku Addai Arhin Appiah, Christian Kofi Gyasi-Sarpong, Edwin M. T. Yenli, Patrick Opoku Manu Maison, Charles Kwame Adofo, George Amoah, Roland Azorliade, Dominic Annor Mintah and Augustina Badu-Peprah

Chapter 56 **Scrotal Skin Metastases Revealing a Prostatic Adenocarcinoma** ... 221
Idriss Ziani, Zayd El Boukili El Makhoukh, Ahmed Ibrahimi, Omar Bellouki, Jihane Benahmed, Yasmine Laraqui, Fouad Zouidia, Hachem El Sayegh, Lounis Benslimane and Yassine Nouini

Chapter 57 **Primary Paratesticular Leiomyosarcoma: A Case Report and Literature Review** ... 226
Zeineb Naimi, Semia Zarraa, Salma Kammoun, Safia Yahyaoui, Maha Driss and Chiraz Nasr

Permissions

List of Contributors

Index

Preface

Every book is initially just a concept; it takes months of research and hard work to give it the final shape in which the readers receive it. In its early stages, this book also went through rigorous reviewing. The notable contributions made by experts from across the globe were first molded into patterned chapters and then arranged in a sensibly sequential manner to bring out the best results.

The urinary system comprises the kidneys, bladder, ureters and urethra. The branch of medicine which focuses on the diagnosis and treatment of conditions related to the urinary system in both males and females is known as urology. It employs a multidisciplinary approach, utilizing medical and surgical interventions, to manage a wide range of urologic disorders such as prostate disorders, erectile dysfunction, urinary tract infections (UTIs), kidney stones, bladder and kidney cancers, urinary tract obstructions, infertility, and congenital abnormalities of the urinary tract. Urology also deals with the diagnosis and treatment of conditions affecting the male reproductive system, such as erectile dysfunction and male infertility. These conditions can be treated through medication, hormonal therapy, minimally invasive procedures, and by surgical interventions. This book provides comprehensive insights into the field of urology. It will serve as a valuable source of reference for graduate and postgraduate students.

It has been my immense pleasure to be a part of this project and to contribute my years of learning in such a meaningful form. I would like to take this opportunity to thank all the people who have been associated with the completion of this book at any step.

Editor

1

Locally Recurrent Leiomyoma of the Bladder Refractory to Visually Complete Transurethral Resection: An Indication for Cystoprostatectomy

Katharina Mitchell,[1] John Barnard ,[2] and Adam Luchey[2]

[1]*West Virginia University School of Medicine, Morgantown, WV, USA*
[2]*West Virginia University, Department of Urology, Morgantown, WV, USA*

Correspondence should be addressed to John Barnard; jbarnar4@hsc.wvu.edu

Academic Editor: Ferdinando Fusco

Leiomyomas are benign smooth muscle tumors that have low malignant potential (0.1%) and can arise in nearly any area of the body. Genitourinary involvement is very rare and represents only 0.05% of all bladder tumors (Mendes et al., 2017; GÖK, 2017). The most common presenting symptoms of bladder leiomyomas are obstructive voiding (49%), irritative voiding (38%), and hematuria (11%) (Goluboff et al., 1994). Treatment involves complete excision, in this case transurethral resection (TUR), and generally results in complete cure with no recurrences noted in the 250 cases reported in the literature for open resection and 18% recurrence rates after TUR which were successfully treated with a repeat TUR in all cases. Herein, we report a case of leiomyoma of the bladder which was refractory to four visually complete transurethral resections and ultimately required radical cystoprostatectomy with ileal conduit urinary diversion.

1. Introduction

Bladder leiomyomas are very rare, representing only 0.05% of all bladder tumors. Worldwide this equates to a 250 cases total ever reported [1, 2]. Equal incidence has been reported between males and females. While leiomyomas of the bladder are benign, they are locally invasive and often symptomatic. The most common presenting symptoms are obstructive voiding (49%), irritative symptoms (38%), and hematuria (11%) [3]. While rare, bladder leiomyomas have historically been cured with surgical extirpation.

2. Case

A 64-year-old male with a past medical history of coronary artery disease, cardiac stent, COPD, HTN, and dyslipidemia presented as a referral for left testicular teratoma and primary bladder leiomyoma. Prior to presenting to our facility, he underwent left radical orchiectomy, and hernia repair due to enlarging left testicle, had a transurethral resection of bladder tumor (TURBT) due to hematuria, and underwent PSA screening. Pathology determined the testicular mass to be a pT1 teratoma without lymphovascular invasion, PSA was found to be elevated (was 4.2 in 2014, now 4.39), and the 40 g of bladder tumor resected during the TURBT was found to be a leiomyoma of the bladder showing no sarcomatoid differentiation. A CT scan was performed which was notable for bilateral pelvic adenopathy with lymph nodes greater than 2 cm and an interaortocaval lymph node of approximately 1.2 cm. Additionally, outside CT scan with IV contrast of abdomen pelvis showed large 6 cm heterogeneous soft tissue mass within the posterior left aspect of the bladder (Figure 1(a)). The mass was causing complete obstruction of the left ureterovesical junction (UVJ), which resulted in severe left sided hydronephrosis and hydroureter. Although the CT findings were highly concerning for metastatic process, the TURBT specimen did not support the diagnosis of metastatic disease from a bladder primary as it had returned leiomyoma of

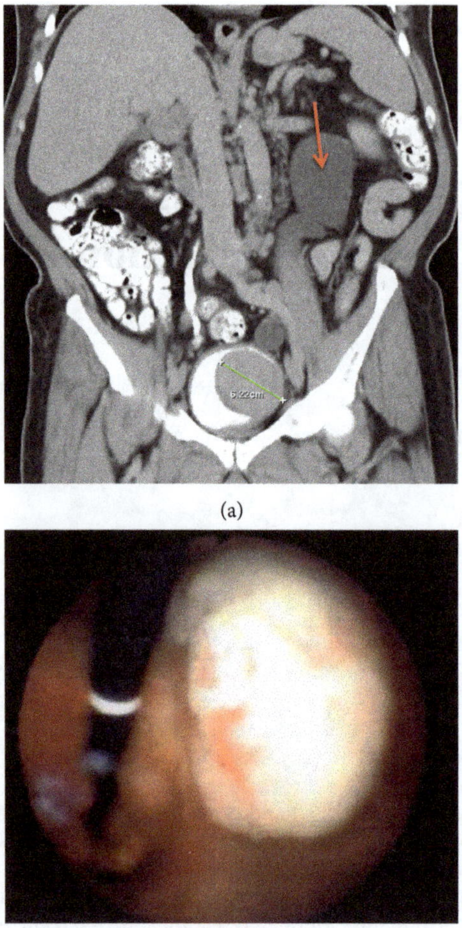

(a)

(b)

Figure 1: (a) CT Urogram, delayed phase, coronal view, showing 6 cm intravesical tumor and left sided hydroureteronephrosis (red arrow) due to mass effect at the level of the left ureteral orifice. (b) Cystourethroscopy revealed a pale white to tan exophytic bladder mass overlying the left ureteral orifice which was obscuring and obstructing the left kidney and ureter.

bladder without sarcomatoid elements. The disparity between imaging findings and pathology results prompted confirmatory testing on both the initial testicular mass and the TURBT specimens. After discussion at multidisciplinary GU tumor board, the consensus recommendation was for CT-guided lymph node biopsy, repeat transurethral resection of bladder tumor, and decompression of the left upper tract via ureteral stent, or nephrostomy. The patient underwent rigid cystourethroscopy, monopolar transurethral resection of bladder tumor (large >5 cm) and monopolar transurethral resection of prostate. During this surgery, a large tumor located on the left wall extending down into the bladder neck and prostatic urethra was resected with an extensive amount of tissue removed (Figure 1(b)). The right ureteral orifice was uninvolved, but the left ureteral orifice was completely obscured by tumor. The bladder neck and prostate were resected down to the level of the verumontanum which was spared. A 3-way foley catheter was placed at the conclusion of the case and the patient was admitted post operatively. He underwent left percutaneous nephrostomy (PCN) placement and IR guided biopsy of the suspicious pelvic lymph nodes prior to discharge.

Following independent pathology review of the outside facility testicular specimen and review of in-house specimens, the previous diagnosis of testicular teratoma was recharacterized as a Leydig cell tumor of the testis and the patient's lymph node biopsy revealed follicular lymphoma. Discussion at multidisciplinary tumor board initially recommended bone marrow transplant, neoadjuvant chemotherapy, and extirpative surgery at a future date depending on the patient's response to chemotherapy. After bone marrow biopsy, his follicular lymphoma was staged as stage 4 with minimal bone marrow involvement. In advanced stage follicular lymphoma there is no survival benefit to early initiation of treatment, therefore serial PET CT scans 6 months apart were recommended by hematology/oncology to follow his lymphoma.

The patient was managed conservatively with nephrostomy tube exchanges every 10–12 weeks and underwent cystoscopy with urodynamic studies after presenting with urinary retention and traumatic foley at approximately 1 year post resection. Cystoscopy revealed a large mass in the left lateral bladder wall extending down into the bladder neck and involving the prostate. He was started on Flomax and discharged without a foley catheter as he was able to void with a normal PVR at the time of the procedure. Due to significant regrowth of leimyoma on cystoscopy, he was encouraged to have repeat debulking of the tumor via transurethral approach as he declined cystoprostatectomy. The patient underwent repeat TURBT with bipolar resectoscope for recurrent left lateral bladder wall, bladder neck, and prostatic mass. The pathology again returned leiomyoma without sarcomatoid differentiation. A month after discharge the patient presented to an outside Emergency Room after developing gross hematuria. He was transferred for continuous bladder irrigation and refractory hematuria which required urgent TURBT to fulgurate bleeding vessels at the left lateral bladder neck and resect additional tumor regrowth.

The patient followed up in clinic 1 month later, and after an in-depth discussion of his clinical course, he decided to undergo surgical extirpation of the bladder and prostate with creation of an ileal conduit urinary diversion. When reviewing the preoperative MRI there was loss of fat plane between the prostate and rectum, therefore colorectal surgery was consulted to assist in rectal dissection. He also underwent preoperative colonoscopy in order to rule out invasion into the rectum and screen the remainder of the colon. The patient underwent open radical cystoprostatectomy with ileal conduit urinary diversion and intraoperative angiogram of the involved bowel segment and omental flap interposition. He had intraoperative proctoscopy by colorectal surgery to ensure no rectal injury was present. He was discharged on postoperative day 4 after progressing without incident. The pathology report from his extirpative surgery revealed a 1.8 cm leiomyoma involving the submucosal bladder wall surrounding the left ureteral orifice. Incidental finding of High Grade Prostatic Intraepithelial Neoplasia was noted on the prostate specimen. The findings did not extend through the bladder wall into the perivesical or periprostatic adipose. Margins were

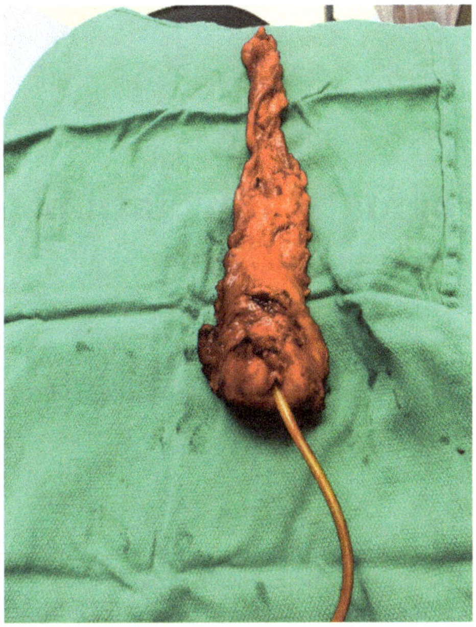

(a)

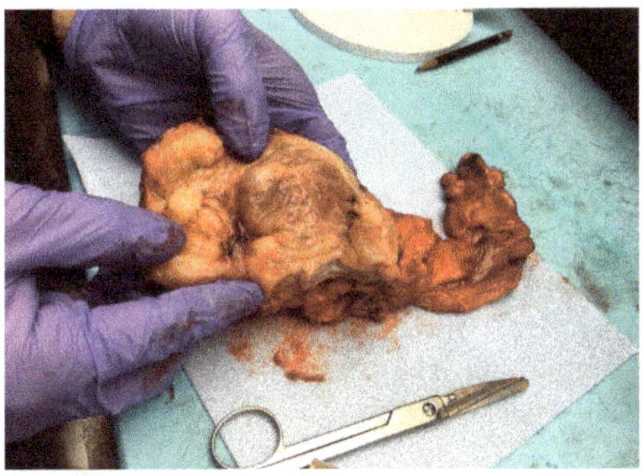

(b)

FIGURE 2: (a) Radical prostatectomy gross specimen. Prostate measured 4 cm from anterior to posterior. Prostate pathology showed high focal intraepithelial neoplasia, acute and chronic inflammation, and previous biopsy site changes. (b) Gross specimen of bivalved bladder. Submucosal leiomyoma measuring 1.8 cm is noted in the area of the left ureteral orifice. The leiomyoma was obstructing the left ureteral orifice. Bladder measured 5 × 5 × 2.5 cm.

negative. The patient was evaluated 8 weeks postoperatively and has had an uncomplicated postoperative course to date. He has been satisfied by his improved functional status and is to be followed with serial renal ultrasound in 6 months to ensure no obstruction at the uretero-ileal anastomoses.

3. Discussion

Leiomyoma of the bladder is a very rare, benign tumor; however, it can be locally invasive and incur significant morbidity if left untreated. Leiomyomas are classified into 3 groups based on location: intravesical, intramural and extravesical [4, 5]. The most common presenting symptoms are obstructive voiding (49%), irritative symptoms (38%), hematuria (11%), and 20% were asymptomatic [6]. The patient in this case presented initially with hematuria prompting initial TURBT revealing leiomyoma of the bladder. The case differs from the previous literature because leiomyoma of the bladder is typically cured by visually complete excision and does not recur. There are around 250 cases of bladder leiomyoma reported [1], and recurrence has never been observed after either complete extirpation of the bladder or complete TUR. Silva-Ramos et al. performed an analysis of 90 cases of leiomyomas. On follow-up of the cases published there has been no recurrence up to 20 years after surgery and no malignant transformation [7]. Our patient's course is in contrast to the published literature because he underwent four visually complete resections endoscopically, but exhibited recurrence after each. After a long course of repeated endoscopic management the patient elected to undergo surgical extirpation of the bladder, prostate, and creation of an ileal conduit urinary diversion. Although only 1.8 cm of residual was noted, it is likely that the unique location of the patient's tumor made it more difficult to completely resect endoscopically which may explain his numerous recurrences (Figure 2(b)). This demonstrates that endoscopic resection of bladder leiomyomas is not always curative even if no gross tumor remains, and bladder leiomyomas can recur after numerous visually complete resections.

Conflicts of Interest

The authors declare that they have no conflicts of interest.

References

[1] J. E. Mendes, A. V. Ferreira, S. A. Coelho, and C. Gil, "Bladder leiomyoma," *Urology Annals*, vol. 9, no. 3, pp. 275–277, 2017.

[2] N. Khater and G. Sakr, "Bladder leiomyoma: presentation, evaluation and treatment," *Arab Journal of Urology*, vol. 11, no. 1, pp. 54–61, 2012.

[3] R. G. Haddad, M. M. Murshidi, N. Abu Shahin, and M. M. Murshidi, "Leiomyoma of urinary bladder presenting with febrile urinary tract infection: a case report," *International Journal of Surgery Case Reports*, vol. 27, pp. 180–182, 2016.

[4] J. J. Wong-You-Cheong, P. J. Woodward, M. A. Manning, and I. A. Sesterhenn, "Neoplasms of the urinary bladder: radiologic-pathologic correlation," *Radiographics*, vol. 26, no. 2, pp. 553–580, 2006.

[5] S. Agrawal, J. Kalathia, S. Chipde, and R. Agrawal, "Total endoscopic management of a large bladder leiomyoma," *Urology Annals*, vol. 7, no. 4, pp. 527–529, 2015.

[6] J. W. Park, B. C. Jeong, S. I. Seo, S. S. Jeon, G. Y. Kwon, and H. M. Lee, "Leiomyoma of the urinary bladder: a series of nine cases and review of the literature," *Urology*, vol. 76, no. 6, pp. 1425–1429, 2010.

[7] H. Erdem, U. Yildirim, A. Tekin, A. Kayikci, A. K. Uzunlar, and C. Sahiner, "Leiomyoma of the urinary bladder in asymptomatic women," *Urology Annals*, vol. 4, no. 3, pp. 172–174, 2012.

2

A Rare Case of Isolated Ureteral Diaphragmatic Herniation: Case Report and Review of Literature

Nassib Abou Heidar,[1] Hussein Elsemesmani,[2] Ahmad Elamine,[2] and Mustafa Natout[2]

[1]*Department of Surgery, Division of Urology, American University of Beirut Medical Center, Beirut, Lebanon*
[2]*Department of Radiology, American University of Beirut Medical Center, Beirut, Lebanon*

Correspondence should be addressed to Mustafa Natout; mn113@aub.edu.lb

Nassib Abou Heidar and Hussein Elsemesmani were contributed equally to the writing of the manuscript.

Academic Editor: Tun-Chieh Chen

Diaphragmatic ureteral hernias are rare causes of ipsilateral renal obstruction. Management strategies varies from conservative to ureteral stenting to operative herniorraphy and reduction. We present a case of a 71-year-old man who was found to have an incidental right ureteral diaphragmatic herniation causing an asymptomatic kidney obstruction. He was managed conservatively with no evidence of increased hydronephrosis on serial imaging and no deterioration of biochemical renal function. We review all similar cases published in the literature and discuss the optimal treatment strategies.

1. Introduction

It is a rarity to encounter ureteral herniation with less than 150 reported in the literature. Common hernia locations are inguinal, femoral, and sciatic locations among others [1]. However, the rarest location for a ureteral herniation is through a defect in the diaphragmatic muscle [2]. Previously, only 12 cases have reported in the literature with varying presentations and management strategies; management varied from conservative to ureteral stenting or surgical repair. On the other hand, the clinical presentation varied from incidental radiographic finding to obstructive pyelonephritis and urosepsis. We hereby present the case of a ureteral diaphragmatic hernia that was incidentally discovered on computed tomography (CT).

2. Case Presentation

A 71-year-old male, with a medical history relevant for uncontrolled hypertension, diabetes mellitus type 2, and chronic kidney disease (baseline creatinine = 1.8 mg/dl), presented to the emergency department with abdominal pain, vomiting and loose stools. The patient denied any new-onset lower tract urinary symptoms, hematuria, fever, or flank pain. His laboratory tests were notable for leukocytosis of 12,000/cu.mm, serum creatinine of 1.9 mg/dl, and negative urinalysis. A CT scan done to rule out an intraabdominal process did not reveal any intraperitoneal pathology; however, a rightsided ureteral diaphragmatic herniation was seen, associated with mild-moderate hydronephrosis and significant blunting of calyceal fornices (Figures 1 and 2). The patient was counselled about his management options which included stenting of the ureter to relieve the obstruction or active surveillance of the hydronephrosis for which he opted. Serial ultrasounds performed every 6 months showed no progression of the hydronephrosis and no renal cortical thinning (Figure 3). Follow-up on serum creatinine showed no change in his baseline levels and was in the 1.8–2 mg/dl range for over 18 months.

3. Discussion

Ureteral hernias are rare entities, with less than 150 cases previously reported. The rarest ureteral herniation reported is thoracic ureteral herniation through a muscular diaphragmatic defect. It is speculated that these types of ureteral herniations are rare because the herniation is occurring through a nondependent space [2]. It is currently unknown if these herniations are acquired or congenital with late presentation.

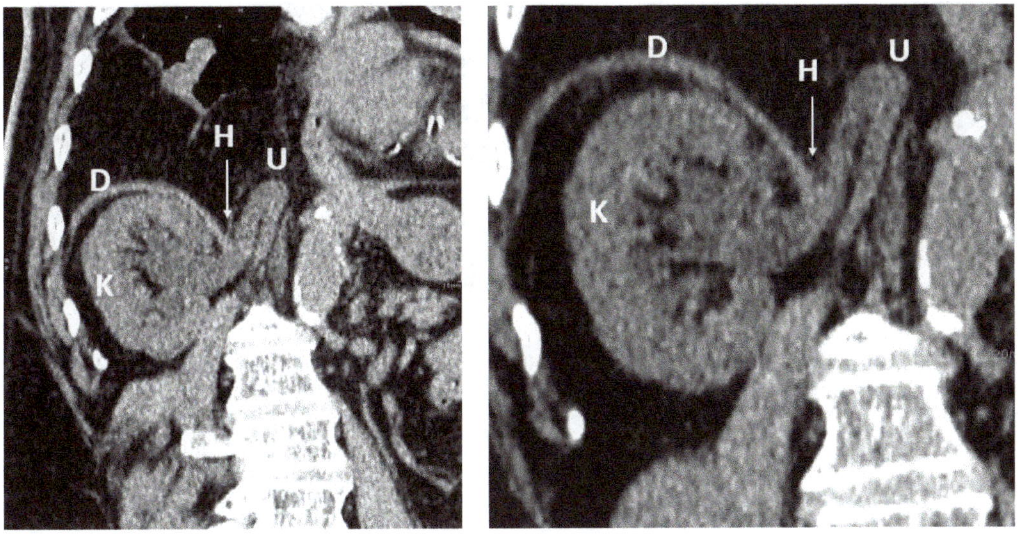

FIGURE 1: Reformatted oblique coronal images of nonenhanced CT scan of the abdomen show the right ureter herniating through a medial diaphragmatic defect causing its obstruction and secondary mild to moderate hydronephrosis. Renal cortical thickness is still preserved. D: right hemidiaphragm. K: right kidney. U: ureter. H: diaphragmatic hernia.

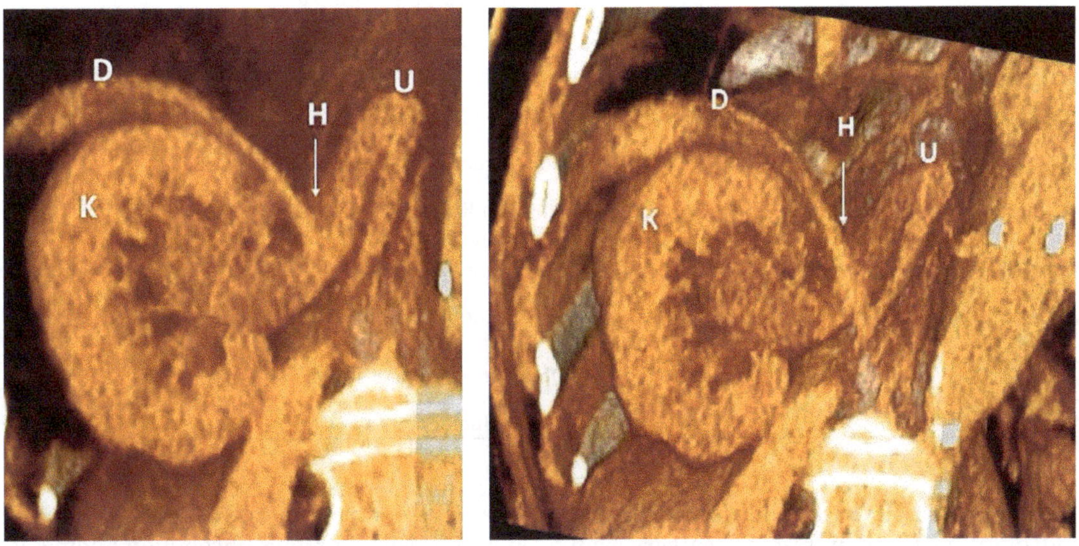

FIGURE 2: 3-D reconstructed images showing the right ureter herniation and the secondary hydronephrosis. D: right hemidiaphragm. K: right kidney. U: ureter. H: diaphragmatic hernia.

A retrospective review of reported cases was done and papers were retrieved from PubMed, Medline, and Scopus. 12 cases were found that had different presentations and management plans ranging from conservative management to ureteral stenting or surgical repair depending on the presentation and the clinical scenario. These were summarized in Table 1.

In the literature, some ureteral herniations are detected incidentally while others presented with symptoms attributable to the ureteral herniation/kidney obstruction. Symptomatic patients presented with flank pain, gross hematuria, renal dysfunction, nephrolithiasis and urosepsis. Among the thoracic ureteral herniations reported in the literature, five presented with right flank pain [2, 3, 5, 6], three were incidental findings in the workup for azotemia [7], contralateral flank pain [8], and PET scan for the workup of a lung nodule [9]. Two cases presented as part of the workup for renal [10] and ureteral [11] stones, one presented as right upper quadrant abdominal pain [12], and one presented as septic obstructive pyelonephritis [13].

Of these reported cases, one was managed conservatively [7], three underwent surgical repair [3, 6, 10], and ureteral stenting [2–4, 11–13]. Among those that underwent stenting, one necessitated a nephrostomy access due to failure of

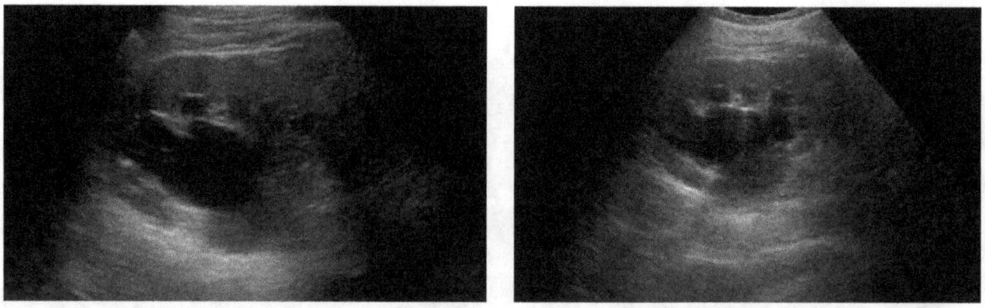

(a) (b)

FIGURE 3: Serial ultrasound images of the right kidney done at 6 month intervals after diagnosis of the kidney obstruction. Showing similar ureteral and pelvicalyceal dilation (a and b) over the span of 6 months with no change in the renal cortex thickness.

TABLE 1: Review of ureteral diaphragmatic herniation.

Authors (Year of publication)	Age/gender	Laterality	Presentation	Management
Swithinbank (1958)	60/F	Right	Right flank pain	Surgical repair
Paterson and Lupton (1989)	75/M	Right	Right flank pain	Surgical repair
Chawla and Mond (1994)	56/M	Right	Incidental on workup for contralateral flank pain	Not mentioned
Catalano et al. (1998)	63/F	Right	Upon workup for renal stones	Surgical repair of the defect
Sukumar et al. (2010)	75/F	Right	Incidental finding on workup for azotemia	Conservative
Balakrishnan and Neerhut (2011)	83/F	Right	Right flank pain	Retrograde ureteral stenting
Song et al. (2011)	75/M	Right	Right upper quadrant pain	Retrograde ureteral stenting
Hatzidakis et al. (2014)	86/F	Right	Septic obstructive pyelonephritis	Nephrostomy drainage followed by ureteral stenting
Almeida et al. (2015)	82/F	Right	Incidental on PET scan for workup of lung nodule	Not mentioned
Dru and Josephson (2016)	94/F	Right	Right flank pain	Retrograde ureteral stenting
Lin et al. (2017)	81/F	Right	Right flank pain	Retrograde ureteral stenting followed by surgical repair
Beland et al. (2019)	84/F	Right	Obstructing ureteral stone	Retrograde intra-renal surgery for stone fragmentation and stenting
Current case	71/M	Right	Incidental	Conservative

retrograde stenting [13], another was followed by surgical repair [2], and one underwent intra-renal surgery with stenting [11]. Two cases did not report management [8, 9]. Most cases occurred in the elderly, with the mean age of diagnosis being 76, and out of the 12 reported cases, 9 were female.

Congenital Bochdalek hernias are a result of failure of fusion of the foramina of the diaphragm. They are usually asymptomatic with prevalence rate reaching 10% [14]. In about 90% of the cases symptoms of Bochdaleck, hernias are left-sided [13]. However, in all reported cases of ureteral herniation, the herniation lateralized to the right-side. This is counterintuitive since the right kidney is higher in location and the liver is right-sided and would occupy a larger space. The authors have no explanation for this observation; however, this observation seems to support the embryologic origin of this diaphragmatic defect. On the other hand, the fact that this seems to be a presentation in the geriatric population discourages the embryologic origin of ureteral herniation.

We report the 13th case of thoracic ureteral herniation to our knowledge, a rather uncommon finding. It further supports the literature in that thoracic ureteral herniations generally occur on the right side. In our case, the herniation was successfully managed conservatively with serial ultrasounds and serum creatinine in order to follow up on the hydronephrosis and renal function, respectively, both done at 6-month-intervals with the former showing no progression of the hydronephrosis and no cortical thinning, and the latter showing no elevations over the period of follow up. This further supports that uncomplicated ureteral herniations can be managed conservatively with surveillance.

Management strategies depend on the clinical context. In cases of obstruction and resultant pain or pyelonephritis, then drainage is imperative. A trial of retrograde ureteral stenting is reasonable and minimally invasive [12] with notable success in the reported cases; however, Hatzidagis et al. reported on failure of double J ureteral stent insertion owing that to the length and tortuosity of the ureter [13]. More importantly, this case encourages that a trial of surveillance of renal function and obstruction is a valid method at management.

4. Conclusion

Ureteral herniations are generally an uncommon entity, with thoracic ureteral herniations being even more exceedingly rare in the literature. Imaging is required to detect, confirm, and follow the herniation for progression. Follow up can take the form of serial ultrasounds and serum creatinine while the patient is managed conservatively. Our case suggests that uncomplicated thoracic ureteral herniations can be managed conservatively without intervention, particularly in patients not amenable to surgery.

Ethical Approval

A written informed consent was obtained from the patient for use of his anonymous clinical and radiological information.

Conflicts of Interest

The authors declare that they have no conflicts of interest.

Authors' Contributions

N. A. H. and H. E. conducted the literature review. M. N. diagnosed the patient and was responsible for retrieval of radiologic images. J. D. and A. E. helped write the manuscript. N. A. H., H. E. and M. N. edited the final version of the manuscript. All authors approved of the final manuscript before submission.

References

[1] L. Bertolaccini, G. Giacomelli, R. Bozzo, E. L. Gastaldi, and M. Moroni, "Inguino-scrotal hernia of a double district ureter: case report and literature review," *Hernia: The Journal of Hernias and Abdominal Wall Surgery*, vol. 9, no. 3, pp. 291–293, 2005.

[2] F. C. Lin, J. S. Lin, S. Kim, and J. R. Walker, "A rare diaphragmatic ureteral herniation case report: endoscopic and open reconstructive management," *BMC Urology*, vol. 17, no. 1, p. 26, 2017.

[3] A. H. Swithinbank, "Intrathoracic deviation of a ureteric loop," *British Journal of Surgery*, vol. 45, no. 192, pp. 379–381, 1958.

[4] V. Balakrishnan and G. Neerhut, "Right sided Bochdalek hernia causing ureteric obstruction," *BJUI*, 2011, http://www.bjui.co.uk/ContentFullItem.aspx?id=769&SectionType=1&title=Right-sided-Bochdalek-hernia-causing-ureteric-obstruction.

[5] C. J. Dru and D. Y. Josephson, "Bochdalek-type diaphragmatic hernia leading to high-grade kidney obstruction," *Urology*, vol. 97, pp. e17–e18, 2016.

[6] I. S. Paterson and E. W. Lupton, "Pelviureteric junction obstruction secondary to renal pelvic incarceration in a congenital diaphragmatic hernia," *British Journal of Urology*, vol. 64, no. 5, pp. 548–549, 1989.

[7] S. Sukumar, P. G. Kumar, and A. Thomas, "Thoracic curlicue: a case of ureteral herniation," *Indian Journal of Urology*, vol. 26, no. 1, pp. 131–132, 2010.

[8] K. Chawla and D. J. Mond, "Progressive Bochdalek hernia with unusual ureteral herniation," *Computerized Medical Imaging and Graphics*, vol. 18, no. 1, pp. 53–58, 1994.

[9] L. Almeida, F. Carvalhaes, A. Bitencourt, and F. Moreira, "Ureteral hernia mimicking retrocrural lymphadenopathy in 18F-FDG PET/CT," *Clinical Nuclear Medicine*, vol. 40, no. 8, pp. e415–e416, 2015.

[10] O. Catalano, A. Nunziata, B. Cusati, and A. Siani, "Retrocrural loop of the ureter: CT findings," *American Journal of Roentgenology*, vol. 170, no. 5, pp. 1293–1294, 1998.

[11] L. E. Beland, M. A. Henry, T. Solomon, and K. Ogan, "Obstructing nephrolithiasis in an 84-year-old Patient with a diaphragmatic herniated ureter," *Urology*, vol. 124, pp. e1–e3, 2019.

[12] Y. S. Song, C. Hassani, and P. M. Nardi, "Bochdalek hernia with obstructive uropathy," *Urology*, vol. 77, no. 6, p. 1338, 2011.

[13] A. Hatzidakis, A. Kozana, D. Glaritis, and C. Mamoulakis, "Right-sided Bochdalek hernia causing septic ureteric obstruction. Percutaneous treatment with placement of a nephroureteral double pigtail," *BMJ Case Reports*, vol. 2014, no. 1, pp. bcr2014207247–bcr2014207247, 2014.

[14] O. Temizöz, H. Gençhellaç, E. Yekeler et al., "Prevalence and MDCT characteristics ofasymptomatic Bochdalek hernia in adult population," *Diagnostic and Interventional Radiology*, vol. 16, no. 1, pp. 52–55, 2010.

3

The Association of Renal Agenesis and Ipsilateral Seminal Vesicle Cyst: Zinner Syndrome Case Report

Mishal AlArifi ,[1] Magdi Al-Gahwary,[2] and Mohamed Gomha[2]

[1] *College of Medicine, Imam Abdulrahman Bin Faisal University, Dammam, Saudi Arabia*
[2] *Department of Urology, King Fahad Specialist Hospital, Dammam, Saudi Arabia*

Correspondence should be addressed to Mishal AlArifi; alarifi.mishal@gmail.com

Academic Editor: Nicola Zampieri

Introduction. Zinner syndrome is a rare congenital malformation characterized by the association of an ipsilateral renal agenesis, ipsilateral seminal vesicle cyst, and ipsilateral ejaculatory duct obstruction. This case is one of the first to be reported in the Kingdom of Saudi Arabia. *Case Presentation.* A 20-year-old Saudi male patient presented complaining of chronic left groin pain radiating to the left testis and the medial aspect of the left thigh for the last 6 years. Patient is also complaining of painful ejaculation with no history of lower urinary tract symptoms, hematuria, or trauma. Physical examination was unremarkable. Ultrasound (US) report from the referring hospital mentioned that there is a left pelvic mass. Computed tomography (CT) and magnetic resonance imaging (MRI) showed diffuse distension of left seminal vesicle (9 X 7 cm) cyst with ipsilateral left renal agenesis which corresponds to Zinner syndrome. Left seminal vesicle cyst excision through a low midline incision was done. The patient was asymptomatic during his follow-up in our clinic with disappearance of the pain. *Conclusion.* The combination of a good clinical history and radiological assays aided in making the diagnosis. Surgical intervention is the mainstay in the management plan in symptomatic patients.

1. Introduction

Zinner syndrome is a rare congenital malformation characterized by the association of an ipsilateral renal agenesis, ipsilateral seminal vesicle cyst, and ipsilateral ejaculatory duct obstruction which was first described by Zinner et al. in 1914 [1]. Zinner syndrome is caused by malformations of the distal portion of the mesonephric duct and is considered the Mayer-Rokitansky-Kuster-Hauser (MRKH) counterpart in males [2]. This case is one of the first to be reported in the Kingdom of Saudi Arabia.

2. Case Presentation

A 20-year-old Saudi male patient not known to have any chronic medical illness was referred to our urology department complaining of chronic left groin pain radiating to the left testis and the medial aspect of the left thigh for the last 6 years. Patient is also complaining of painful ejaculation with no history of lower urinary tract symptoms, hematuria, or trauma. Physical examination was unremarkable. Laboratory tests were ordered including complete blood count and renal function tests which all were within normal ranges. Ultrasound (US) report from the referring hospital mentioned that there is a left pelvic mass. Computed tomography (CT) and magnetic resonance imaging (MRI) showed diffuse distension of left seminal vesicle (9 X 7 cm) cyst (Figure 1) with ipsilateral left renal agenesis (Figure 2) which corresponds to Zinner syndrome. Left seminal vesicle (SV) cyst excision through a low midline incision was done. After general anesthesia and drabbing, a low midline incision was done with a transperitoneal approach, then retracting the intestine exposing and dissecting the right seminal vesicle cysts with release of the adhesion from the pelvic side wall reaching the level of the vas then ligations of both the distal end of SV and vas while preserving the contralateral vas and SV. Haemostasis was done with the insertion of a pelvic drain and closure of the wound in layers. The patient was asymptomatic during his follow-up in our clinic with disappearance of the pain.

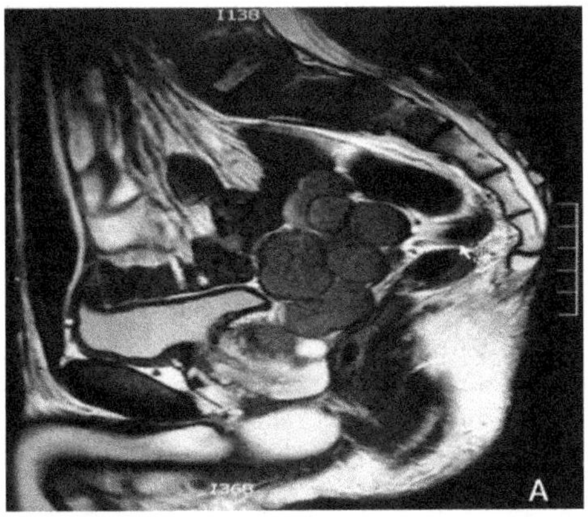

(a)

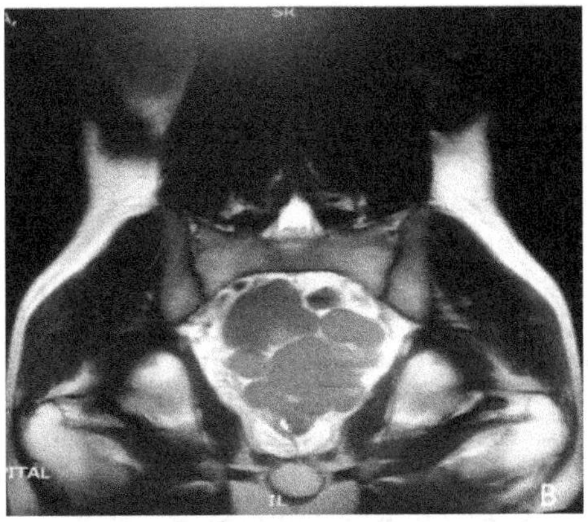

(b)

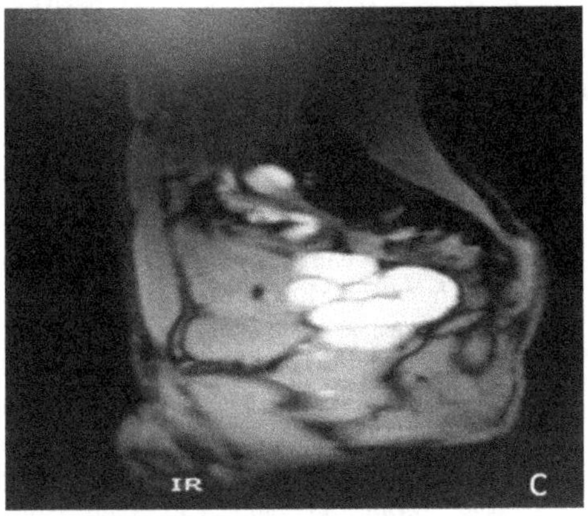

(c)

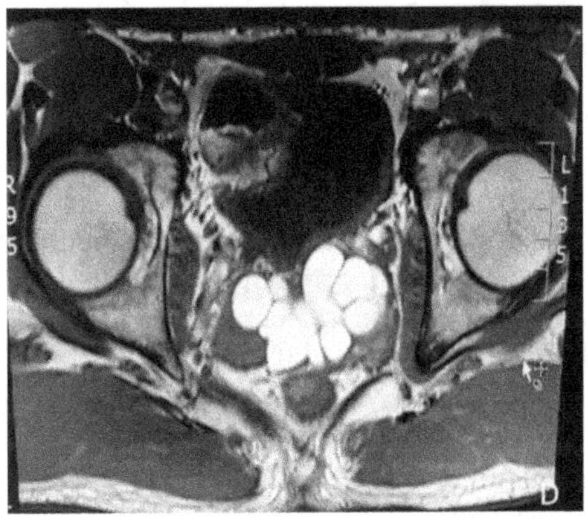

(d)

FIGURE 1: (a) MRI sagittal section T2, (b) MRI coronal section T2, (c) MRI sagittal section T1, and (d) MRI axial section T1. (a)-(b) showed diffuse dilatation of left seminal vesicles with low signal intensity, and (c)-(d) showed diffuse dilatation of left seminal vesicles with high signal intensity.

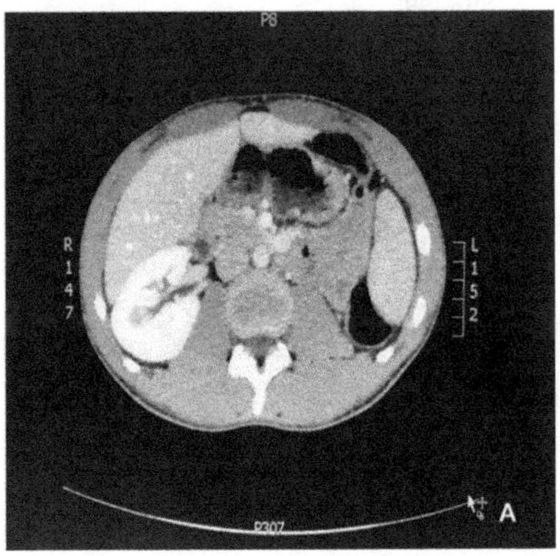

(a)

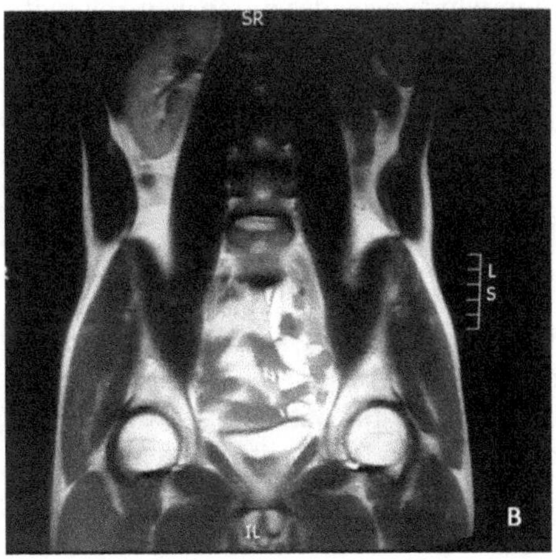

(b)

FIGURE 2: (a) CT axial section showed left renal agenesis. (b) MRI coronal section showed left renal agenesis.

3. Discussion

Zinner syndrome is one of the rarest congenital anomalies of the urogenital tract and is usually discovered and diagnosed in the 2nd-4th decade of life [3]. The frequency of this condition is reported to be 0.0046% according to Farooqui et al. [4]. Patients with this syndrome are usually asymptomatic but they can present with dysuria, frequency, perineal pain, or epididymitis [3].

The embryological origin of the kidneys and seminal vesicles is similar; the kidney is formed by the metanephric blastema which is induced by ureteral bud that originates from the dorsal aspect of the distal mesonephric duct. The mesonephric duct gives rise to most of the genital tract including epididymis, vas deferens, ejaculatory duct, and seminal vesicle [5]. Any malformation of the ureteral bud or mesonephric duct can cause Zinner syndrome.

Radiological modalities have a significant role in diagnosing and evaluating Zinner syndrome including US, CT, and MRI. US is a quick imaging modality that is used mainly in this condition to detect the absence of the ipsilateral kidney or to show some anechoic structures in the pelvis resembling the obstructed ejaculatory duct [3, 6]. CT findings might include an ipsilateral kidney agenesis in addition to a retrovesicular periprostatic cystic mass [3, 7]. MRI is considered to be the imaging modality of choice in diagnosing this condition due to its high resolution properties in evaluating the seminal vesicles cysts and the ejaculatory ducts [3].

Management of the seminal vesicles cysts depends on the presentation and the presence of symptoms, and asymptomatic patients are usually observed until they start to complain of symptoms. Surgical intervention can be carried out by different modalities and techniques reported in the literature. First option is open surgical excision, and minimally invasive surgeries including the laparoscopic and robotic-assisted approaches are considered the best option due to their better outcomes, less blood loss, and shorter hospitalization [8–11]. Another option is simple cyst drainage or transrectal aspiration which provides a transient relief of symptoms but both are associated with greater chance of recurrence.

4. Conclusion

The association of ipsilateral renal agenesis and ipsilateral seminal vesicle cyst is a rare unique congenital presentation that is called Zinner syndrome. The combination of a good clinical history and radiological assays aided in making the diagnosis. Surgical intervention is the mainstay in the management plan in symptomatic patients. Relieving the patient symptoms and improving his quality of life were our main goal which was accomplished.

Disclosure

The authors have no ethical conflicts to disclose.

Conflicts of Interest

The authors declare no conflicts of interest.

References

[1] A. Zinner, "Ein fall von intravesikaler Samenblasenzyste," *Wiener Medizinische Wochenschrift*, vol. 64, article 605, 1914.

[2] S. Khanduri, G. Katyal, H. Sharma et al., "Unique association of multiple seminal vesicle cysts with contralateral renal agenesis: a rare variant of zinner syndrome," *Cureus*, vol. 9, no. 7, article e1415, 2017.

[3] S. Mehra, R. Ranjan, and U. C. Garga, "Zinner syndrome—a rare developmental anomaly of the mesonephric duct diagnosed on magnetic resonance imaging," *Radiology Case Reports*, vol. 11, no. 4, pp. 313–317, 2016.

[4] A. Farooqui, L. AlDhahir, and A. B. Mahfooz, "Massive seminal vesicle cyst with ipsilateral renal agenesis - Zinner syndrome in a Saudi patient," *Urology Annals*, vol. 10, no. 3, pp. 333–335, 2018.

[5] A. Slaoui, S. Regragui, A. Lasri et al., "Zinner's syndrome: report of two cases and review of the literature," *Basic and Clinical Andrology*, vol. 26, no. 10, 2016.

[6] J. Trigaux, B. Van Beers, and F. Delchambre, "Male genital tract malformations associated with ipsilateral renal agenesis: sonographic findings," *Journal of Clinical Ultrasound*, vol. 19, no. 1, pp. 3–10, 1991.

[7] P. J. Kenney and M. D. Leeson, "Congenital anomalies of the seminal vesicles: spectrum of computed tomographic findings," *Radiology*, vol. 149, no. 1, pp. 247–251, 1983.

[8] E. Kord, A. Zisman, A. E. Darawsha, N. Dally, P. H. Noh, and A. Neheman, "Minimally invasive approach for treatment of seminal vesicle cyst associated with ipsilateral renal agenesis," *Urologia Internationalis*, vol. 99, no. 3, pp. 338–342, 2017.

[9] D. Van den Ouden, J. H. M. Blom, C. Bangma, and A. H. V. De Spiegeleer, "Diagnosis and management of seminal vesicle cysts associated with ipsilateral renal agenesis: a pooled analysis of 52 cases," *European Urology*, vol. 33, no. 5, pp. 433–440, 1998.

[10] V. A. Politano, R. W. Lankford, and R. Susaeta, "A 9 transvesical approach to total seminal vesiculectomy: a case report," *The Journal of Urology*, vol. 113, no. 3, pp. 385–388, 1975.

[11] B. O. Okoye, D. J. Jones, M. J. Lancashire, E. F. Brown, and A. W. S. Ritchie, "Transvesical endoscopic drainage of a seminal vesicle cyst," *British Journal of Urology*, vol. 76, no. 6, pp. 810-810, 1995.

4

Subcutaneous Dorsal Penile Vein Thrombosis or Penile Mondor's Disease: A Case Report and Literature Review

Adama Ouattara,[1] Abdoul Karim Paré,[1] Aristide F. Kaboré,[2] Clotaire Yaméogo,[2] Gnimdou Botcho,[1] Désiré Ky,[2] Abdoul Aziz Ouédraogo,[1] Amidou Bako,[1] Rigobert Kiba,[1] Zakari Nikiéma,[3] and Timothée Kambou[1]

[1]*Division of Urology, Souro Sanou University Teaching Hospital, Bobo-Dioulasso, Burkina Faso*
[2]*Division of Urology, Yalgado Ouedraogo University Teaching Hospital, Ouagadougou, Burkina Faso*
[3]*Division of Radiology and Imaging, Souro Sanou University Teaching Hospital, Bobo-Dioulasso, Burkina Faso*

Correspondence should be addressed to Adama Ouattara; adamsouatl@hotmail.com

Academic Editor: Giorgio Carmignani

A 34-year-old man, trader, and married with four wives, otherwise healthy, without any remarkable medical history, was admitted in urology ward in emergency with superficial venous thrombosis of the penis known also as Penile Mondor's Disease (PMD), a rare nosologic entity of the penis associated with pain and an indurated dorsal cord of the root of the penis. The patient receives nonsteroidal anti-inflammatory drugs and coagulation and platelet aggregation inhibitors drugs. Healing and total recovery occur after eight weeks without any complications.

1. Introduction

Mondor's Disease (MD) is a rare nosologic entity, most often localized in the anterolateral thoracic wall and mammary region. It was first described by Henri Mondor in 1939 [1]. It is a superficial venous thrombosis occurring in a healthy vein but regress spontaneously. The thoracic and abdominal wall, abdominal wall, penis, upper arm, and other parts of the body may also be involved by the disease penile localization, known as Penile Mondor's Disease (PMD) which was first described by Braun Falco in 1955 [2] and then by Helm and Hodge in 1958 [3]. It is a rare and underreported benign genital condition and its clinical aspects are common and etiologies and risk factors are various. Nowadays, there are no standard strategy treatments of PMD and sometimes the management can combine several means. Usually, patient presents redness and swelling of the penis accompanied by painful palpable venous thrombosis of the penis. Pathogenesis is not well known but it is believed by most authors that it is due to pulling and torsion of the dorsal vein of the penis following microtrauma or during laborious sexual intercourse [4]. We present our first observation of this benign genital condition in our urology division in a young man who was admitted with this disease and was treated with success.

2. Case Presentation

A 34-year-old man, married with four women, trader, with no known past medical history, was admitted in emergency in the urology division at Souro Sanou University Teaching Hospital of Bobo-Dioulasso (Burkina Faso) for a painful swelling penis following laborious sexual intercourse. This symptomatology began nine (9) days later with progressive painful swelling at the balanopreputial ring just after sexual intercourse. The patient consulted previously in a private clinic and was given some medication without success, and then he is admitted in emergency in our urology ward because of the generalized involvement of the entire penis with painful oedema. Medical history does not find any recent trauma or use of any medication; no urinary tract symptoms were reported but recent intense sexual intercourse was noted. The patient reported that he is married to four women and regularly having vigorous sexual intercourse

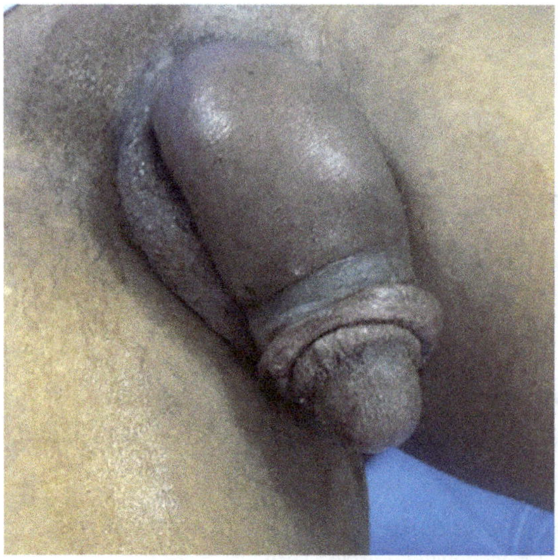

FIGURE 1: Generalized swelling of the penis.

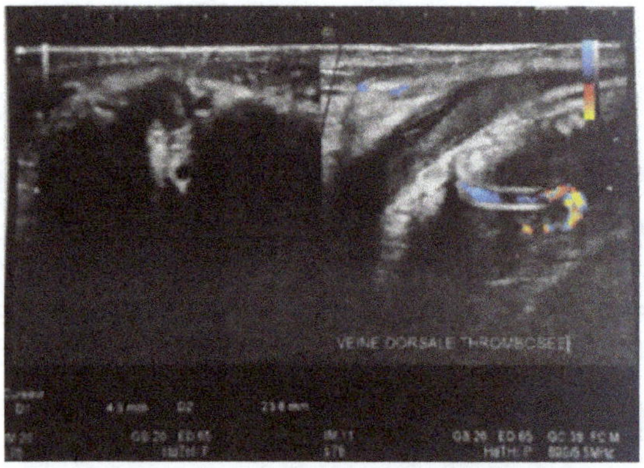

FIGURE 2: Doppler coupled with USS showing an intraluminal thrombosis (weight arrow) of the dorsal vein of the penis.

activities. Physical examination found an indurated subcutaneous filiform and painful cord, palpated at the dorsal root of the penis with soft swelling of the whole penis (Figure 1).

Examination of genito-urinary system was normal. Standard investigations (blood and urine) requested were normal, and blood cell count, urea, and creatinine were without anomalies. Urine analysis does not reveal any infection. Suspicion of penile fracture was made but anamnesis does not find a popping sound or hearing a cracking or losing an erection suddenly during sexual intercourse. Secondary, diagnosis of thrombosis of the superficial dorsal penile vein was made. An ultrasonography coupled with Doppler of the penis was requested and revealed a thrombosis of the superficial dorsal vein of the penis with the presence of the intravascular blood clot thrombosis (Figure 2).

To be sure to excluded penile fracture, penile magnetic resonance imaging (MRI) was performed and do not reveal any traumatic lesion of cavernous and spongious bodies (Figure 3).

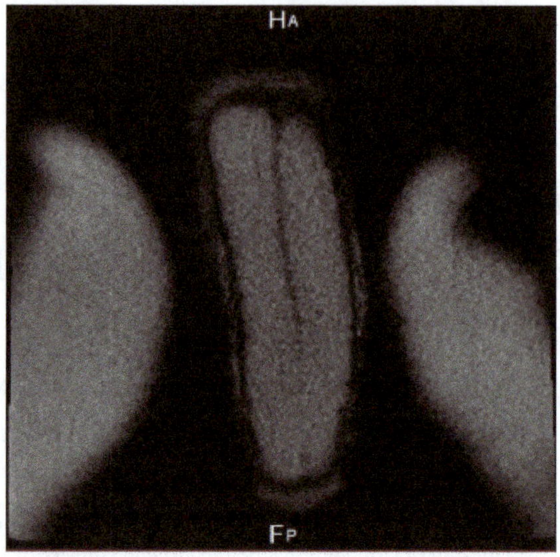

FIGURE 3: MRI of the penis showing the integrity of the cavernous bodies.

Conservative treatment was done with nonsteroidal anti-inflammatory drugs (NSAID) and acetyl salicylic acid stick (100mg/day) for thrombosis prevention by coagulation and platelet aggregation inhibition. The patient was informed about the necessity of sexual abstinence till disappearance of all symptoms. The evolution was marked by quick and favorable recovery with disappearance of pain in eight weeks, reduction of the swelling, and complete and total recovery of the penis. At six months of follow-up, no evidence of reoccurrence was observed.

3. Discussion

Penile Mondor's Disease (PMD) by superficial venous thrombosis of the dorsal vein of the penis described the first time by Braun Falco in 1955 is a benign genital condition [2]. It affects men with active sexual activities. Etiopathogenesis is not well known; many risks factors are being described. The main risk factor is excessive sexual activities, but also implicated are trauma, sexual abstinence, local infections as sexual transmitted disease, pelvic tumours, or use of vasoconstrictive drugs, bladder overdistension, use of vacuum erection device, and so on. Association of PMD with some urologic tumours as bladder cancer or prostate cancer has been reported and this pathology has been described as a first unusual manifestation of the metastatic pancreatic adenocarcinoma [5]. In our case, intense sexual activity was identified as a main risk factor. Our patient was married with four women, and he reported an intense sexual activity during the period when PMD have occurred. However Penile Mondor's Disease can occur without a clearly determined aetiology. Sickle cell disease could be also a risk factor as reported by some authors [6]. In fact, Nachmann and colleagues in their study on Penile Mondor's Disease argued that, during sickle cell disease crisis, PMD can occurr regarding possibility of the genesis of thrombus [7]. Diagnosis of Penile Mondor's Disease is usually made on clinical findings; thorough taking of the medical history and a correct physical examination are essential for diagnosing. A cord-like lesion with few centimeters in length can be easily recognized on inspection, and a hard induration can be palpated beneath the skin [3]. Sometime the lesion can extended cranially to the suprapubic region, and the vein will appear distended and erythematous like in the case of our patient. Laboratories tests and invasive diagnostic tool are not always mandatory to make the PMD diagnosis. The thrombosed superficial veins should first be detected with a gray-scale sonogram. Doppler coupled with ultrasound can be helpful in certain situations when the diagnosis is not evident. Doppler and US can be also used for follow-up, showing the recanalization of the endoluminal thrombosis vein after the total recovery of the patient. In our patient Doppler couple with Ultrasound, Magnetic Resonance Imaging of the penis was requested to ensure that there are no lesions in the cavernous and spongious bodies and thus the diagnosis of the superficial venous thrombosis was retained. Differential diagnosis of the painful swelling deforming penis may include penile fracture, Peyronie disease, which is a painful deviation of the shaft during erection, without palpation of the indurated dorsal cord like in PMD. The treatment of the superficial dorsal venous thrombosis of the penis varied from simple observation, conservative therapy, and anticoagulation drugs administration to radical treatment with surgery including thrombectomy and dorsal vein resection. General measures must be observed as sexual abstinence and treatment of underlying disease if present. In reported cases, where patient received no treatment, healing occurs after 6 or 8 weeks with recanalization of the thrombosed vein [7]. In acute state, proposed therapies are variable: antiplatelet aggregate agents, NSAID, heparin drugs for preventive and curative treatment for 15 days. In case where medical treatment was not effective or PMD which not responding to medical treatment, surgical thrombectomy of the superficial dorsal vein can be attempted [8]. Sasso F and colleagues distinguished three types of treatment according to the clinical stage. None of the proposed method has shown a significant reduction in the healing duration. [4]. For Walsh and colleagues, Penile Mondor's Disease is a benign condition with common presentation but an uncommon disease but its treatment is primarily symptomatic but may vary depending on possible underlying disease processes [9]. However antibiotics drug administration is associated when there is cellulitis or sexually transmitted diseases (STD) till remission of symptoms. Nazir SS and colleagues found that the local infiltration of anesthetics (bupivacaine 0.5%) around the thrombosed area considerably retrieved the pain [10]. Our patient received a nonsteroidal anti-inflammatory and antiplatelet aggregate drug and total resolution was achieved in 8 weeks.

4. Conclusion

Mondor's Disease localized in the penis is a rare and benign pathology that the pathogenesis is not yet clear and well known. The diagnosis is based on clinical findings and the investigations by Doppler coupled with ultrasound can contribute to the diagnosis. Conservative therapy with observation or NSAID anticoagulation agent administration and temporary sexual abstinence can occur healing with total recovery. Surgical treatment can be indicated when there is persistence of thrombosis after a long-term medical treatment.

Disclosure

The authors would like to state that an earlier version of this case report was presented at "59th Annual scientific congress of West African College of Surgeons", Dakar, 2019.

References

[1] H. Mondor, "Subcutaneous tronculitis of the anterolateral thoracic wall," *Mémoires. Académie de chirurgie*, vol. 65, pp. 1258–1271, 1939.

[2] O. Braun-Falco, "Zur Klinik, histologie, und pathogenese der strangformigenoberflachlichen phlebitiden," *Dermatol Wochenschr*, vol. 132, pp. 705–715, 1955.

[3] J. D. Helm and I. G. Hodge, "Thrombophlebitis of a dorsal vein of the penis; report of a case treated by phenylbutazone (butazolidin)," *The Journal of Urology*, vol. 79, no. 2, pp. 306-307, 1958.

[4] F. Sasso, G. Gulino, M. Basar, A. Carbone, P. Torricelli, and E. Alcini, "Penile Mondors' disease: an underestimated pathology," *BJU International*, vol. 77, no. 5, pp. 729–732, 1996.

[5] E. Desportes, A. Rabii, R. Dautry et al., "Superficial venous thrombosis of the penis (Penile Mondors Disease). A case report and literature review," *Annales Françaises de Médecine d'Urgence*, vol. 3, pp. 337–339, 2013.

[6] G. Botcho, K. Tengué, T. M. Kpatcha et al., "Superficial venous thrombosis of the penis (Penile Mondor's Disease). A case report and literature review," *Uro'Andro*, vol. 1, no. 6, pp. 294–296, 2016.

[7] M. M. Nachmann, J. S. Jaffe, P. C. Ginsberg, M. M. Horrow, and R. C. Harkaway, "Sickle cell episode manifesting as superficial thrombophlebitis of the penis," *The Journal of the American Osteopathic Association*, vol. 103, no. 2, pp. 102–104, 2003.

[8] H. Zidani, M. Foughali, and J.-P. Laroche, "Superficial venous thrombosis of the penis: Penile Mondor's disease ? A case report and literature review," *Journal des Maladies Vasculaires*, vol. 35, no. 6, pp. 352–354, 2010.

[9] J. C. Walsh, S. Poimboeuf, and D. S. Garvin, "A common presentation to an uncommon disease. penile mondor's disease: A case report and literature review," *International Medical Case Reports Journal*, vol. 7, pp. 155–157, 2014.

[10] S. S. Nazir and M. Khan, "Thrombosis of the dorsal vein of the penis (Mondor's Disease): A case report and review of the literature," *Indian Journal of Urology*, vol. 26, no. 3, pp. 431–433, 2010.

5

Penile Fracture: Delayed Presentation, Primary Urethral Repair and Satisfactory Outcome

Bashir Yunusa,[1] Kalamon Wullie,[1] Soeghen E. Willie,[1] Solomane Konneh,[1] Swaliho Sherriff,[1] Ayun Cassell ,[2] and Edit Ikpi[1]

[1]*Department of Surgery, Liberia College of Physicians and Surgeons, Monrovia, Liberia*
[2]*Département d'Urologie et d'Andrologie, Hôpital Général de Grand Yoff, Dakar, Senegal*

Correspondence should be addressed to Ayun Cassell; ayuncasselliii@gmail.com

Academic Editor: David Duchene

Penile fracture is a relatively rare condition warranting emergency intervention. The commonest etiological factor remains coital activities, which explains why it is being underreported. Presentation is usually delayed and up to 38% of cases present with associated urethral injury. Prompt surgical intervention and primary urethral repair are associated with a good outcome. We present a 30-year-old male with unilateral penile fracture and associated urethral injury following sexual intercourse.

1. Introduction

Penile fracture is defined as the rupture of the tunica albuginea of the corpus cavernosum caused by blunt trauma to the erect penis [1]. The condition is relatively rare and under reported [2], but its occurrence requires emergency intervention. There are several etiological factors, but blunt trauma from coitus accounts for most causes [3]. Others include falls, forceful manipulation or masturbation [4, 5] or rolling over an erect penis [6], and Penile curvature (chordae) [7]. Penile fractures usually present with a 'popping' sound with concomitant sudden swelling and ecchymosis of the penis followed by rapid detumescence [2]. A significant number of cases come with associated urethral injury, ranging from 3% to 38% in different literatures [8, 9]. Before now, we do not know whether delay in presentation or surgical intervention may affect the outcome of repair or risk recurrence [10].

We present here a case of 30-years-old man who presented two weeks after he sustained penile fracture from rigorous sexual intercourse to the ER of John F. Kennedy Medical Centre, Monrovia, Liberia.

A 30-years-old Liberian male presented with painful swollen penis following sexual intercourse for 2 weeks. Patient was involved in sexual activity in the male dominant position when his penis slipped out and hit the inner thigh of his partner with immediate excruciating pain along the shaft of his penis, slow detumescence ranging 3–5 minutes, swelling of the right side of his penis, and left curvature. He denied the use of sex enhancing drugs and did not admit penile curvature prior to the trauma. He presented within 2 weeks to the emergency room following increasing painful micturition and hematuria where he had successful catheterization prior to urological review.

All other examinations were normal except the area of pathology. The distal half of the penis, including the glans, was tilted to the left, the penile shaft appeared edematous without apparent discoloration. There was neither associated scrotal nor perineal swelling, urethral catheter in situ draining bloody urine. There was tenderness on palpation of the penile shaft with the point of maximum tenderness on the right mid-third of the shaft. He was diagnosed of penile fracture with possible urethral injury and prepared for surgery.

1.1. Intraoperative Findings. A degloving incision was made through the skin, the Dartos fascia found intact and then separated, and the deep penile (Buck) fascia was found to have a bulging hematoma on the right mid shaft and an approximate 4 cm transverse defect on the ventral surface of the right tunica albuginea with complete urethral defect at the same spot were seen. Tunical defect was repair in two layers with PDS 3/0

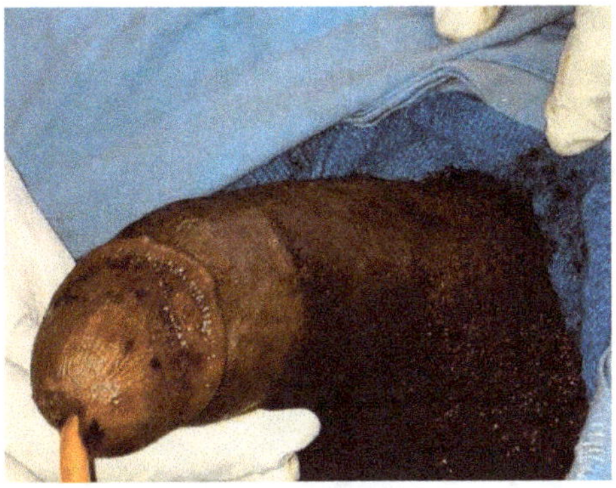

FIGURE 1: The penis preoperatively, with left curvature and right mid shaft swelling.

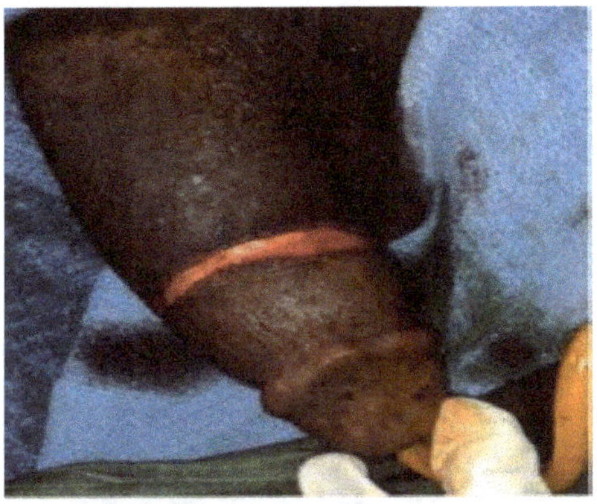

FIGURE 2: Degloving incision at the beginning of surgery.

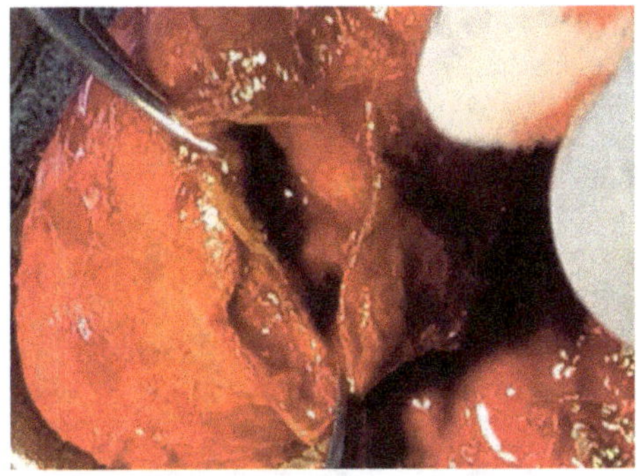

FIGURE 3: The right exposed tunica albuginea with a 4 cm transverse defect.

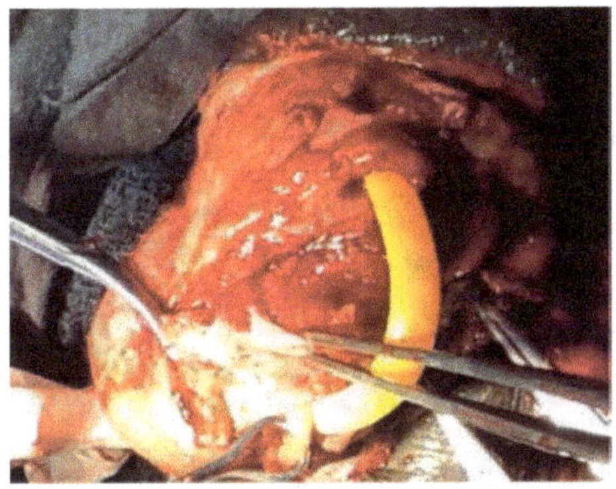

FIGURE 4: The completely disrupted urethra and part of the exposed erectile bodies.

suture and the urethra spatulated and anastomosed with vicryl 3/0 over the indwelling catheter. The Buck's and Dartos fascia and the penile skin closed in layers in a simple interrupted fashion. Saline induced erection demonstrated leak free repair. Patient admitted having morning tumescence. Catheter was removed after 2 weeks of repair and rigid cystoscopy revealed intact urethra with visible suture lines.

2. Discussion

A penile fracture typically occurs in the setting of blunt penile trauma to the erect penis, most often during sexual intercourse or masturbation. The characteristic symptoms of penile fracture are a "snapping" or "popping" sound, penile pain, and immediate detumescence followed by ecchymosis and swelling of the penile shaft [11]. Distinguishing penile ecchymosis from a true penile fracture, or a rupture through the tunical albuginea, can be a challenging clinical conundrum, most especially in patients like ours, who presented up to 2 weeks after the trauma and denied the typical popping sounds, with a relatively long time of 3–5 minutes for penile collapse but admitted painful urine and hematuria.

Physical examination findings may vary significantly in patients with a history suggestive of penile fracture, especially in late presentation, and the severity of the penile ecchymosis frequently does not correlate with the presence or absence of tunical rupture. History and physical examination may be inaccurate in 15% of patients with a suspected penile fracture [11], as non-sex related rupture has also been described [12]; but the typical history of slipping and striking the perineum made us suspect the fracture. With the history of late presentation, we did not find ultrasound or retrograde urethrography (RUG), necessary, since, further delay can increase risk of infection and probable suture dehiscence [13, 14].

The patient presented with swollen right sides and deviation of the phallus to the left as shown in (Figure 1), suggestive of ipsilateral/unilateral fracture. Unilateral fractures are common in 89.7% of cases in some series and very rarely bilateral cases in up to 1.9% [14]. Where isolated fractures occur, right fracture is more frequently documented, up to 53.2% than left 45.2% [15]. With unilateral rupture suspected due to the curvature to the left, painful hematuria and no history of curvature before trauma, a carvenosogram could have been done to rule out bilateral rupture. However, due to delayed presentation, suspected increased risk of infection and absent radiological facilities and expertise in our centre, we did not consider the study. RUG would have shown partial or complete disruption of the urethra. Although, complete urethral disruption, would have been more associated with bilateral rupture, prior catheterization might have caused the complete injury seen intraoperatively.

Penile fractures are common among young adults, with average age of 38 years, who are sexually very active, with

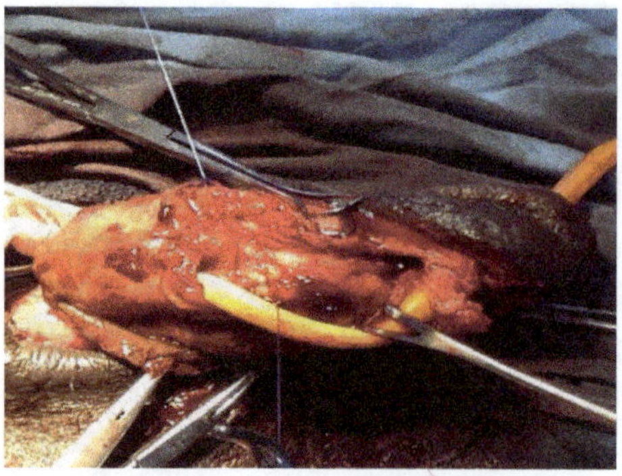

FIGURE 5: Repaired right tunica albuginea first layer.

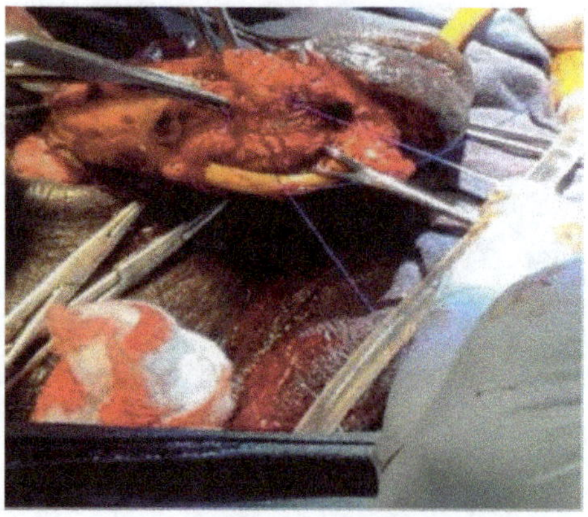

FIGURE 6: Repair of tunica albuginea of the right corpus Cavernosum, second layer.

aggressive sexual behaviors, and the tendency to use sex enhancing drugs for various reasons as described by Tang et al. [15]; further describing summer seasons with highest admission due to penile fracture, when young adults are more likely to have high sexual contacts. But, in Africa, where these adults may be close to or under the care of the parents, may feel ashamed to disclose the ailment to other family members or even hospital staff, leading to delayed presentation; and the concomitant lack of urologist may lead to delayed repair due to time taken for referrals.

Subcoronal skin incision [14] gives good access for degloving and is cosmetically appealing as shown in (Figure 2). Our findings included bulging hematoma on the right Bucks' fascia and a 4 cm transverse tear on the tunica mid shaft (Figure 3) with complete disruption of the urethra at the same level (Figure 4). Associated urethral injuries are documented in up to 38% of cases [15, 16]. The defect was repaired in two layers with PDS 3/0 suture (Figures 5 and 6). The approach was based on knowledge of the clinical application of the two layered anatomy of the tunica albuginea of the corpus caversosum as reported by Hsu et al. [17]. Thus, the repair of the outer longitudinal layer was considered a determinant factor of the surgical success in this tunical surgery regardless of the strength of the suture, even with our choice of PDS suture [17].

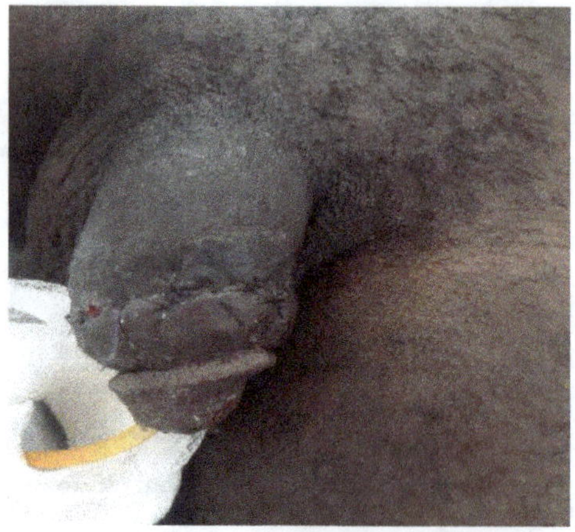

FIGURE 7: Penile straightened after repair.

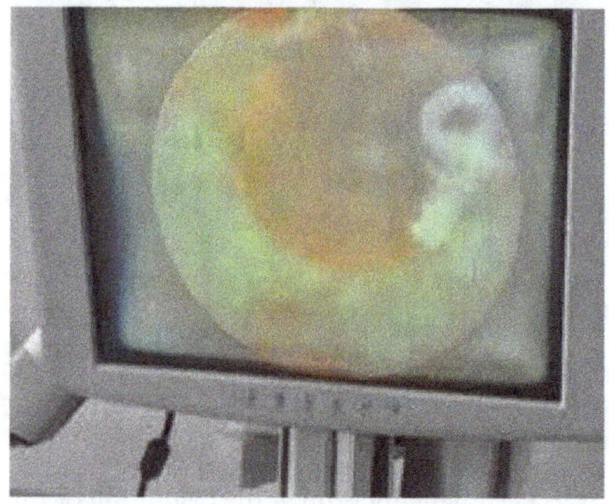

FIGURE 8: Rigid cystoscopy revealed intact urethra with some yet to be absorbed vicryl.

The urethra was repaired primarily, spatulated, and anastomosed with vicryl 3/0 over the indwelling catheter with continuous suture [18, 14]; although interrupted suture repairs are most documented [19]. The postoperative outcome was satisfactory within two weeks; as primary repair has been proven to have a good outcome in some reports [16]. Hsu and colleagues documented curvature correction after some series of repair (7), but we could not find reasons for subsequent repair of curvature, as there was no previous history of curvature or demonstrable postoperative curvature. We obtained a good outcome with continuous sutures on top of delayed presentation. Delayed presentation and or repair have been documented to have satisfactory outcome. There was immediate straightening of the penis after the repairs (Figure 7) and an intact urethra was demonstrated by rigid cystoscopy (Figure 8) two weeks postoperatively.

3. Conclusion

Penile fracture is either rare or under reported, patients in our resource depleted environment tend to conceal or delay presentation, but delayed presentations and primary urethral repair do have satisfactory outcome.

Conflicts of Interest

The authors declare that they have no conflicts of interest.

References

[1] P. Kasaraneni, P. Mylarappa, R. Desi Gowda, S. Puvvada, and D. Kasaraneni, *Archivio Italiano di Urologia e Andrologia*, vol. 90, no. 4, pp. 283–287, 2018.

[2] I. Anastasiou, A. Anastasiou, I. Katafigiotis, D. Tsavdaris, and C. Constantinides, "Isolated corpus spongiosum injury after sexual intercourse," *Archivio Italiano di Urologia e Andrologia*, vol. 90, no. 4, pp. 295–296, 2018.

[3] I. Alnadhari, O. A. Abdeljaleel, V. R. Pai Sampige, A. Abdulmuhsin, and A. Shamsodini, "Penile fracture: simultaneous complete urethral rupture with bilateral corpora cavernosa rupture," *Case Reports in Urology*, vol. 2018, Article ID 4929518, 3 pages, 2018.

[4] F. M. da Silva Barroso, C. S. Paiva, J. E. R. Rodriguez, B. T. F. Cabral, H. D. de Araujo, and P. M. de Souza, "Recurrent bilateral penile fracture: Case report," *Urology Case Reports*, vol. 21, pp. 32–33, 2018.

[5] L. Dell'Atti, S. Scarcella, G. Argalia, L. Montesi, G. M. Giuseppetti, and A. B. Galosi, "Rupture of the cavernous body diagnosed by contrast-enhanced ultrasound: presentation of a clinical case," *Archivio Italiano di Urologia e Andrologia*, vol. 90, no. 2, pp. 143–144, 2018.

[6] F. A. Gulmi, "Penile Fracture, NYU Case of the Month, Early February 2018," *Reviews in Urology*, vol. 20, no. 1, pp. 41–42, 2018.

[7] G. L. Hsu, C. H. Hsieh, H. S. Wen, and C. T. J. Han-Sun, "Curvature correction in patients with tunical rupture: a necessary adjunct to repair," *The Journal of Urology*, vol. 167, no. 3, pp. 1381–1383, 2002.

[8] A. Kandemir, M. Balasar, N. Poyraz, and M. M. Piskin, "Penile fracture with urethral injury: radiological evaluation," *Eurasian Journal of Medicine*, vol. 49, pp. 217–219, 2017.

[9] R. Barros, M. I. S. Silva, V. Antonucci, L. Schulze, L. Koifman, and L. A. Favorito, "Primary urethral reconstruction results in penile fracture," *The Annals of the Royal College of Surgeons of England*, vol. 100, pp. 21–25, 2018.

[10] B. Nascimento, G. B. Guglielmetti, E. P. Miranda et al., "Recurrent penile fracture—case report and alternative surgical approach," *Sexual Medicine*, vol. 6, pp. 263–266, 2018.

[11] I. S. Metzler, A. B. Reed-Maldonado, and T. F. Lue, "Suspected penile fracture: to operate or not to operate?" *Translational Andrology and Urology*, vol. 6, no. 5, pp. 981–986, 2017.

[12] Z. Bayraktar and S. Albayrak, "Non sex-related subtotal rupture of the corpus cavernosum without urethral injury: a case report and literature review," *Archivio Italiano di Urologia e Andrologia*, vol. 88, no. 3, pp. 233–234, 2016.

[13] M. A. Hassali, A. I. Nouri, A. A. Hamzah, and A. K. Verma, "Role of penile doppler as a diagnostic tool in penile fracture," *Journal of Medical Ultrasound*, vol. 26, no. 1, pp. 48–51, 2018.

[14] E. Rajih, A. Alenizi, and A. El-Hakim, "Penile fracture with two ipsilateral corporal tears and delayed presentation: a case report," *Canadian Urological Association Journal*, vol. 9, no. 9–10, 741 pages, 2015.

[15] Z. Tang, L. Yang, Q. Wei et al., "Management and outcomes of penile fracture: a retrospective analysis of 62 cases with long-term assessment," *Asian Journal of Andrology*, vol. 20, no. 4, pp. 412–413, 2018.

[16] R. Barros, M. Guimarães, C. Nascimento Jr., L. R. A., L. Koifman, and L. A. Favorito, "Penile refracture: a preliminary report," *International Brazilian Journal of Urology*, vol. 44, no. 4, pp. 800–804, 2018.

[17] G.-L. Hsu, "Hypothesis of human penile anatomy, erection hemodynamics and their clinical applications," *Asian Journal of Andrology*, vol. 8, no. 2, pp. 225–234, 2006.

[18] M. Rahman, M. S. Faridi, N. Mibang, and R. S. Singh, "Penile manipulation: the most common etiology of penile fracture at our tertiary care center," *Journal of Family Medicine and Primary Care*, vol. 5, no. 2, pp. 471–473, 2016.

[19] M. S. Faridi, N. Agarwal, P. Saini, N. Kaur, and A. Gupta, "Myriad presentations of penile fracture: report of three cases and review of literature," *Journal of Family Medicine and Primary Care*, vol. 4, no. 2, pp. 273–275, 2015.

6

A Paratesticular Angiolipoma: A Case Report of a Rare Benign Scrotal Mass and Review of Literature

Mohamed Ali Nouioui,[1] Tarek Taktak,[1] Seif Mokadem,[1] Faten Gargouri,[2] Houssem Mediouni,[1] Ramzi Khiari,[1] and Samir Ghozzi[1]

[1]*Department of Urology, Military Hospital of First Instruction of Tunis, Tunisia*
[2]*Department of Pathology, Military Hospital of First Instruction of Tunis, Tunisia*

Correspondence should be addressed to Mohamed Ali Nouioui; mednouiouimed@gmail.com

Academic Editor: Tun-Chieh Chen

We report a rare case of paratesticular angiolipoma in a young male. The patient is a 21-year-old male who presented with a palpable firm right intrascrotal mass of 21 mm. Ultrasound findings demonstrated that it is a solid mass. Under the diagnosis of an intrascrotal solid mass, a right inguinal radical orchiectomy was performed. Histopathological examination concluded to a paratesticular angiolipoma. Angiolipoma is a rare benign form of paratesticular tumour and its diagnosis is based on histological findings of the surgical specimen with no recurrence risk. This mesenchymal tumour should be distinguished from liposarcoma, which has malignant or aggressive clinical course.

1. Introduction

Angiolipoma is an extremely rare form of paratesticular tumour observed in urologic clinical practice [1]. A search of the Medline database revealed few rare cases of such lesion, usually confirmed by the microscopic pathologic evaluation of the surgical specimen. Tumours occurring in the paratesticular region may be clinically indistinguishable from intratesticular tumours, thus resulting in initial misdiagnosis. The preoperative distinction between the benign and malignant lesion is rarely made which results in difficulty in diagnosis and management [2] such as in the case reported herein.

2. Case Presentation

A 21-year-old male with a history of one episode of right orchitis well treated with antibiotics two years ago presented to the urology outpatient department with a painless swelling of the right hemiscrotum without any associated other symptoms. Local examination revealed a palpable firm right testicular mass with atrophy of the whole testis. The left testis was palpated in the scrotum and is of normal size with no suspicious mass. His laboratory findings including Germ Cell Tumour serum markers were within the normal range (Alpha-fetoprotein (AFP): 0,86 μg/L, Beta human chorionic gonadotrophin (β-HCG) < 0,5 mIU/mL, and lactate dehydrogenase (LDH): 241 UI/ml).

Scrotal ultrasound (Figure 1) demonstrated a suspicious solid well-defined mass within the right epididymis, measuring 21 x 14 mm. The mass was slightly heterogeneous with hyperechoic appearance and regular smooth contour. Distinct from the lesion, the right testis appeared smaller in size measuring 23 x 12 x 15 mm. Imaging of the contralateral scrotum revealed no anomaly. A radical right orchiectomy was performed via an inguinal incision. Recovery was uneventful. The surgical specimen consisted of the right testis measuring 3.5x2.5x1 cm in size and of the spermatic cord measuring 5 cm in length. Sectioning of the specimen (Figure 2) revealed a single well circumscribed nodular tissue with multiple foci of hemorrhage. Microscopic examination of the nodular tissue (Figure 3) showed an admixture of mature lobulated adipose tissue and numerous dilated and thicken walled blood vessels with no signs of malignancies such as germ cell atypia or intraepithelial germ cell neoplasm. Thus a diagnosis of paratesticular angiolipoma was made.

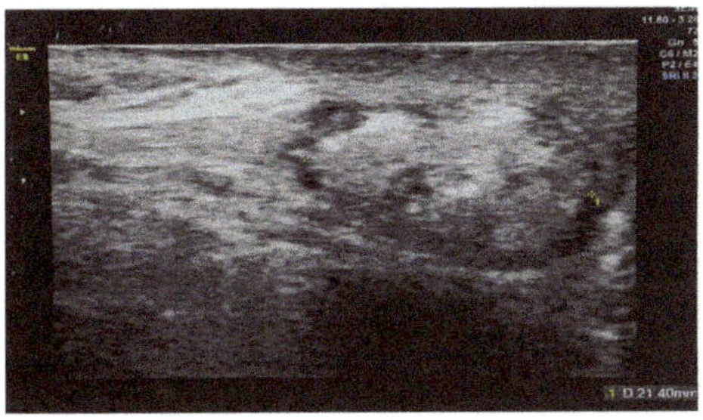

FIGURE 1: US demonstrating a solid 21 mm mass within the right epididymis.

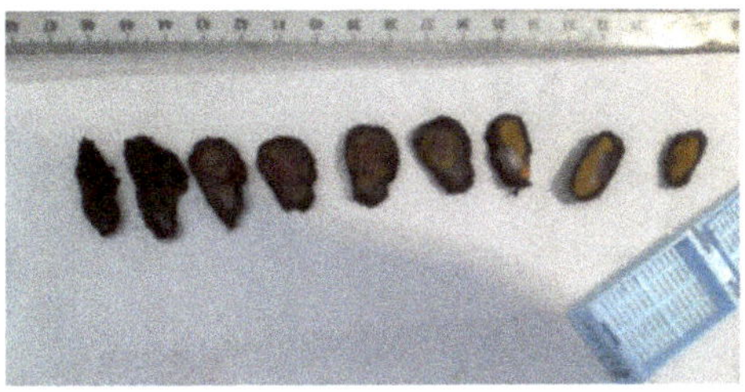

FIGURE 2: Sectioning of the specimen revealing a single well circumscribed nodular tissue.

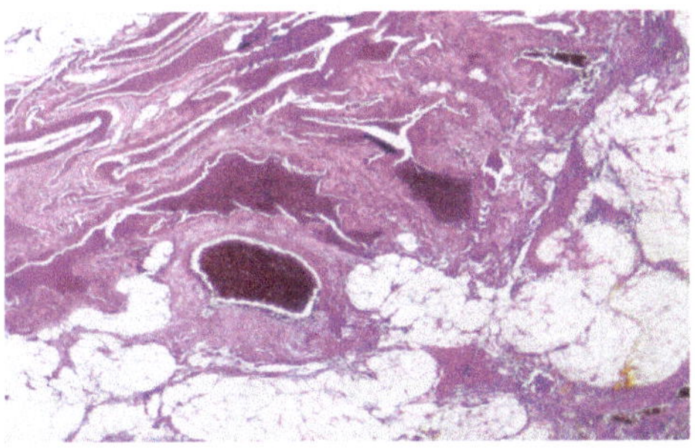

FIGURE 3: Microscopic examination showing a mature lobulated adipose tissue and numerous dilated and thicken walled blood vessels.

3. Discussion

The paratesticular region is a complex anatomical area which includes the contents of the spermatic cord, testicular tunics, epididymis, and vestigial remnants. Histogenetically, this area is composed of a variety of epithelial, mesothelial, and mesenchymal elements and neoplasms arising from this region, therefore form a heterogeneous group of tumours with different behavioural patterns [3]. While 95% of intratesticular lesions are malignant, most of paratesticular masses are benign [4]. Lipoma accounts for approximately 90% of benign paratesticular soft tissues tumours. Variants of lipoma, including fibrolipoma and angiolipoma, may arise in the testis such in our case [5]. Usually the most common clinical manifestations include vague scrotal discomfort or heaviness leading to a physical examination that discovers a painless firm scrotal mass. Because of the availability, ease of use, and high resolution of ultrasonography (US), it is the imaging modality of choice for testicular pathologies and characterisation of testicular masses [6] with high sensitivity regarding the detection, localization, and sizing of such lesions. However, it shows low specificity in differentiating benign from malignant type [7]. This makes an inguinal testicular exploration necessary because the diagnosis of paratesticular angiolipoma can only be made by histological evaluation of the surgical specimen. One of the top differential diagnoses of angiolipoma is well differentiated liposarcoma which is a malignant mesenchymal neoplasm showing adipocytic differentiation with completely different management recommendations and prognosis.

Less than 5% of soft tissue sarcomas arise from the genitourinary tract, accounting for only 1–2% of all malignant genitourinary tumours [8].

Liposarcoma accounts for 20 to 56% of sarcomas at this anatomical site in adults and most paratesticular liposarcomas are well differentiated [2, 9].

Due to the rarity of this type of tumour, clinical research regarding this disease is difficult.

Both benign lipoma and liposarcoma present as a nonspecific painless paratesticular, sometimes inguinal, firm mass.

On gross examination, lipoma-like well differentiated liposarcoma resembles mature fat which makes it difficult for initial intraoperative assessment by surgeons, thus mistreated with initial marginal resection of the lesion which is largely insufficient for such an aggressive tumour. Histologic features are important in the assessment of these lesions because well differentiated liposarcoma consists of mature adipocytes with marked variation in cell size, nuclear atypia such as enlarged hyperchromatic nuclei, and a variable number of scatted lipoblasts, all not found in benign adipocytic lesions [10].

Immunohistochemically, the most useful diagnostic markers are MDM2 and CDK4, which allow distinguishing well differentiated liposarcoma from benign lipomatous lesions [11].

The clinical course of well differentiated liposarcoma has tendency for local recurrence after inadequate resection, whereas distant spread is rare but common for high grade tumours. Local recurrence is often repeated and may involve the inguinal canal, pelvis, and scrotum [12, 13].

Thus, the recommended treatment policy for liposarcoma includes aggressive local management consisting of surgery and RT for most patients [14].

Appropriate surgery consists of radical inguinal orchiectomy and wide excision of the prior scar and tumour bed if initially excised including removal of all the soft tissues in the inguinal canal with high ligation of the spermatic cord at the level of the inguinal ring. Hemiscrotectomy should be performed in cases where the scrotum was violated by prior biopsy or excision or if there was direct involvement of the scrotum by tumour [12].

However, angiolipoma has a favourable prognosis with no recurrence rate if well excised.

4. Conclusion

Angiolipoma is an uncommon benign tumour that is rarely found in the scrotum but need to be considered when assessing a patient with scrotal mass. Ultrasound findings can be indecisive. An inguinal surgical approach provides a suitable exposure for complete resection. Histopathological examination is the only way to provide the definitive diagnosis to distinguish it from a lipoma-like well differentiated liposarcoma, thus determining the appropriate course of treatment.

References

[1] A. L. Folpe and S. W. Weiss, "Paratesticular soft tissue neoplasms," *Seminars in Diagnostic Pathology*, vol. 17, no. 4, pp. 307–318, 2000.

[2] B. Khoubehi, V. Mishra, M. Ali, H. Motiwala, and O. Karim, "Adult paratesticular tumours," *BJU International*, vol. 90, no. 7, pp. 707–715, 2002.

[3] T. F. Lioe and J. D. Biggart, "Tumours of the spermatic cord and paratesticular tissue. a clinicopathological study," *British Journal of Urology*, vol. 71, no. 5, pp. 600–606, 1993.

[4] Ş. Başal, E. Malkoç, E. Aydur et al., "Fibrous pseudotumors of the testis: The balance between sparing the testis and preoperative diagnostic difficulty," *Turk Uroloji Dergisi*, vol. 40, no. 3, pp. 125–129, 2014.

[5] V. Vagnoni, E. Brunocilla, R. Schiavina et al., "Inguinal canal tumors of adulthood," *Anticancer Reseach*, vol. 33, no. 6, pp. 2361–2368, 2013.

[6] V. S. Dogra, R. H. Gottlieb, M. Oka, and D. J. Rubens, "Sonography of the scrotum," *Radiology*, vol. 227, no. 1, pp. 18–36, 2003.

[7] T. Auer, T. De Zordo, C. Dejaco et al., "Value of multiparametric US in the assessment of intratesticular lesions," *Radiology*, vol. 285, no. 2, pp. 640–649, 2017.

[8] A. Jemal, R. Siegel, E. Ward et al., "Cancer statistics, 2008," *CA: A Cancer Journal for Clinicians*, vol. 58, no. 2, pp. 71–96, 2008.

[9] Z. A. Dotan, R. Tal, D. Golijanin et al., "Adult genitourinary sarcoma: the 25-year memorial Sloan-Kettering experience," *The Journal of Urology*, vol. 176, no. 5, pp. 2033–2039, 2006.

[10] C. N. Johnson, A. S. Ha, E. Chen, and D. Davidson, "Lipomatous soft-tissue tumors," *Journal of the American Academy of Orthopaedic Surgeons*, vol. 26, no. 22, pp. 779–788, 2018.

[11] M. R. Clay, A. P. Martinez, S. W. Weiss, and M. A. Edgar, "MDM2 and CDK4 immunohistochemistry: should it be used in problematic differentiated lipomatous tumors?: a new perspective," *The American Journal of Surgical Pathology*, vol. 40, no. 12, pp. 1647–1652, 2016.

[12] M. J. Khandekar, C. P. Raut, J. L. Hornick, Q. Wang, B. M. Alexander, and E. H. Baldini, "Paratesticular liposarcoma: unusual patterns of recurrence and importance of margins," *Annals of Surgical Oncology*, vol. 20, no. 7, pp. 2148–2155, 2013.

[13] J. Levay, B. O'sullivan, C. Catton et al., "Outcome and prognostic factors in soft tissue sarcoma in the adult," *International Journal of Radiation Oncology • Biology • Physics*, vol. 27, no. 5, pp. 1091–1099, 1993.

[14] M. T. Ballo, G. K. Zagars, P. W. Pisters, B. W. Feig, S. R. Patel, and A. C. Von Eschenbach, "Spermatic cord sarcoma: outcome, patterns of failure and management," *The Journal of Urology*, vol. 166, no. 4, pp. 1306–1310, 2001.

7

Organ-Sparing Surgery for a Giant Verrucous Carcinoma of the Penile Shaft: A Case Report and Review of the Literature

Prodromos Philippou[1,2], Christos Kitsios,[1,2] Maria Miliatou,[1,2] Christiana Poullou,[3,4] and Pavlos Konstantinou[3,4]

[1] *St George's Medical School, University of Nicosia, Nicosia, Cyprus*
[2] *Apollonion Hospital, Nicosia, Cyprus*
[3] *Histopathology and Cytology Laboratory Services, Nicosia, Cyprus*
[4] *School of Medicine, European University of Cyprus, Cyprus*

Correspondence should be addressed to Prodromos Philippou; brucemed@hotmail.com

Academic Editor: Ferdinando Fusco

Verrucous Carcinoma is a rare but well-differentiated variant of penile squamous cell carcinoma. Its clinical presentation is usually that of an exophytic cauliflower-like lesion with a broad-based growth pattern. We herein report the case of a 61-year-old man who presented with a giant verrucous carcinoma occupying the dorsal surface of the penile shaft. The patient underwent penile-sparing surgery, achieving both disease control and organ preservation. We discuss relevant issues, including clinical features, diagnosis, surgical management, and prognosis and we review the rather sparse literature regarding this rare lesion.

1. Introduction

Penile carcinoma is a rare malignancy in the West, with an incidence of 0.1-0.9 cases per 100.000 adult males in Europe [1, 2]. A significant geographical variation of this malignancy is noted, as the incidence may be as high as 19 cases per 100.000 males in some parts of Asia, South America, and Africa [1, 2].

Verrucous carcinoma (VC) is a relatively rare and well-differentiated variant of penile squamous cell carcinoma. Its biological behavior is that of a well-differentiated tumor with an extremely low metastatic potential [3–5]. Penile VC may, however, exhibit a pattern of aggressive local growth and occasionally presents as locally advanced disease [6, 7]. Historically, in the vast majority of patients presenting with penile carcinomas, the primary lesion was managed by either radical surgery (partial or total penile amputation) or radiotherapy, but the current trend is for a less aggressive (i.e., organ-sparing) surgical approach [8–10]. In the case of VC, due to the rarity of the disease, solid data on optimal management are lacking.

We herein report the case of a 61-year-old man who presented with a large VC occupying the penile shaft and was successfully managed by penile-preserving surgery.

2. Case Presentation

A 61-year-old policeman, with no previous urological history, presented with a large exophytic, cauliflower-like, and partially ulcerated lesion, measuring 7x4 cm located at the dorsal surface of the penile shaft (Figure 1). The patient reported a past medical history of hypertension but was otherwise fit and healthy. He was sexually active, denied erectile dysfunction, and had never smoked. On palpation, the lesion was large but mobile and did not appear to invade the corpora cavernosa. Physical examination confirmed the absence of palpable inguinal nodes, and routine laboratory tests (including Alkaline Phosphatase and Calcium levels) were within normal limits. After excluding infections, including sexually transmitted diseases, an incisional biopsy of the lesion revealed the presence of low-grade squamous cell carcinoma and the absence of lymphovascular invasion. Staging

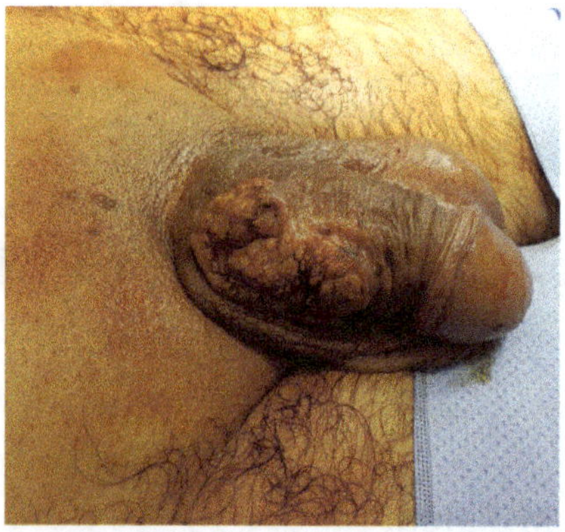

Figure 1: A large exophytic, cauliflower-like, and partially ulcerated lesion, measuring 7x4 cm located at the dorsal surface of the penile shaft.

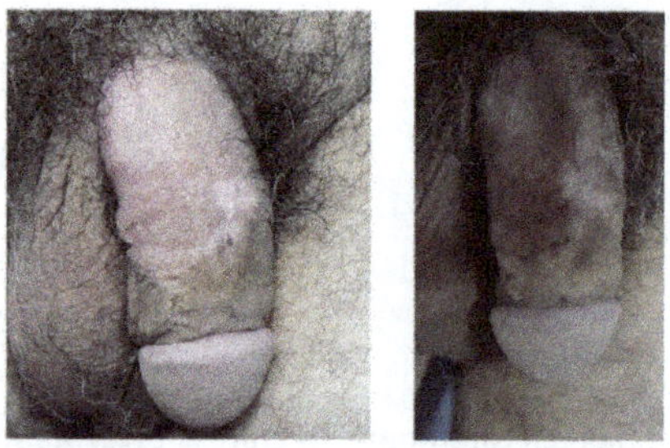

Figure 2: A satisfactory cosmetic result was recorded at 3 months (left) and 6 months (right) postoperatively.

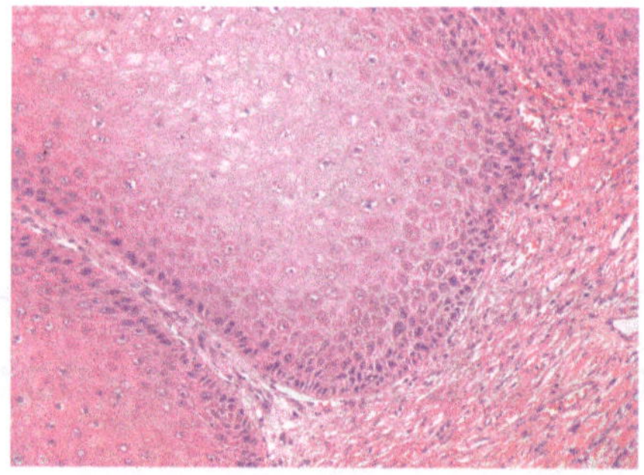

Figure 3: On microscopy, the tumor front is broad-based and pushes the subepithelial tissues [haematoxylin-eosin stain, original magnification x200].

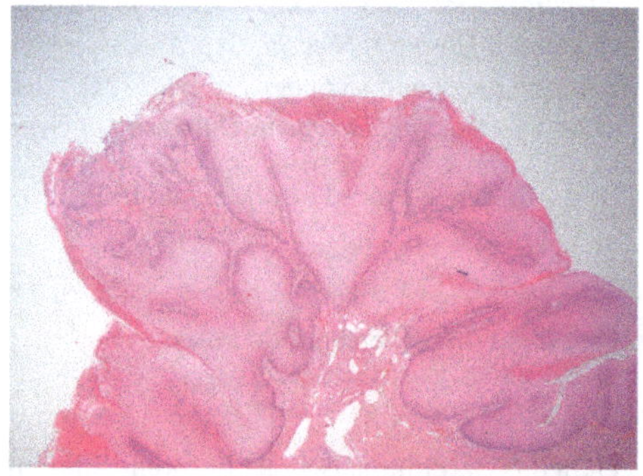

Figure 4: The tumor is characterized by prominent papillomatosis and acanthosis [haematoxylin-eosin stain, original magnification x20].

CT of the chest, abdomen, and pelvis did not demonstrate metastatic disease or enlarged lymph nodes.

After discussion, further surgical management was decided, including excision of the primary lesion and reconstruction of the tissue gap. The patient underwent wide local excision of the affected area of skin in the penile shaft, and intraoperative frozen section analysis was used to confirm margin negativity. A circumcision was also performed, and the penis was grafted with a partial-thickness skin graft. In particular, a 0.4 mm split-skin graft was harvested from the lateral thigh with an air dermatome and was used to cover the tissue defect. The graft was quilted using 5–0 interrupted polyglactin sutures. The patient made an excellent recovery with resolution of symptoms and restoration of sexual function. A satisfactory cosmetic result was recorded at 3 and 6 months postoperatively (Figure 2).

Histological examination confirmed the presence of a very well-differentiated neoplasm with sharp delineation at the tumor-stroma junction. On microscopy, the tumor exhibited hyperkeratosis, papillomatosis, and acanthosis. The tumor front was broad-based and pushed the subepithelial tissues. Small foci of clear-cut infiltration of subepidermal connective tissue, however, were also present. The neoplastic cells were well-differentiated, with minimal deviation from normal squamous cells and small, bland, round, or vesicular nuclei. Cellular atypia was focal and minimal, while mitoses were rare (Figures 3 and 4). The morphological findings were consistent with verrucous carcinoma of the penis. Lymphovascular invasion or perineural invasion was not identified (pT1a disease).

Based on final histology, the patient was classified as low risk for nodal involvement and was managed with surveillance for recurrence at the primary site and the groin areas as per current guidelines. Clinical examination and follow-up imaging up to 3 years postoperatively showed no locoregional recurrence or distant metastases.

3. Discussion

In 1925, Buschke and Löwenstein described 'carcinoma-like condylomata acuminata' as a locally invasive, rapidly growing tumor [11]. Buschke-Löwenstein tumor is classified as a verrucous carcinoma. The term 'verrucous carcinoma' was first introduced by Ackerman in 1948 and has been reported in the oral cavity, anus, penis, and female genitalia [12]. Buschke-Löwenstein tumor is generally considered as verrucous carcinoma involving the genital regions, but in some reports the lesions are regarded as distinct entities [12, 13]. It is a less common variant of penile squamous cell carcinoma, accounting for 3-8% of all penile tumors [13].

The exact etiology of verrucous carcinoma is yet to be clarified. Human Papilloma Virus types 6 and 11 have been linked with the pathogenesis of this tumor, but other studies have shown that HPV infection is not a universal finding in VC [5]. Risk factors for VC are low socioeconomic status, drug abuse, sexually transmitted diseases, diabetes, and smoking [12]. A mechanism related to impaired immune response has been proposed, and anogenital VC in association with HIV infection has been described [14].

Macroscopically, it is challenging to identify penile VC due to the gross similarities with condyloma acuminatum. It usually involves the glans as the common squamous cell carcinoma and presents as a cauliflower- or wart-like painless lesion. Verrucous carcinoma, however, grows slowly and may invade the glans or even the shaft. If left untreated, certain verrucous carcinomas evolve to giant masses which may be foul-smelling, painful, and ulcerated [7].

The literature on verrucous carcinoma mostly focuses on case reports and rarely on large-scale studies. Nevertheless, surgical treatment for penile verrucous carcinoma has been generally accepted as the mainstay for treatment. Since penile VC exhibits nonaggressive biological behavior, organ-sparing surgery, if possible, is an acceptable treatment option to avoid mutilating surgery and maintain the appearance and function of the penis [3, 8, 10]. VC, a well-differentiated tumor, is ideal for a wide range of conservative excisional and reconstructive techniques. A low threshold for intraoperative frozen section analysis of excision margins is recommended to balance oncological safety and preservation of functional penile length, especially if the macroscopic margin is under question [9, 10]. Despite the lack of metastatic potential, the chance of local recurrence is not to be overlooked, but rates vary between studies and appear to be significantly lower compared to the aggressive perianal VC [7, 15].

The optimal technique for penile skin reconstruction remains a point of debate and appropriate selection of graft type depends on the size and location of the defect. Some surgeons prefer full-thickness skin grafts, due to their greater elasticity and less primary contraction after harvesting. Split-thickness skin grafts, however, require less ideal conditions for survival and have lower incidence of graft failure. We apply the latter, harvested from the thigh in order to minimise donor-site morbidity and to achieve adequate cosmetic and functional results [8, 16].

Systemic or intralesional chemotherapy (with 5-fluorouracil or cisplatin) and intralesional interferon have been suggested, as alternative monotherapies or as an adjunct to surgery [6, 7]. Intra-aortic infusion chemotherapy (with methotrexate or mitomycin C plus 5-fluorouracil) has been used in a small series of patients with advanced penile VC and the results appear promising but large-scale data are lacking [6]. Radiotherapy remains controversial, due to the concern for radiation-induced anaplastic transformation of the primary verrucous carcinoma [6, 7]. Carbon dioxide laser ablation has also been tried with positive results in younger patients with smaller lesions confined to the glans [17, 18].

According to the limited amount of available evidence, local excision of VC with negative margins results in favorable long-term prognosis [19]. In previous case series, inguinal lymphadenectomy was performed in some patients but there was no nodal involvement [3, 15, 19]. Thus, inguinal lymphadenectomy is not recommended. One should note, however, that according to the findings of Shimizu et al. [20], foci of invasive squamous cell carcinoma were found in ~30% of verrucous carcinomas and the possibility of progression to other types of invasive squamous cell carcinoma is not to be excluded. This finding is relevant in the context of counselling and close follow-up of patients who undergo penile-conserving surgery. In the case presented herein, the presence of subepithelial invasion (pT1a disease) is of concern in regard to the increased risk of local recurrence [10]. Since local recurrence is more likely after organ-sparing surgery, commitment to a strict follow-up schedule according to the EAU guidelines should be ensured [1].

4. Conclusion

Penile verrucous carcinoma is a rare clinical entity with distinct clinical and histological characteristics. Organ-sparing excisional surgery with appropriate reconstruction achieves adequate disease control with excellent cosmesis. A well-structured approach, based on clinical and histological features, is essential, to avoid possible diagnostic pitfalls and overtreatment. The lack of clear recommendations based on evidence, however, underscores the need for multicenter studies with adequate sample size and follow-up.

References

[1] O. W. Hakenberg, E. M. Compérat, S. Minhas et al., "EAU guidelines on penile cancer: 2014 update," *European Urology*, vol. 67, no. 6, pp. 142–150, 2015.

[2] M. R. Pow-Sang, U. Ferreira, J. M. Pow-Sang, A. C. Nardi, and V. Destefano, "Epidemiology and natural history of penile cancer," *Urology*, vol. 76, no. 2, pp. S2–S6, 2010.

[3] D. G. Hatzichristou, A. Apostolidis, V. Tzortzis, K. Hatzimouratidis, E. Ioannides, and K. Yannakoyorgos, "Glansectomy: an alternative surgical treatment for Buschke-Löwenstein tumors of the penis," *Urology*, vol. 57, no. 5, pp. 966–969, 2001.

[4] S. Mannweiler, S. Sygulla, E. Winter, and S. Regauer, "Two major pathways of penile carcinogenesis: HPV-induced penile cancers overexpress p16ink4a, HPV-negative cancers associated with dermatoses express p53, but lack p16ink4a overexpression," *Journal of the American Academy of Dermatology*, vol. 69, no. 1, pp. 73–81, 2013.

[5] N. Fujimoto, G. Nakanishi, H. Ushida et al., "Penile verrucous carcinoma arising in HPV-negative condylomatous papules," *European Journal of Dermatology*, vol. 21, no. 3, pp. 436–438, 2011.

[6] M.-C. Sheen, H.-M. Sheu, M.-Y. Jang, C.-Y. Chai, Y.-W. Wang, and C.-F. Wu, "Advanced penile verrucous carcinoma treated with intra-aortic infusion chemotherapy," *The Journal of Urology*, vol. 183, no. 5, pp. 1830–1835, 2010.

[7] M. Nomikos, P. Barmpoutis, E. Papakonstantinou et al., "A giant verrucous carcinoma of the penis presenting with urinary sepsis and angina," *Case Reports in Medicine*, vol. 2014, Article ID 207026, 3 pages, 2014.

[8] Y. Smith, P. Hadway, O. Biedrzycki, M. J. A. Perry, C. Corbishley, and N. A. Watkin, "Reconstructive surgery for invasive squamous carcinoma of the glans penis," *European Urology*, vol. 52, no. 4, pp. 1179–1185, 2007.

[9] S. Minhas, O. Kayes, P. Hegarty, P. Kumar, A. Freeman, and D. Ralph, "What surgical resection margins are required to achieve oncological control in men with primary penile cancer?" *BJU International*, vol. 96, no. 7, pp. 1040–1043, 2005.

[10] P. Philippou, M. Shabbir, P. Malone et al., "Conservative surgery for squamous cell carcinoma of the penis: Resection margins and long-term oncological control," *The Journal of Urology*, vol. 188, no. 3, pp. 803–808, 2012.

[11] A. Buschke and L. Löwenstein, "Uber carcinomahnliche condylomata acuminata des penis," *Klinische Wochenschrift*, vol. 4, no. 36, pp. 1726–1728, 1925.

[12] F. T. Kraus and C. Perez-Mesa, "Verrucous carcinoma. Clinical and pathologic study of 105 cases involving oral cavity, larynx and genitalia," *Cancer*, vol. 19, no. 1, pp. 26–38, 1966.

[13] A. Chaux and A. L. Cubilla, "Advances in the pathology of penile carcinomas," *Human Pathology*, vol. 43, no. 6, pp. 771–789, 2012.

[14] C. Grodner, A. Henn, J.-D. Lelièvre, and S. Gallien, "Successful improvement of Buschke-Löwenstein tumour in an HIV-infected patient with antiretroviral therapy alone," *BMJ Case Reports*, vol. 2016, 2016.

[15] W. Gelders, P. Vanstraelen, and P. van Erps, "Giant penile tumour: a case report," *Acta Chirurgica Belgica*, vol. 109, no. 1, pp. 114–116, 2009.

[16] H. J. Thakar and D. D. Dugi, "Skin grafting of the penis," *Urologic Clinics of North America*, vol. 40, no. 3, pp. 439–448, 2013.

[17] J. Ayer, S. Matthews, N. Francis, N. P. J. Walker, M. Dinneen, and C. B. Bunker, "Successful treatment of Buschke-Lowenstein tumour of the penis with carbon dioxide laser vaporization," *Acta Dermato-Venereologica*, vol. 92, no. 6, pp. 656-657, 2012.

[18] A. Frega, P. Stentella, A. Tinari, A. Vecchione, and M. Marchionni, "Giant condyloma acuminatum or Buschke-Lowenstein tumor: review of the literature and report of three cases treated by CO2 laser surgery. A long-term follow-up," *Anticancer Reseach*, vol. 22, no. 2, pp. 1201-1204, 2002.

[19] F. Li, Y. Xu, H. Wang et al., "Diagnosis and treatment of penile verrucous carcinoma," *Oncology Letters*, vol. 9, no. 4, pp. 1687–1690, 2015.

[20] A. Shimizu, A. Tamura, and O. Ishikawa, "Invasive squamous cell carcinoma arising from verrucous carcinoma: Recognition of verrucous carcinoma of skin as an in situ carcinoma," *European Journal of Dermatology*, vol. 16, no. 4, pp. 439–442, 2006.

Perinephric Hematoma with Active Arterial Hemorrhage following Extracorporeal Shockwave Lithotripsy

Edward Assaf,[1] Rawad Abou Zahr,[1] Elie Ghabi,[2] and Imad Ghantous[1]

[1] *Urology Department, St George Hospital University Medical Center, University of Balamand, Beirut, Lebanon*
[2] *Faculty of Medicine and Medical Sciences, St George Hospital University Medical Center, University of Balamand, Beirut, Lebanon*

Correspondence should be addressed to Imad Ghantous; drimadghantous@gmail.com

Academic Editor: Tun-Chieh Chen

Subcapsular hematoma is an exceedingly rare complication of extracorporeal shockwave lithotripsy (ESWL) for renal stones with cases demonstrating evidence of active arterial bleeding even more so. A 49-year-old male presented with acute onset right flank pain two hours following ESWL. CT scan with contrast revealed active contrast extravasation consistent with arterial bleeding. The patient was managed with arterial embolization and recovered uneventfully following a 4-day hospitalization.

1. Introduction

Since its first application by Chaussy et al., extracorporeal shockwave lithotripsy (ESWL) has been a safe, noninvasive, and successful technique for the management of renal calculi [1]. Complications, however, are possible, range from benign and self-limited to catastrophic, and have been recognized for several years [2, 3]. Renal hematoma is one such injury [3–11]. Ultrasound screening reveals an incidence of renal hematoma formation post-ESWL ranges from 0.1% to 0.6% [4], whereas magnetic resonance (MR) screening reveals an incidence of 20–25% [3]. The incidence of clinically significant hematoma is reported to be <1%; however, newer generation imaging modalities determine its ranges from 3% to 12% [9]. Documented cases of renal hematoma following ESWL were benign and self-limited, successfully managed with conservative therapy [4–8] or percutaneous drainage [10, 11]. Only few cases of active arterial hemorrhage (reported by Silberstein [9] among others) exist in the literature, making the occurrence exceedingly rare in an already rare phenomenon. The following case report is of a 49-year-old patient who developed perinephric hematoma with evidence of active arterial extravasation on computed tomography (CT) scan and arterial angiography that was successfully treated with arterial embolization and follow-up supportive care. By highlighting this occurrence, we hope to increase clinical suspicion of active bleeding when patients present with acute onset flank pain following EWSL.

2. Case Presentation

A 49-year-old male presented to our hospital for severe pain in his right flank of 2 hours duration following Extracorporeal Shockwave Lithotripsy (ESWL) performed on the same day for a stone in his right kidney. His past medical history includes nephrolithiasis, for which he underwent ESWL 3 years prior to presentation. At presentation, the patient was afebrile and hemodynamically stable with normal vital signs. Examination revealed exquisite tenderness over the right costovertebral angle. Laboratory studies revealed a hemoglobin value of 14.9g/dL, a hematocrit of 43.9%, creatinine of 1.03 mg/dL, and BUN of 30 mg/dL. An abdominal CT with contrast revealed 17x13x11 cm right perinephric hematoma with evidence of active contrast extravasation in the arterial phase (Figure 1). A decision was made to send the patient for emergent arteriography. Catheterization was performed with a 5F Cobra catheter and contrast injection revealed active extravasation arising from the small branches of the middle subsegmental posterior renal artery (Figure 2). The subsegmental branches were cannulated using a 2.7F Cobra catheter, and contrast injection revealed two bleeding branches from the posterior capsule. Embolization with

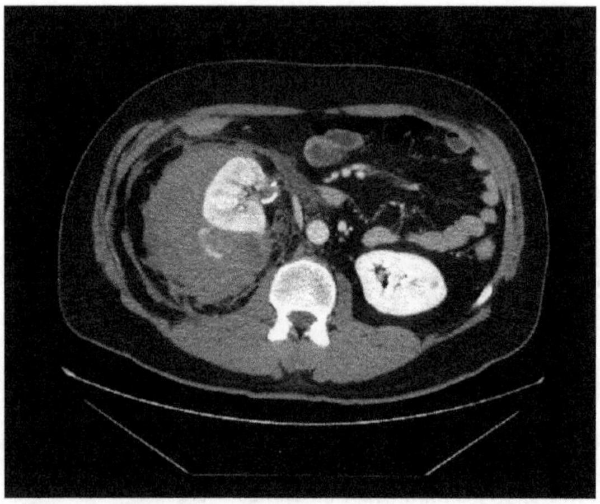

FIGURE 1: Active contrast extravasation from the right kidney on computed tomography.

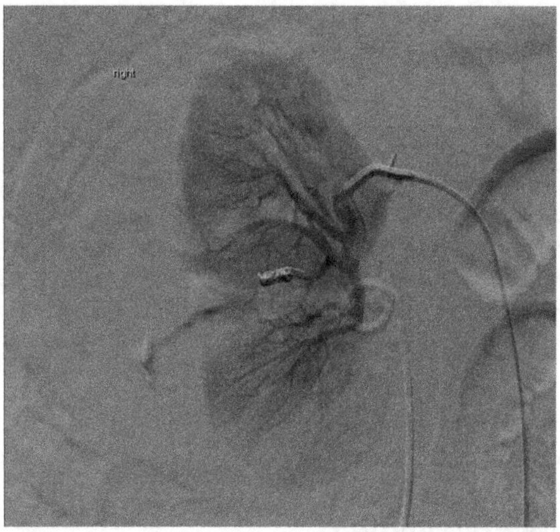

FIGURE 2: Active contrast extravasation on arteriography.

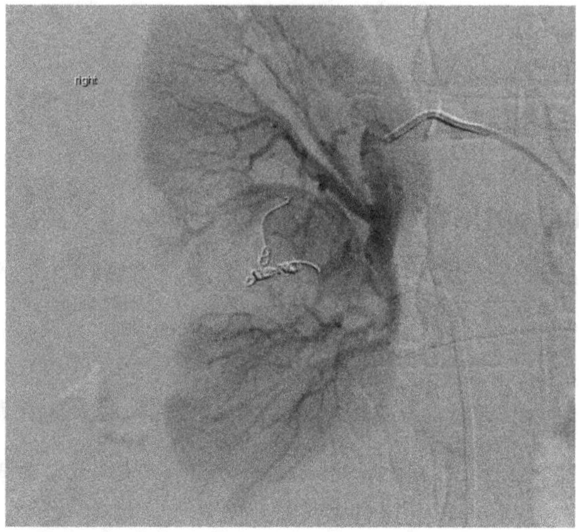

FIGURE 3: Successful arterial embolization demonstrating no signs of active contrast extravasation.

0.018 microcoils was performed and subsequent contrast injection did not show evidence of extravasation (Figure 3). The patient was admitted for monitoring and supportive care. Serial complete blood count revealed a steady decline of hemoglobin concentration to reach 9.3g/dl on the 3rd day of hospitalization. At the time, the patient had nausea, fatigue, pallor, and tachycardia. He was successfully managed with transfusion of 1 unit of packed red blood cells and IV hydration. A follow-up CT scan revealed a slight reduction in the size of the hematoma to measure 16x12x10cm. Throughout his hospitalization, the patient's renal function was intact as determined by a stable creatinine value of 0.8 mg/dL (estimated GFR = 105ml/min/1.73m^2 as calculated by CKD-EPI). Following hemodynamic stabilization and symptom resolution, the patient was discharged after a 4-day hospitalization and was followed up on an outpatient basis.

3. Discussion

Though major complications of ESWL are rare, several complications are frequently observed, most commonly microhematuria due to microtrauma to the kidney. Other complications include acute pyelonephritis, acute kidney failure, and ureteric obstruction due to stone fragments [3]. Nonrenal complications also occur with reports of myocardial injury, abdominal aneurysmal rupture, venous thrombosis, and subcapsular hepatic hematoma, though these occurrences are rare [3, 9, 12]. Renal subcapsular and perinephric hematoma is a recognized complication with an incidence ranging from 0.1 to 0.6% as detected by ultrasound [3] and between 20 and 25% as detected by MR or CT [4]. A retrospective study between 1987 and 1996 revealed the incidence of renal hematoma to be 0.28% relative to the number of patients (10,953) and 0.14% relative to the number of sessions (21,699) with the most common presenting symptom (74%) being lower back pain [4]. Several risk factors were found to be predispose to renal hematoma formation, particularly preexisting hypertension [9]. Knapp et al. also report that the incidence of hematoma increased from 0.66% to 2.5% in hypertensive patients and to 3.8% in patients with poorly controlled hypertension [13]. Furthermore, a multivariate analysis revealed no association between mean arterial blood pressure and the incidence of renal hematoma [9]. Other risk factors include diabetes mellitus, atherosclerosis, obesity, bleeding diathesis, male gender, and age with a 1.67 times increased risk for every 10-year increase in age [3, 4, 9]. Moreover, the number of shocks and frequency of shock delivery were found to be a significant predisposing factor to hematoma formation [9]. Patient presentation varies, though the most common complaints at presentation were lower back pain and flank pain. Gross hematuria is a common complaint, usually significant of renal injury but not to the extent of renal damage. Patients presenting with gross hematuria were found to have benign renal injury and impairment that resolved within 12 hours [9]. Patients who develop hematoma are generally managed conservatively; however a high index of suspicion for active bleeding, renal or otherwise, should be present.

In our case, the patient presented with flank pain, a relatively common symptom after ESWL, and he was hemodynamically stable. However, the severity of the pain along with nonresponsiveness to analgesia raised the suspicion of a more severe pathology, thus warranting further investigation by CT scan.

It is not common practice to order CT scans for every patient presenting for flank pain after ESWL, since most of these patients will respond to analgesia and the pain is usually a classic renal colic type pain.

4. Conclusion

Renal hematoma following ESWL for renal calculi is a rare but generally benign condition only requiring conservative management. Few serious complications occur requiring more invasive therapy. A hematoma due to an active arterial bleed is exceedingly rare but should be suspected in patients presenting with lower back or flank pain acutely after ESWL, especially in patients who are unresponsive to intravenous analgesics. Active bleeding, though rare, should be considered despite hemodynamic stability, thereby warranting further investigation.

Consent

Written consent was obtained from the patient for this case report.

References

[1] C. Chaussy, E. Schmiedt, D. Jocham, W. Brendel, B. Forssmann, and V. Walther, "First clinical experience with extracorporeally induced destruction of kidney stones by shock waves," *The Journal of Urology*, vol. 127, no. 3, pp. 417–420, 1982.

[2] C. M. Williams, J. V. Kaude, R. C. Newman, J. C. Peterson, and W. C. Thomas, "Extracorporeal shock-wave lithotripsy: Long-term complications," *American Journal of Roentgenology*, vol. 150, no. 2, pp. 311–315, 1987.

[3] A. Skolarikos, G. Alivizatos, J. de la Rosette, and E. N. Liatsikos, "Extracorporeal shock wave lithotripsy 25 years later: complications and their prevention," *European Urology*, vol. 50, no. 5, pp. 981–990, 2006.

[4] A. C. Serra, J. H. Pérez, F. M. G. De Vicuña, A. R. Barón, F. I. De La Torre, and J. V. Rodríguez, "Renal hematoma as a complication of extracorporeal shock wave lithotripsy," *Scandinavian Journal of Urology*, vol. 33, no. 3, pp. 171–175, 1999.

[5] B. H. Jeon, J. H. Jang, J. H. Oh et al., "Kidney rupture after extracorporeal shockwave lithotripsy: report of a case. of Emergency Medicine," *Journal of Emergency Medicine*, vol. 37, no. 1, pp. 13-14, 2009.

[6] D. E. Maziak, A. Ralph-Edwards, M. Deitel, J. Wait, H. J. Watt, and A. Marcuzzi, "Massive perirenal and intra-abdominal bleeding after shock-wave lithotripsy: Case report," *Canadian Journal of Surgery*, vol. 37, no. 4, pp. 329–332, 1994.

[7] T.-B. Kim, H.-K. Park, K.-Y. Lee, K.-H. Kim, H. Jung, and S.-J. Yoon, "Life-threatening complication after extracorporeal shock wave lithotripsy for a renal stone: A hepatic subcapsular hematoma," *Korean Journal of Urology*, vol. 51, no. 3, pp. 212–215, 2010.

[8] A. P. Labanaris, R. Kühn, G. E. Schott, and V. Zugor, "Perirenal hematomas induced by Extracorporeal Shock Wave Lithotripsy (ESWL). Therapeutic management," *The Scientific World Journal*, vol. 7, pp. 1563–1566, 2007.

[9] J. Silberstein, C. M. Lakin, and J. K. Parsons, "Shock wave lithotripsy and renal hemorrhage," *Reviews in Urology*, vol. 10, no. 3, p. 236, 2008.

[10] Y. B. Jang, K. P. Kang, S. Lee et al., "Treatment of subcapsular haematoma, a complication of extracorporeal shock wave lithotripsy (ESWL), by percutaneous drainage," *Nephrology Dialysis Transplantation* , vol. 21, no. 4, pp. 1117-1118, 2006.

[11] S. Hallmann, J. Petersein, J. Ruttloff, and T. H. Ecke, "Successful evacuation of large perirenal hematoma after extracorporeal shock wave lithotripsy (ESWL)-step 1 of the IDEAL recommendations of surgical innovation," *Clinical Case Reports*, vol. 5, no. 2, pp. 123–125, 2017.

[12] J. Gordetsky, S. Hislop, M. Orloff, M. Butler, and E. Erturk, "Subcapsular hepatic hematoma with right hepatic vein thrombosis: A complication of shock wave lithotripsy," *Canadian Urological Association Journal*, vol. 2, no. 1, pp. 61–63, 2008.

[13] P. M. Knapp, T. B. Kulb, J. E. Lingeman et al., "Extracorporeal shock wave lithotripsy-induced perirenal hematomas," *The Journal of Urology*, vol. 139, no. 4 I, pp. 700–703, 1988.

9

Unusual Mechanisms of Penile Amputation

Julian Fazi, David Adkins, Jennifer Knight, and Adam Luchey

Department of Urology, West Virginia University, Morgantown, WV 26505, USA

Correspondence should be addressed to Julian Fazi; juf0001@mix.wvu.edu

Academic Editor: David Duchene

Penile amputation is an uncommon and highly morbid injury. Many mechanisms have been reported ranging from self-mutilation and domestic violence to traumatic circumcisions. We present two unusual cases of traumatic penile amputation. An older gentleman endured extensive perineal trauma after being trapped underneath an industrial-sized lawnmower, and a young adolescent was bitten by an English bulldog and suffered amputation of the glans of his penis. These unique and very different cases of penile amputation highlight differences in operative managements, complications, and reconstructive possibilities.

1. Introduction

Penile amputation can present as an isolated injury or as part of an extensive perineal trauma requiring intensive care unit admission. Nevertheless this serious injury has major functional and psychological consequences [1]. Penile amputation injuries are rare, making it difficult to develop standardized management guidelines. The most common causes of penile amputations in adults are self-mutilation, domestic violence, and trauma. The most common causes in pediatrics are traumatic circumcision and automobile accidents [2, 3].

The original approach for penile replantation, which was first described in the late 1920's by Ehrich, was a macrosurgical technique that focused on aligning the major structures of the penis including the urethra, corpora spongiosa, corpora cavernosa, and glandular epithelium [4, 5]. This approach is dependent on the corporal sinusoidal blood flow [4]. The first microsurgical approach was completed in the late 1970's. This approach focuses on realigning smaller structures such as the dorsal neurovascular structures and the cavernosal arteries [1, 4]. The macrosurgical technique has higher rates of complications including skin necrosis, sensation deficits, erectile dysfunction, urethral strictures, and fistula formation when compared with the microsurgical approach [2–4]. Nonetheless, a variety of factors and situations help to determine if replantation is possible. These include degree of contamination, preservation of amputated segment, mechanism of injury, and ischemic time [2].

We report two unique cases of penile amputation. A 69-year-old man who rolled his industrial-sized lawnmower and experienced significant perineal trauma with near complete penile amputation after he became trapped underneath the lawnmower blade. The second case is a 12-year-old boy who had his glans bitten off by a dog. These rare and unusual mechanisms of penile amputation highlight differences in the management, complications, and reconstructive possibilities.

2. Case Presentations

2.1. Case One. The first case is a 69-year-old male who was found underneath an industrial-sized lawn mower in a rural area. The lawnmower had tipped as he was ascending a hill, and he was trapped underneath for an indeterminate amount of time. The patient suffered avulsion of his penis, scrotum, and testicles along with sustaining gaping perineal and left lower extremity wounds (Figure 1). He arrived in hemorrhagic shock. After resuscitation his immediate surgical management included hemostatic control, a descending loop colostomy, open J tube placement, and irrigation and debridement (I and D) of his perineal wound. His prostatic urethra was deemed intact and he had 4 cm of corpora cavernosa remaining bilaterally. A 16 French (Fr) Foley catheter was inserted into the urethra stump to empty the bladder and to prevent urine from further contaminating an already dirty surgical field. Bleeding was identified from the corporal stumps prompting ligation with

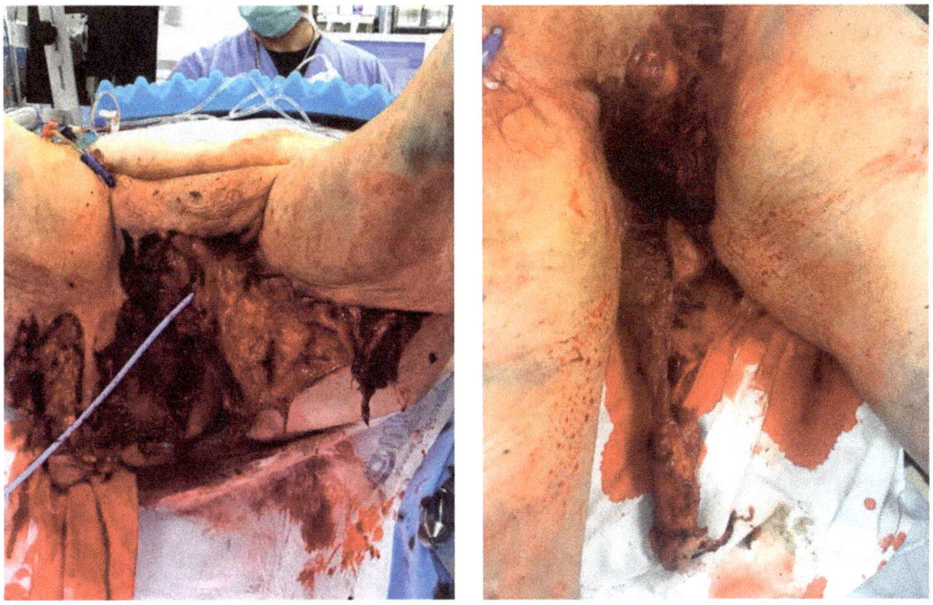

(a) (b)

Figure 1: (a) The gaping perineal wound while lying in lithotomy position status post penectomy. A Foley catheter was inserted into the urethral stump. (b) Anterior view of perineal wound showing near complete amputation of the phallus.

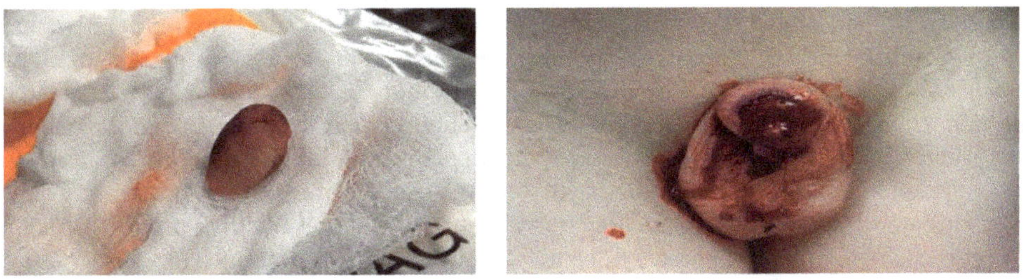

(a) (b)

Figure 2: (a) The amputated glans. (b) The phallus proximal to the amputation.

3-0 Vicryl horizontal mattress sutures. On the following day, his perineal and lower extremity wounds were irrigated and debrided. A 16 Fr suprapubic catheter was placed 2 centimeters proximal to the pubic symphysis allowing for urinary diversion from the large perineal wound. The remaining corporal stumps were found to be nonviable, prompting a total penectomy. The 4 cm corpora cavernosa stump was resected at the base of the penis, divided with LigaSure and suture ligated with 2-0 Vicryl. The corpora spongiosum and bulbomembranous urethra were ligated using interrupted vertical mattress with 0 Vicryl.

The patient returned to the operating room every other day for the next few weeks for I and D of his perineal wound. He underwent numerous nonurologic operations in the following months including open reduction and internal fixation of his left fibula, cephalomedullary nail insertion into his femur, and grafting of his perineal wound. Since the operations, the patient has returned for exchange of his suprapubic catheter, bladder spasms that are managed with anticholinergics, and urinary tract infections. The patient was most recently seen in the clinic two years following his initial injury. He is able to ambulate but continues to have intermittent bladder spasms controlled with oxybutynin. His suprapubic catheter is exchanged on a monthly basis.

2.2. Case Two. Patient two is a 12-year-old male who presented to the emergency department (ED) after his glans had been bitten off by an English bulldog (Figure 2). After hemorrhage control and gauze placement on the penile stump, the glans was wrapped in gauze and put in a bag of saline which was put in another bag of slush ice water. The patient was taken to the operating room, and it was determined that his corpora cavernosa were intact bilaterally. The operative team failed to identify any neurovascular structures conducive to microvascular repair. Hemorrhage control was attained using a vessel loop. Nonviable tissue was debrided from the distal shaft, and the distal shaft and glans were irrigated with copious amounts of normal saline and bacitracin. A 10 Fr Foley catheter was threaded through the penile meatus on the amputated glans and the urethra on the distal shaft to approximate, realign, and replant the glans. Immediate return of urine was noted when the catheter was advanced to the bladder. The urethral anastomosis was completed with 4-0 Vicryl sutures.

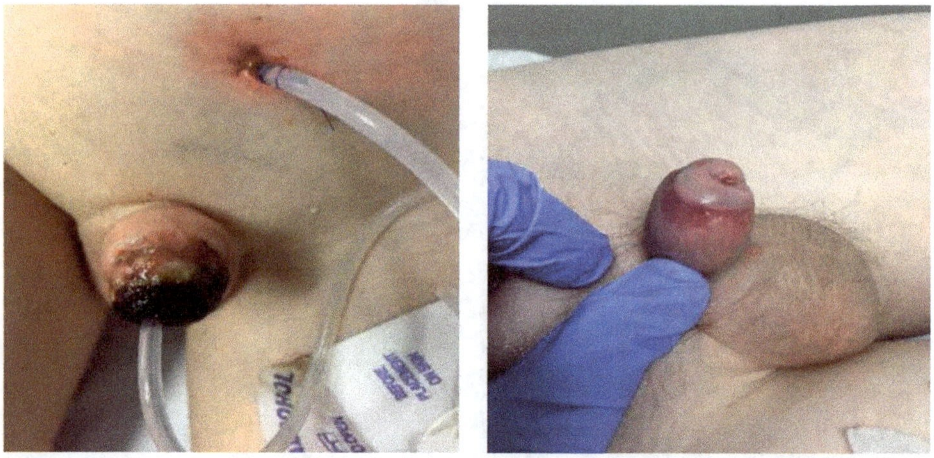

(a) (b)

FIGURE 3: (a) Replantation of glans with suprapubic cystostomy tube. (b) Postoperative week ten with suprapubic and urethral catheters removed.

The glans was reapproximated, with a macrosurgical approach, to the distal penile shaft with 4-0 Vicryl, and the glandular epithelium was reapproximated with 4-0 Monocryl sutures. The vessel loop was released. The glans was noted to be pink and purple without evidence of necrosis immediately following surgery. The patient was prescribed oral Augmentin for five days, Oxybutynin and Tamsulosin postoperatively. Mild superficial glans necrosis was noted two weeks postoperatively (Figure 3(a)) but the majority of the glans remained viable (Figure 3(b)). He was taken back to the operating room for placement of a 12 Fr suprapubic catheter and upsizing of his transurethral Foley catheter to 14 Fr to alleviate urinary retention and UTIs (Figure 3(a)). Cystoscopy noted a fibrotic urethra from the point of transection distally, without evidence of stricture. The Foley catheter was removed 6 weeks later. The patient performed clean intermittent catheterization (CIC) for one year postoperatively with the goal of preventing urethral stricture. CIC frequency was tapered down over the course of the year from every three-four hours initially to every eight hours, and he eventually was performing CIC on a weekly basis. Two years postoperatively the patient has a patent and nonstenotic urethra and meatus with a partially atrophic glans that is acceptable in size and cosmetic look. His urinary stream is normal and straight without any issues. The patient also reports that he is able to achieve erections and has sensation in the distal aspects of the penis.

3. Discussion

Penile amputation is a rare and devastating injury with a variety mechanisms reported. Some of the more common mechanisms include self-mutilation, domestic violence, trauma, and failed circumcision [2, 4, 6, 7]. Less common injuries include boating accidents, animal bites, agricultural machinery accidents among others [8–10]. A series of penile amputations in Thailand were maliciously performed in the 1970's by wives of unfaithful husbands [11]. Morrison et al. report that most amputations are complete amputations, and after replantation a majority of people have normal urinary function (97.4%), erections (77.5%), and sensation (68.4%) [2]. The most common complications after repair are skin necrosis (54.8%) and venous congestion (20.2%) [2].

Certain situations and factors make replantation more likely than others in the preoperative and operative settings. For example, success is very dependent on the length of ischemia that the amputated segment has endured; warm ischemia has a worse prognosis than cold ischemia [3]. Replantation has been reported after 16 hours of ischemia, and Jezior et al. suggest attempting replantation within 24 hours [1]. Other positive prognostic signs preoperatively are minimal contamination and preservation of the amputated segment [2]. Intraoperatively there is a greater chance of graft survival and preservation of erectile and urinary function with less postoperative complications if the microsurgical technique is used instead of the macrosurgical. Good venous outflow and return of normal color are good intraoperative and postoperative indicators of lasting tissue survival [2–4]. Furthermore, patients should be medically and psychologically stable before attempting replantation [1]. In our first case, reimplantation was not attempted given the severity of the trauma, lack of any clean margins, wound contamination, and the patient's hemodynamic instability.

In the setting of distal penile amputation involving only the glans, situations where vasculature cannot be identified or when instrumentation for microscopic surgery is not available, macroscopic replantation may be the only reconstructive option besides completion of a stump plasty [2, 12]. Amputation of only the glans is less common than more proximal amputations with one study citing glans amputations at 3.7% of total amputations [13]. Two adult cases of amputation at the glans, reported by Terayama et al., were repaired with stump plasty and experienced minimal postoperative complications. Normal urinary function, erectile function, and ability to have intercourse were ultimately achieved with one brief episode of urinary difficulty. One patient had reduced frequency of intercourse due to the shorter phallus causing an inferiority complex [13].

4. Conclusion

These cases contrast each other in mechanism, circumstances, and operative management. The 69-year-old male highlights a case where contamination, prolonged time of warm ischemia, severity of other injuries, and a poorly preserved phallus make replantation via a microsurgical or macrosurgical approach impossible. It also presents a unique mechanism of penile and perineal trauma not commonly cited. The 12-year-old male demonstrates a rare case of an amputation only involving the glans that was able to be macrosurgically replanted due to short time of cold ischemia and good tissue preservation.

References

[1] J. R. Jezior, J. D. Brady, and S. M. Schlossberg, "Management of penile amputation injuriess," *World Journal of Surgery*, vol. 25, no. 12, pp. 1602–1609, 2001.

[2] S. D. Morrison, A. Shakir, K. S. Vyas et al., "Penile replantation: a retrospective analysis of outcomes and complications," *Journal of Reconstructive Microsurgery*, vol. 33, no. 4, pp. 227–232, 2017.

[3] A. R. Babaei and M. R. Safarinejad, "Penile replantation, science or myth? A systematic review," *Urology Journal*, vol. 4, no. 2, pp. 62–65, 2007.

[4] S. Garg, S. V. Date, A. Gupta, and A. S. Baliarsing, "Successful microsurgical replantation of an amputated penis," *Indian Journal of Plastic Surgery*, vol. 49, no. 1, pp. 99–105, 2016.

[5] W. S. Ehrich, "Two unusual penile injuries," *The Journal of Urology*, vol. 21, no. 2, pp. 239–241, 1929.

[6] N. Fernando, J. Facio, L. C. Spessoto et al., "Penile replantation after five hours of warm ischemia," *Urology Case Reports*, vol. 3, no. 3, pp. 77–79, 2015.

[7] T. Patial, G. Sharma, and P. Raina, "Traumatic penile amputation: a case report," *BMC Urology*, vol. 17, no. 1, p. 93, 2019.

[8] S. Elmaraghi, T. J. Chen, J. E. Heckman et al., "Functional penile replantation after traumatic avulsion amputation below the pubis: a case report," *Microsurgery*, pp. 1–4, 2019.

[9] P. N. Dogra, G. Gautam, and M. S. Ansari, "Penile amputation and emasculation: hazards of modern agricultural machinery," *International Urology and Nephrology*, vol. 36, no. 3, pp. 379–380, 2004.

[10] C. M. Gomes, L. Ribeiro-Filho, A. M. Giron, A. I. Mitre, E. R. Figueira, and S. Arap, "Genital trauma due to animal bites," *Journal of Urology*, vol. 165, no. 1, pp. 80–83, 2001.

[11] K. Bhanganada, T. Chayavatana, C. Pongnumkul et al., "Surgical management of an epidemic of penile amputations in Siam," *The American Journal of Surgery*, vol. 146, no. 3, pp. 376–382, 1983.

[12] Y. E. El harrech, N. Abaka, O. Ghoundale, and D. Touiti, "Genital self-amputation or the Klingsor syndrome: successful non-microsurgical penile replantation," *Urology Annals*, vol. 5, no. 4, pp. 305–308, 2013.

[13] T. Terayama, T. Sakamoto, and H. Ikeuchi, Y. Tanaka, "Self-penile glans amputation: a report of two cases," *Acute Medicine and Surgery*, vol. 42, no. 1, pp. 101–104, 2017.

Tumefactive Fat Necrosis with Multinucleate Giant Cell Reaction Mimicking Recurrent Renal Cell Carcinoma following Percutaneous Renal Cryoablation

Amanda E. Kahn,[1] **Kevin J. Wu**,[2] **and David D. Thiel**[1]

[1]*Department of Urology, Mayo Clinic, Jacksonville, FL, USA*
[2]*Department of Pathology, Mayo Clinic, Jacksonville, FL, USA*

Correspondence should be addressed to David D. Thiel; thiel.david@mayo.edu

Academic Editor: David Duchene

Multinucleate Giant Cell (GC) reaction is a biological response that occurs secondary to infection, an implanted foreign body, tissue injury, or inflammation. In rare instances GC reactions have been reported following tissue ablation. Multinucleate GC reactions and tumefactive fat necrosis both have the ability to mimic cancer recurrence or metastasis and can appear as enhancing masses. We discuss a case of a surgically resected retroperitoneal perinephric mass thought to be recurrent renal cell carcinoma (RCC) that was pathologically confirmed as tumefactive fat necrosis with multinucleate GC reaction 2 years following percutaneous cryoablation of a small renal mass.

1. Introduction

Multinucleate Giant Cell (GC) reaction is typically a biological response to infection, tissue injury, or inflammation and can be noted following implantation of biomaterials or medical devices [1]. The GC reaction occurs when the immune system is activated causing merging of histiocytes, monocytes, and macrophages to become multinucleate cells that surround the foreign material or inflamed tissue [1–3]. Although multinucleate GC reactions are typically secondary to tissue damage and immune system activation, some GC reactions have been observed following ablation for the treatment of renal and liver lesions [4, 5]. We report our observation of a single patient that developed a delayed onset perinephric mass following percutaneous cryoablation that was pathologically noted to be multinucleate GC reaction with tumefactive fat necrosis following resection.

2. Case Presentation

A 60-year-old male had incidentally discovered bilateral renal masses identified on computed tomography (CT) imaging. Robotic assisted partial nephrectomy of the right renal lesion was completed on a 4-centimeter Furman Grade 2, pT1a clear cell RCC with negative surgical margins. Due to the posterior location of the 2-centimeter mass on the left kidney (Figure 1(a)), the patient opted for percutaneous cryoablation of the mass 4 months following the right robotic partial nephrectomy (Figure 1(b)). Follow-up cross-sectional imaging revealed no evidence of cancer recurrence in either kidney over a 2-year period (Figure 1(c)). A new contrast-enhancing lesion was noted in the perinephric fat of the left kidney 2 years following therapy (Figure 2(a)). Magnetic resonance imaging (MRI) scans also demonstrated a 2-centimeter enhancing and restricting ill-defined soft tissue focus in the left kidney region where previous cryoablation was performed. Biopsy was foregone due to the new rapid development, consistency, and location of the lesion. The patient underwent open subcostal partial nephrectomy with complete perinephric fat removal (Figure 2(b)). Surgical pathology revealed the resected renal mass to contain organized tumefactive fat necrosis with multinucleate GC reaction (Figure 3(a)) without evidence of clear cell RCC recurrence (Figures 3(c) and 3(d)). Immunohistochemistry

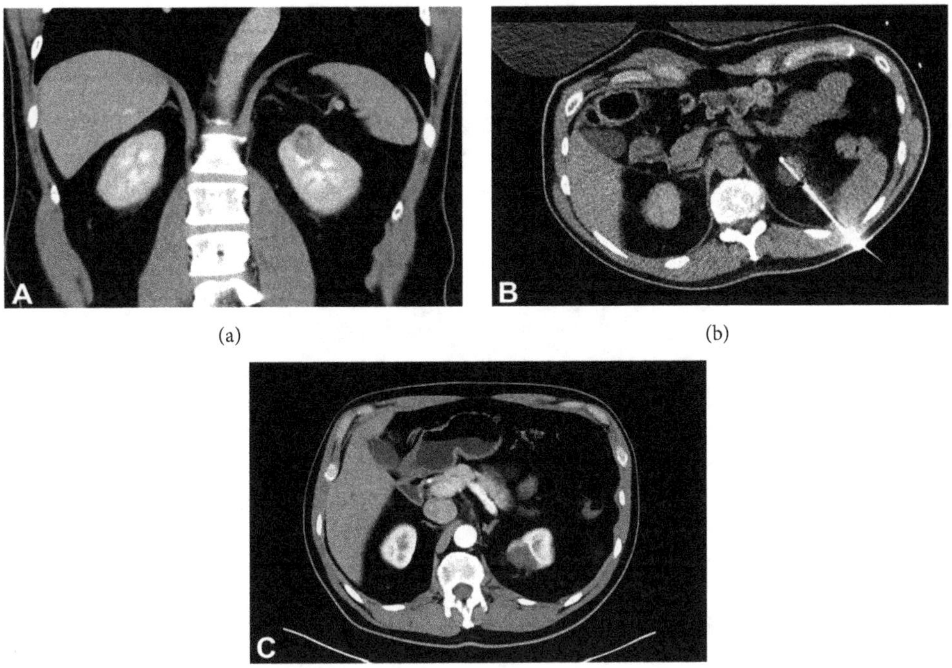

(a) (b) (c)

FIGURE 1: Patient imaging. (a) Contrast enhanced CT scan prior to ablation displaying 2-centimeter left renal mass in the upper pole. (b) An intra-therapy image of CT-guided left renal cryoablation probe displaying the tract of needle. (c) Contrast enhanced CT 1 year following cryoablation of left renal mass demonstrating absence of mass enhancement.

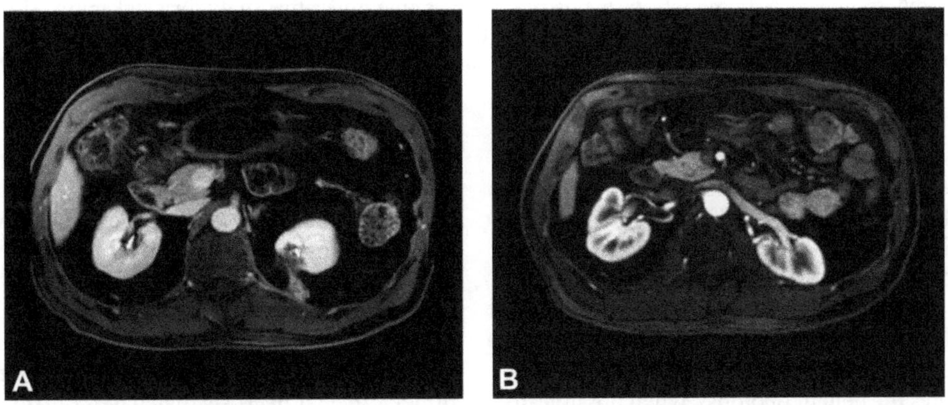

(a) (b)

FIGURE 2: Patient imaging following cryoablation. (a) Contrasted MRI 2 years following cryoablation of left renal mass demonstrating new lesion development described as an ill-defined 2-centimeter focus of soft tissue highly suspicious for disease recurrence. The lesion appears to follow the cryoablation tract path. (b) Contrasted MRI 2-year status-post-partial nephrectomy of left renal lesion with full excision of perinephric fat displaying stable changes of bilateral partial nephrectomy without evidence of local recurrence.

studies (Figures 3(a) and 3(b)) demonstrated an inflammatory reaction characterized by abundant histiocytes and multinucleate giant cells that were positive for CD68 (KP1). Cytokeratin AE1/AE3 and PAX-8 immunohistochemistry were both negative (Figures 3(c) and 3(d)). The patient is 2 years removed from surgery without cancer or disease recurrence.

3. Discussion

Cryoablation is a favorable nephron-sparing treatment for certain renal lesions secondary to its ability to treat small, complex lesions in a minimally invasive fashion [4]. Our report describes a case of tumefactive fat necrosis with multinucleate GC reaction presented as a distinct mass in

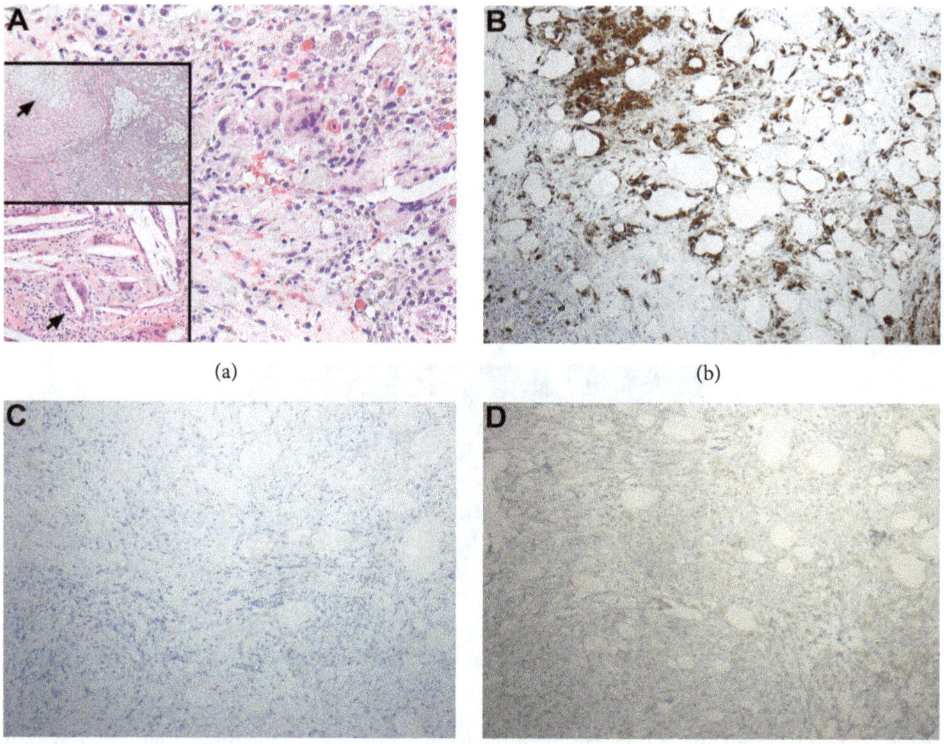

(a) (b) (c) (d)

FIGURE 3: Pathology of lesion following partial nephrectomy. (a) Pathology of lesion showing area with prominent hemosiderin laden macrophages and multinucleate giant cells (H/E, 20X). Lower inset demonstrating foci of giant cells associated with cholesterol clefts (arrow) (H/E, 20X). Upper inset shows necrotic fat (arrow) with surrounding inflammatory reaction (H/E, 4X). (b) CD68 (KP1) immunohistochemistry (10X). CD68 is highly expressed by monocytes, macrophages, and histiocytes and is positive in numerous histiocytes and macrophages in adipose tissue. (c) Immunohistochemistry demonstrating a negative study for cytokeratin AE1/AE3 confirming no recurrence of renal cell carcinoma (10X). (d) Immunohistochemistry demonstrating a negative study for PAX-8 confirming no recurrence of renal cell carcinoma (10X).

the perinephric tissue concerning for cancer recurrence. Our finding of tumefactive fat necrosis following cryoablation of a renal mass has been similarly reported by Durack et al. [6]. They describe 2 patients who presented with RCC, underwent cryoablation, and developed what looked like RCC recurrence. The patients underwent biopsy which confirmed both lesions as benign soft-tissue nodules with fat necrosis, fibrosis, inflammation, and histiocytes present [6]. The case demonstrates the benefit of biopsy, when possible, to avoid unnecessary excision of benign renal masses. This case study differs from our findings due to its lack of GC reaction but similarly reports patients who developed a delayed onset of fat necrosis following cryoablation.

The cellular disturbances that occur during cryoablative therapy can contribute to the development of a multinucleate GC reaction due to tissue damage, necrosis, and creation of cellular debris which stimulates an immune response [1]. A GC reaction in renal tissue has previously been observed by Johnson et al. who identified a patient that presented with RCC, underwent radiofrequency ablation, and developed a firm cortex at the site of ablation. A nephrectomy was performed 11 months following treatment secondary to the atrophic nature of the kidney revealing a granulomatous, foreign body GC reaction not detected on CT [4].

Also notable in our case was the presence of abundant fat necrosis. A study by Lokken et al. found that necrotic fat and inflammatory nodules have the ability to mimic tumor seeding or recurrence following cryoablation with delayed presentation in 2.7% of cases [7]. These nodules typically present in the tract of the cryoprobe and can display as an enhancing lesion on contrast-enhanced CT or MRI [7]. The unique combination of both multinucleate GC reaction and tumefactive fat necrosis may have contributed to the delayed presentation on imaging in our case allowing the reaction to mimic RCC recurrence in the cryoablative tract.

The histological appearance of our patient's radiographic abnormality following partial nephrectomy and perinephric fat excision is characterized by extensive tumefactive fat necrosis and multinucleate GC reaction at the site of previous ablative therapy (Figure 3(a)). As seen in Figure 3(b), CD68 stain is positive showing numerous histiocytes and macrophages, which is typical in GC reactions. It is important to note the keratin and PAX8 stains were both negative demonstrating the absence of RCC recurrence as shown in Figures 3(c) and 3(d), respectively.

GC reactions have been noted to be enhanced on both contrast-enhanced CT and MRI thereby mimicking cancer recurrence [8] (Figure 2(a)). Various GC reactions mimicking recurrent or metastatic cancer have also been observed in bone and brain tissues as primary tumors and in colon tissue secondary to hemicolectomy [9–11]. For these reasons, patients can benefit from biopsy or fine needle aspiration prior to resection when suspicious lesions develop. The literature is void of substantial reports noting the frequency of GC reactions following ablation therapy of other organs.

4. Conclusion

Our report describes the delayed presentation of tumefactive fat necrosis and multinucleate GC reaction following cryoablation of clear cell RCC. This case demonstrates the importance of considering every possibility when presented with a patient that develops new perinephric abnormalities following ablation. This knowledge, combined with thorough evaluation, may aid in avoiding unnecessary invasive treatments for suspicious but nonmalignant lesions following ablation treatments.

Abbreviations

CT: Computed tomography
GC: Giant cell
MRI: Magnetic resonance imaging
RCC: Renal cell carcinoma.

References

[1] W. G. Brodbeck and J. M. Anderson, "Giant cell formation and function," *Current Opinion in Hematology*, vol. 16, no. 1, pp. 53–57, 2009.

[2] J. Lloreta, O. Bielsa, A. Munné et al., "Renal cell carcinoma with syncytial giant cell component," *Virchows Archiv*, vol. 440, no. 3, pp. 330–333, 2002.

[3] J. M. Anderson, A. Rodriguez, and D. T. Chang, "Foreign body reaction to biomaterials," *Seminars in Immunology*, vol. 20, no. 2, pp. 86–100, 2008.

[4] D. B. Johnson, M. H. Saboorian, D. A. Duchene, K. Ogan, and J. A. Cadeddu, "Nephrectomy after radiofrequency ablation-induced ureteropelvic junction obstruction: Potential complication and long-term assessment of ablation adequacy," *Urology*, vol. 1453, no. 2, pp. 351-352, 2003.

[5] S. N. Goldberg, G. S. Gazelle, C. C. Compton, P. R. Mueller, and K. K. Tanabe, "Treatment of intrahepatic malignancy with radiofrequency ablation: radiologic-pathologic correlation," *Cancer*, vol. 88, no. 11, pp. 2452–2463, 2000.

[6] J. C. Durack, B. Richioud, J. Lyon, and S. B. Solomon, "Late emergence of contrast-enhancing fat necrosis mimicking tumor seeding after renal cryoablation," *Journal of Vascular and Interventional Radiology*, vol. 25, no. 1, pp. 133–137, 2014.

[7] R. P. Lokken, D. A. Gervais, R. S. Arellano et al., "Inflammatory nodules mimic applicator track seeding after percutaneous ablation of renal tumors," *American Journal of Roentgenology*, vol. 189, no. 4, pp. 845–848, 2007.

[8] A. Bandyopadhyay, S. Bhattacharya, B. Maiti, and K. Bose, "Calcified amyloid tumor of neck with exuberant giant cell reaction," *Journal of Laboratory Physicians*, vol. 7, no. 1, p. 61, 2015.

[9] W. Li and Z. Maleki, "Giant cell tumor of bone mimicking metastatic renal cell carcinoma: A case report," *Diagnostic Cytopathology*, vol. 40, no. 2, pp. E169–E171, 2012.

[10] C. C. Moran, S. T. Vakili, K. S. Caldemeyer, and R. R. Smith, "Foreign body giant cell reaction associated with epidermoid tumor: Ct and mr findings," *Journal of Computer Assisted Tomography*, vol. 19, no. 4, pp. 628–630, 1995.

[11] P. B. Tripathi, S. Kini, and A. D. Amarapurkar, "Foreign body giant cell reaction mimicking recurrence of colon cancer," *Trop Gastroenterol*, pp. 30–219, 2009.

11

Plexiform Schwannoma of the Penis: A Rare Subtype of Genital Schwannoma

Chrysovalantis Gkekas,[1] Vasileios Kalyvas,[1] Evangelos N. Symeonidis,[1] Apostolos Malioris,[1] Michail Papathanasiou,[1] Nikolaos Kalinderis,[2] Kyriakos Moisidis,[2] and Konstantinos Hatzimouratidis[2]

[1] *Department of Urology, 424 General Military Hospital of Thessaloniki, Thessaloniki, Greece*
[2] *2nd Department of Urology, Aristotle University of Thessaloniki, Thessaloniki, Greece*

Correspondence should be addressed to Chrysovalantis Gkekas; valantisgekas@yahoo.gr

Academic Editor: Mohamed A. Ghoneim

Schwannomas are benign, encapsulated neurogenic tumors which present in diverse histological subtypes despite the limited variety of their cellular constituents. These include the cellular, ancient, cystic, epithelioid, melanotic, psammomatous, schwannoma with pseudoglandular elements, and plexiform varieties. The plexiform schwannoma (PS) represents 4.3% of all schwannomas. These lesions are commonly encountered in the head and neck region and are extremely rare in the penis. To the best of our knowledge only 34 cases of penile schwannomas have been reported and this is the 3rd case of plexiform penile schwannoma. A 39-year-old patient presented to our andrology outpatient clinic complaining for two painful penile nodules. The lesions were located on the dorsum of the penile shaft. His medical history was insignificant for penile trauma and sexual transmitted diseases. The masses measured 2x1 cm and 0.5x1 cm. After sonographic and magnetic resonance evaluation the patient was admitted to theatre and underwent topical resection of the lesions. Histopathology revealed plexiform schwannoma. Postoperatively, penile tenderness and hyperesthesia ensued which was managed with pregabalin administration and topical corticosteroids. Plexiform schwannomas are rare in the penile region. Surgical excision is inevitably the only way to diagnose and treat the lesions. They must be differentiated by a variety of malignant and benign clinical conditions. Topical excision suffices for oncological control and allows for acceptable functional outcomes.

1. Background

Plexiform schwannomas (PS) represent a rare subtype of schwannomas. External genitalia are a relatively unusual landing location for this type of lesions and can pose a diagnostic and therapeutic challenge. We hereby report the case of a 39-year-old patient with penile PS, its diagnostic approach, and definitive treatment.

2. Introduction

Schwannomas are benign, encapsulated neurogenic tumors originating from the Schwann cells of the peripheral nerve sheath [1]. Plexiform schwannoma represents a unique variant, accounting for 4.3% of all schwannomas. These lesions are commonly encountered in the head and neck region [2]. Despite the extensive innervation of genitalia, neurilemmomas (Schwannomas) are exceedingly rare in the penis. Two recent reviews have identified 34 cases of penile schwannomas published in the English literature and this represents the 3rd characterized PS variant isolated to the penis [3–5].

Although their benign behavior is a fundamental feature of PS they can easily be confused with plexiform neurofibromas. The latter are pathognomonic of Von Recklinghausen's disease and have malignant potential [4, 6].

Plexiform schwannomas on the contrary can occur even in the absence of Von Reckligausen's genotype and malignant transformation has never been described [6].

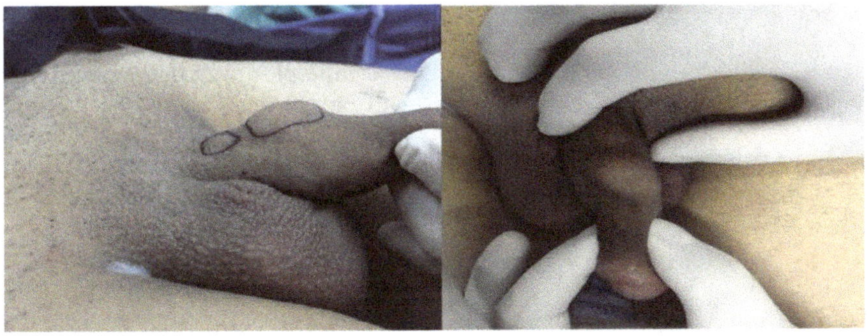

FIGURE 1: Two separate lumps on the dorsolateral aspect of the penis.

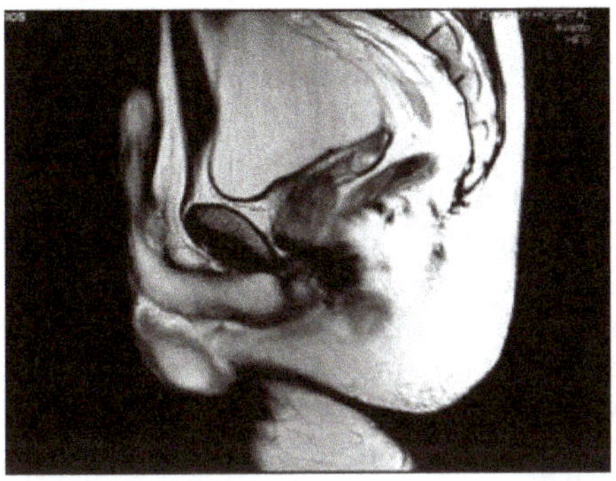

FIGURE 2: MRI of the penis T2 sagittal, demonstrating a distinct nodule on the dorsal aspect of the penis.

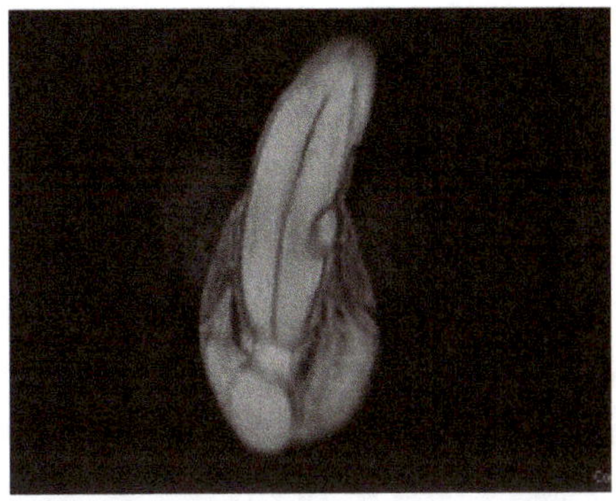

FIGURE 3: MRI of the penis T2 coronal. Dorsolaterally located nodule: clearly separate from tunica albuginea but included in Buck's fascia.

3. Case Presentation

A 39-year-old patient presented to our andrology clinic complaining of two gradually enlarging penile lumps. The lesions were located on the dorsum of the penile shaft having enlarged within a 2-year period. He complained of mild dorsal deviation of the shaft on erection and reported occasional pain during intercourse. He had not had any history of penile trauma or any sexually transmitted disease. Clinically, two distinct, soft, and painless nodules with a smooth contour could be identified on the dorsum of the penis. They were not fixed in place, yet not completely mobile (Figure 1). Artificial erection excluded penile curvature. Blood tests and urinalysis were insignificant. Sonographically, the lesions appeared hypoechoic and contained within a hyperechoic capsule, exhibiting diffuse central and peripheral blood flow. Magnetic resonance imaging depicted two well-capsulated masses ensheathed within Buck's fascia measuring 2x1 cm and 0.5x1cm each (Figures 2 and 3).

The larger and peripherally located lesion was removed via a 2 cm dorsal midline shaft incision under local anesthetic infiltration and penile block. The incision was restricted to the dorsal shaft without the need for circumcision. Macroscopically, the specimen appeared to be a 2.3cm spindle-shaped, elastic mass (Figure 4). In cross-section it had a soft, elastic texture and a yellow-tanned tinge. Histopathology reported a PS with strongly positive S-100 immunostain consistent with the neural origin of the tumor cells, the characteristic Antoni A and B areas, and the nuclear palisading (Figures 5 and 6). At this point it is worth mentioning that the patient had no physical findings of neurofibromatosis (NF), i.e., no café-au-lait spots, no Lisch nodules, no freckles, no osseous malformations, and no family history of NF.

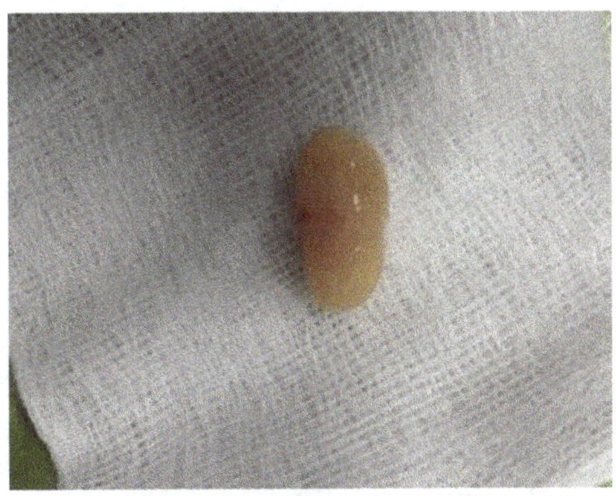

FIGURE 4: Penile plexiform schwannoma. Surgical specimen after excision: yellowish, spindle-shaped, and elastic in consistency.

Postoperatively, there was tenderness of the dorsal shaft and granular hyperesthesia with intermittent tingling and burning sensation. The symptoms attenuated after 6 months upon administration of low dose oral pregabalin and topical corticosteroids. This combination treatment was deemed

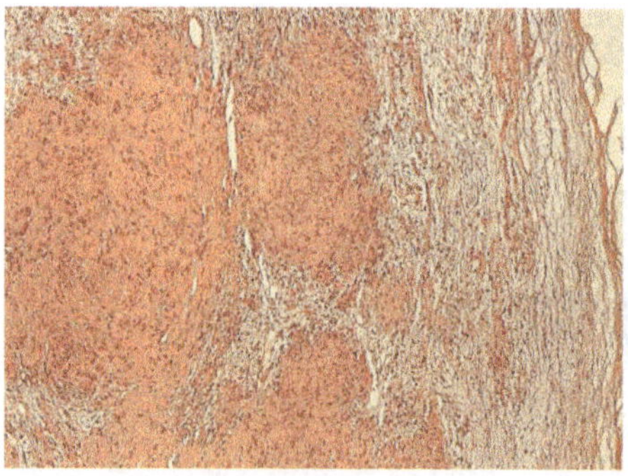

FIGURE 5: Small plexiform nodules with elongated, spindle-shaped tumor cells with no atypia or mitoses: Antoni A (left). Haphazard, scarce cellular arrangement in a loose stroma: Antoni B (right). E&H stain x10.

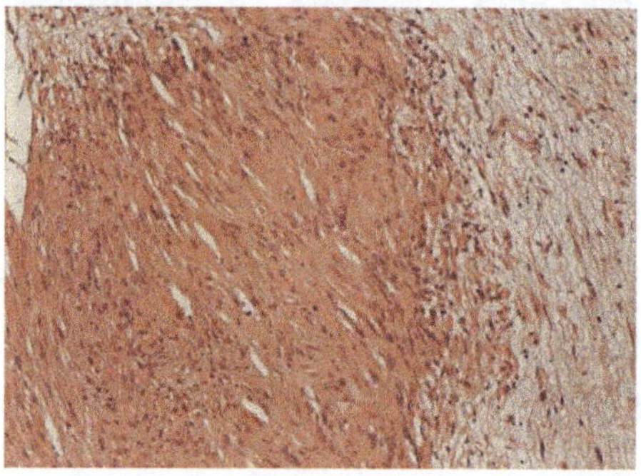

FIGURE 6: Antoni A area on the left with dense cellularity and nuclear palisading. Antoni B area on the right demonstrating loose array of the cells. E&H stain x20.

necessary after the initial failure of simple analgesics for the relief of the neuropathic penile pain resulting from surgery and postop scarring. The patient returned to his preoperative sexual status at 6 months after the operation and upon resolution of his numbness and dysesthesia.

Nine months after the removal of the first lesion the patient underwent excision of the second and more proximal lesion. It was less mobile and firmly attached to the neurovascular bundle and due to its proximal position was marginally out of the area covered by the penile block. It was removed under general anesthesia. Histology confirmed multifocal PS and due to its firm attachment to the neurovascular bundle the patient experienced dysesthesia of the glans and developed a dorsal cicatricial band causing discomfort during erection. Once again it was treated with pregabalin and long-term topical steroids with slow improvement.

4. Discussion

Harkin et al. reported the first 6 cases of plexiform schwannoma in 1978 and distinguished them from plexiform neurofibroma [7]. Most lesions were solitary and sporadic. Multifocality was usually associated with neurofibromatosis type 2. Despite PS being considered benign, recurrences have been reported in cases of incomplete resection [7]. They are usually located in the head and neck region (23%), the upper (22%) and lower extremities (22%), and the trunk (18%) [2].

Penile plexiform schwannomas are extraordinarily rare with only 2 cases having been identified so far out of the 34 published cases of penile schwannomas. Recently, in 2017, Kumar U et al. reported an uncommon presentation of sizeable penile schwannoma mimicking a scrotal mass in a 16-year-old boy [8].

Despite considered painless, penile schwannomas have been associated with painful intercourse, erectile dysfunction, and penile curvature[2]. Differential diagnosis includes Peyronie's disease, fibrosis after intracavernosal injections, lipomas, leiomyomas, sarcomas, and the other schwannoma subtypes [9]. Histopathology is the only safe means to distinguish them from other benign lesions [10, 11]. They demonstrate the key histopathological features of schwannomas such as the densely cellular Antoni A areas where nuclear palisading and whorling patterns predominate and the hypocellular Antoni B areas with the loose hypocellular stroma. Plexiform schwannomas are usually superficial, occurring typically in the dermis and subcutaneous tissue.

Malignant peripheral nerve sheath tumors (MPNST) have been described in the penis and require wide excision due to their risk of recurrence and their aggressive behavior [11, 12]. Although plexiform schwannomas have not been associated with malignant transformation, plexiform neurofibromas can progress into MPSNT and therefore identifying PS is essential due to their different biological behavior. S-100 immunostaining could be helpful since it is weakly expressed (or even not at all) in MPNSTs whilst PSs exhibit strong expression of the specific protein. Another differentiating feature is the increased number of mitoses and cellular atypia observed in MPNSTs in comparison to PSs as well as the fact that they are usually deep seated rather than superficial which is the case for most PSs.

Sexual dysfunction is the patient's primary concern and should be taken into consideration in the decision making. However, extensive surgery such as penectomy may be required in patients with advanced malignant disease along with adjuvant radiotherapy [3, 11, 12]. Surgical excision is the only method to differentiate and treat the condition. The rarity of the specific entity and the lack of extensive experience impede the construction of an evidence based treatment algorithm. Every reported case adds on the growing body of evidence.

References

[1] R. Asci, M. Danaci, S. Gur, E. Akdeniz, and Y. S. Baris, "Complete resection of penile schwannoma without sexual dysfunction," *Turkish Journal of Urology*, vol. 36, no. 2, pp. 207–210, 2010.

[2] J. C. Berg, B. W. Scheithauer, R. J. Spinner, C. M. Allen, and I. G. Koutlas, "Plexiform schwannoma: a clinicopathologic overview with emphasis on the head and neck region," *Human Pathology*, vol. 39, no. 5, pp. 633–640, 2008.

[3] A. H. Nguyen, M. L. Smith, E. L. Maranda, and S. Punnen, "Clinical features and treatment of penile schwannoma: a systematic review," *Clinical Genitourinary Cancer*, vol. 14, no. 3, pp. 198–202, 2016.

[4] D. Sato, T. Kase, M. Tajima et al., "Penile schwannoma," *International Journal of Urology*, vol. 8, no. 2, pp. 87–89, 2001.

[5] L. Wang, A. Arachchi, and A. Makris, "A rare case of concurrent penile and spinal schwannomas," *Urology Annals*, vol. 8, no. 2, pp. 233–235, 2016.

[6] M. Megahed, "Plexiform schwannoma," *American Journal of Dermatopathology*, vol. 16, no. 3, pp. 288–293, 1994.

[7] J. H. Harkin, J. H. Arrington, and R. J. Reed, "Benign plexiform schwannoma: a lesion distinct from plexiform neurofibroma," *Journal of Neuropathology & Experimental Neurology*, vol. 37, no. 5, p. 622, 1978.

[8] U. Kumar and N. Jha, "Schwannoma of the penis, presenting as a scrotal mass, rare entity with an uncommon presentation," *Urology Annals*, vol. 9, no. 3, p. 301, 2017.

[9] J. M. Woodruff, M. L. Marshall, T. A. Godwin, J. W. Funkhouser, N. J. Thompson, and R. A. Erlandson, "Plexiform (multinodular) schwannoma. A tumor simulating the plexiform neurofibroma," *The American Journal of Surgical Pathology*, vol. 7, no. 7, pp. 691–697, 1983.

[10] K. Malhotra, S. Shukla, N. Husain, A. Gupta, N. Awasthi, and 1. Dhayal, "Penile neurilemmoma: Utility of fine-needle aspiration cytology in diagnosis of a rare entity," *Journal of Cytology*, vol. 31, no. 3, p. 176, 2014.

[11] N. Parekh, E. Cockrell, and D. McMahon, "Malignant peripheral nerve sheath tumor of the penis: a case report and review of the literature," *Urology*, vol. 81, no. 5, pp. 1067-1068, 2013.

[12] J. Kaur, R. Madan, L. Singh et al., "Malignant peripheral nerve sheath tumour of penis," *Andrologia*, vol. 47, no. 3, pp. 333–335, 2015.

12

Necrotizing Epididymo-Orchitis: A Rare Manifestation of COVID-19

Ali Tavoosian, Sana Ahmadi, and Seyed Mohammad Kazem Aghamir

Urology Research Center, Tehran University of Medical Sciences, Tehran, Iran

Correspondence should be addressed to Seyed Mohammad Kazem Aghamir; mkaghamir@tums.ac.ir

Academic Editor: Tun-Chieh Chen

Epididymo-orchitis is an infection of the epididymis and testis, one of the most common urogenital infections. It can be seen at any age. It is caused by sexually transmitted microorganisms and nonsexual transmitted pathogens. Viruses such as mumps and cytomegalovirus can also cause epididymo-orchitis. During the COVID-19 pandemic, in case of abnormal clinical manifestations of COVID infection and inadequate therapeutic response to the routine therapies, this disease with unusual manifestations should be considered. The case introduced in this paper is a 55-year-old man referred to a urology clinic with typical clinical presentations of epididymo-orchitis. Diagnosis by color Doppler examination and ultrasound also confirmed epididymo-orchitis. The patient underwent appropriate and routine treatment for epididymo-orchitis. Because of the lack of adequate clinical response and the continuation of fever and the development of scrotal lesions and the results of the control ultrasound, which suggested rupture of the tunica albuginea capsule, he underwent surgical exploration and subsequent orchiectomy. Due to the unconventional conditions and the usual culture and pathology, COVID-19 PCR was also performed on the tissues. The PCR showed tissue infection with COVID-19. The patient's clinical condition improved with an orchiectomy, the fever stopped, and he was discharged in a good general condition. It should be noted that before referral to the urology clinic and during hospitalization, evaluation, and treatment, the patient had no evidence in favor of respiratory tract infection with the coronavirus.

1. Introduction

In the last days of 2019, coronavirus disease 2019 (COVID-19), first identified in China, became a worldwide pandemic. Respiratory compromise is the most important feature of the disease. Soon, the COVID-19 outbreak became a world challenge [1, 2]. The common symptoms of COVID-19 are cough, fever, and fatigue [3].

Epididymo-orchitis is a common urological condition that occurs at any age. The most common cause of epididymo-orchitis in young adults is sexually transmitted pathogens, such as Chlamydia trachomatis and Neisseria gonorrhoeae. In older men, epididymo-orchitis is most often caused by nonsexually transmitted Gram-negative bacteria causing urinary tract infections, which rarely occur without concomitant epididymitis [4–6]. Orchitis, especially in young males, can be caused by a virus such as mumps (which is the most common cause of viral orchitis), rubella, coxsackievirus, varicella, echovirus, and cytomegalovirus. Widespread MMR vaccination decreased the frequency of mumps orchitis [4, 5].

During the past two years of COVID-19 pandemic, many presentations and complications such as several genitourinary disorders have been reported worldwide [5, 7].

2. Case Presentation

A 55-year-old gentleman was referred to a urologist due to the right hemiscrotal pain and swelling four days ago, and fever started two days ago. He reported some irritative symptoms of the lower urinary tract such as dysuria and frequency. There was no obstructive symptom. There was no history of unprotected sexual contact. He agreed on orchiectomy and report his case by signing the written informed consent, and the case report is based on CARE guideline. On initial examination, 101.3°F (38.5°C) oral fever, erythema of right hemiscrotal skin was founded, and the skin of the

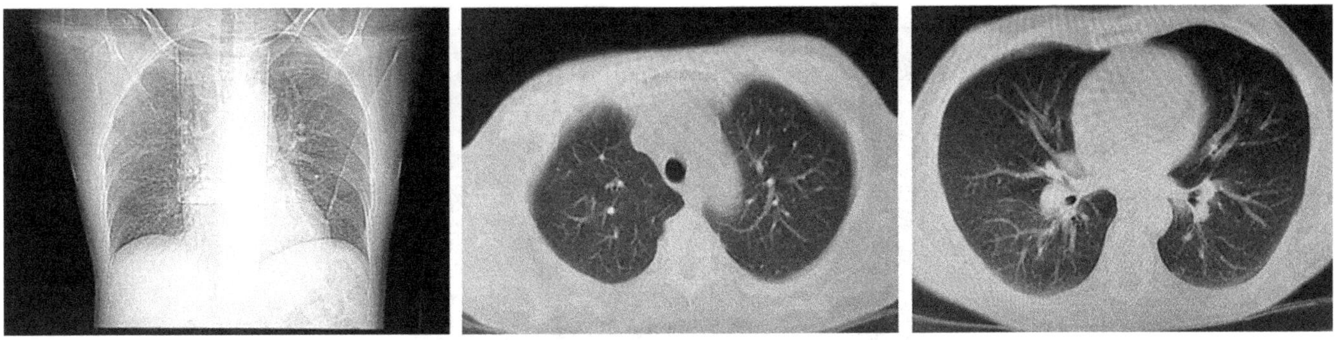

FIGURE 1: (a) First sonographic image. (b) Second sonographic images.

right hemiscrotal was edematous. We found no evidence of a sexually transmitted disease (such as purulent discharge) on examination. On palpation, enlargement of the right testicle and stiffness and induration of the right epididymis were evident. On touch, the testicle had tenderness, which, based on an examination, was suggested to be a right epididymo-orchitis.

In color Doppler ultrasound performed from the testis (Figure 1), the left testicle was normal, the skin of the right scrotum was edematous, with increasing the size of the right testicle and its echo was heterogeneous and decreased. An increase in the size of the right epididymis and an increase in the arterial flow of the right epididymis and testis, along with mild hydrocele with internal debris, have also been reported. The patient had no history of medication, and the patient's complete history indicates no illness and past medical problems and no history of unsafe sex. Also, he had no history of exposure to the COVID-19 for more than his last two weeks. His complete blood count (CBC) to evaluate his overall health detects WBC: 9200, neutrophil: 54, lymphocyte: 36, RBC: 10-12, BAC: rare, and negative nitrite. His chest CT-scan images are presented in Figure 2. The above items in the ultrasound report confirmed the right epididymo-orchitis. With the mentioned diagnosis, the patient is admitted to the urology department and underwent the following treatment:

(1) Complete bed rest

(2) Ciprofloxacin 400 mg IV/BID

(3) Tablet of Ibuprofen 400 mg PO/TDS

(4) Testis elevation

(5) Testis cold compression

Despite 48 hours of intravenous antibiotic treatment, the patient's fever continued, and the scrotal swelling increased sharply. The scrotal skin was severely edematous on the second ultrasound (Figure 1), and severe hydrocele was reported in the right hemiscrotal with no abscess formation. The right testicle continues to increase in size, and its echo has heterogeneity and increased vascular flow.

The patient did not have any upper respiratory symptoms before referring to the urology clinic with a mentioned urological manifestation and during the hospital stay. Due to the persistence of fever and the consult with an infectious disease specialist, a request was made for nasopharyngeal secretions tests and high-resolution computed tomography (HRCT) of the chest to rollout the COVID-19. There was no change in the patient's IV antibiotic regimen. HRCT showed no evidence of COVID 19-induced pulmonary involvement, and the nasopharyngeal test was negative for COVID19. During the 96 hours since admission, the patient remained feverish. The testicular pain increased sharply. On examination of the right hemiscrotal, tenderness, severe scrotal skin edema, and severe hydrocele were evident. The patient underwent color Doppler ultrasound of the testicles again (Figure 1), ruptured of the tunica albuginea capsule, and exudation of the intratesticular tissues to outside the tunica albuginea capsule was reported.

The patient was a candidate for exploratory surgery. By transverse incision on the right hemiscrotal, we entered the space between the tunica-vaginalis and the tunica-albuginea, and about 800 ml of fluid (which was pyocele) was drained. Extensive rupture of the tunica albuginea in the middle bridge of the right testicle was evident, along with extensive necrosis of the internal tissues of the right testicle. The decision was made for a right orchiectomy. Extracted tissues were sent for pathology, culture, antibiogram, and PCR of testicular tissue for COVID-19. After orchiectomy, the patient's general condition has improved. And within 12 hours of surgery, the patient's fever stops. We ordered PCR test of the testicle tissue. Twenty-four hours after the tests, PCR of the testicular tissue submitted was positive for COVID 19.

The patient was treated with remdesivir based on the infectious disease specialist recommendation for five days based on infectious counseling. The patient had no upper or lower respiratory tract infection symptoms during this time. Finally, the patient was discharged in a good general condition without fever and significantly reduced swelling and scrotal edema.

3. Discussion

Although COVID-19 in some patients can be presented without fever, and many of the patients did not have abnormal radiological findings, other rare results were found in some of them, such as urogenital signs and symptoms [1, 7]. Urogenital involvement of coronavirus is rare and limited with some case reports [4, 8, 9]. Some of the urogenital

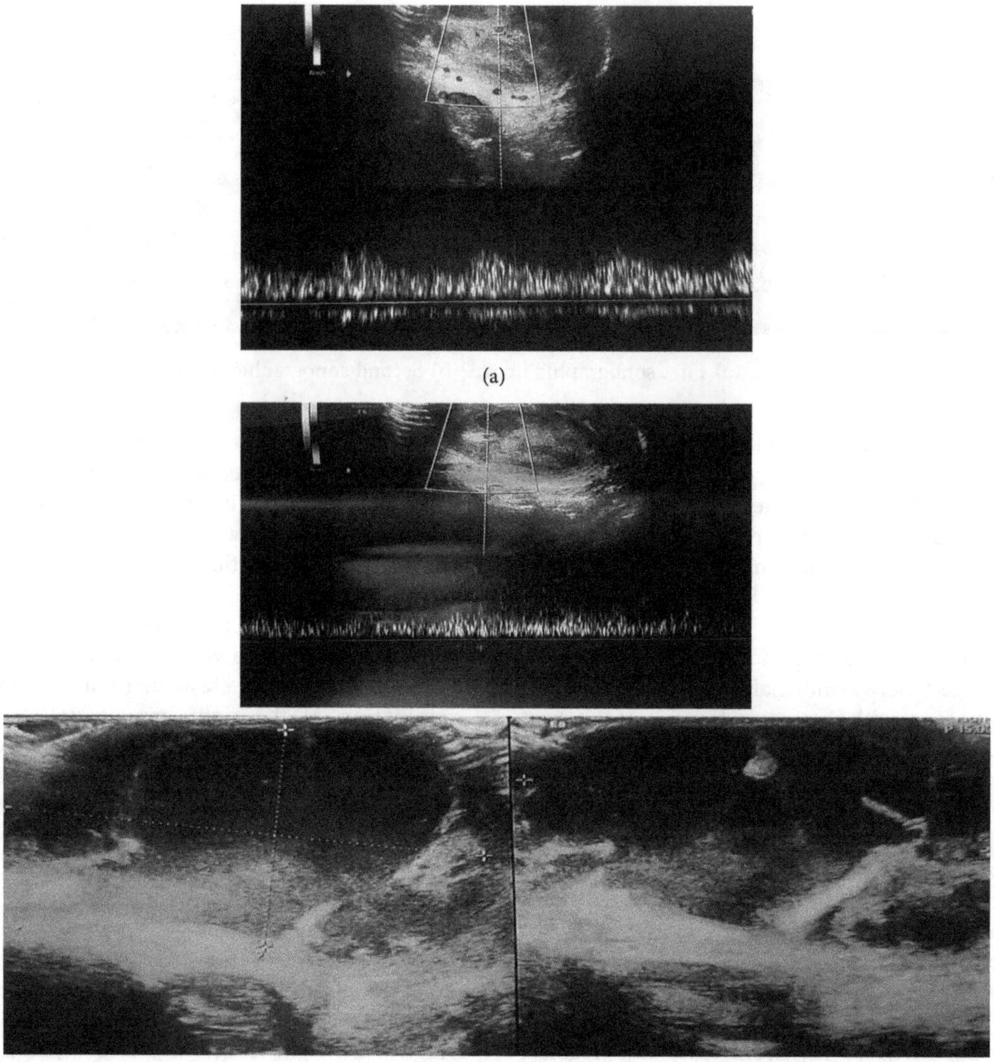

(a)

(b)

Figure 2: (a) Chest CT and (b) Sonography report.

complications caused by COVID-19 have been secondary to hypercoagulable states [5]. There are some case reports regarding patients with epididymo-orchitis symptoms such as abdominal, testicular, and back pain; bilateral testicular warmth, testicular discomfort, swelling, pain, and erythema; and concurrent COVID-19, without any respiratory symptom [5, 6, 10–13]. These studies reported NSAID or antibiotic therapy would be successful in all patients with testicular pain, and no patient required more invasive procedures [4, 6, 14, 15].

In our study, we describe a case of a gentleman with no symptom of coronavirus disease and negative respiratory tests for COVID-19, who was referred to our clinic with epididymo-orchitis symptoms. The question is how can the coronavirus infect the testicles?

The mechanism of the COVID-19 infection is binding to Angiotensin-Converting Enzyme 2 (ACE2). This is known as the main pathway of influencing host cells [16]. ACE2 is expressed in many tissues in the genitourinary system. Today, we know that the testis presents some conditions that might favor COVID-19 infection, such as the expression of ACE2, and the fact that Leydig cells of the testis receptors can act as the ACE2 receptor. This finding could explain the COVID-19 passage into the testicular microcirculation where reduced blood flow and presence of its receptor (ACE2) could enhance testicular infection [5, 13, 17–21].

4. Conclusion

This paper presents a case of epididymo-orchitis who was infected by a coronavirus. We also tried to answer the question of how the testicles become infected with the coronavirus by perusing other similar cases presented all around the world. Further studies are needed to determine exactly how the coronavirus infects the genitourinary tract and what the effects of the infection will be in the future.

Ethical Approval

The patient agreed on orchiectomy and report his case by signing the written informed consent, and the case report is based on CARE guideline.

Consent

Informed consent was obtained in both written and verbal format from the patient to report this case.

Acknowledgments

The authors would like to thank the patient and the Urology research center at Sina hospital.

References

[1] W. J. Guan, Z. Y. Ni, Y. Hu et al., "China medical treatment expert group for COVID-19," *Clinical characteristics of coronavirus disease*, vol. 382, no. 18, pp. 1708–1720, 2019.

[2] A. S. Fauci, H. C. Lane, and R. R. Redfield, "COVID-19—navigating the uncharted," *New England Journal of Medicine*, vol. 382, no. 13, pp. 1268-1269, 2020.

[3] W.-j. Guan, Z.-y. Ni, Y. Hu et al., "Clinical characteristics of coronavirus disease 2019 in China," *New England Journal of Medicine*, vol. 382, no. 18, pp. 1708–1720, 2020.

[4] C. Ediz, H. H. Tavukcu, S. Akan et al., "Is there any association of COVID-19 with testicular pain and epididymo- orchitis?," *International Journal of Clinical Practice*, vol. 75, no. 3, article e13753, 2021.

[5] R. E. Bridwell, D. R. Merrill, S. A. Griffith, J. Wray, and J. J. Oliver, "A coronavirus disease 2019 (COVID-19) patient with bilateral orchitis," *The American Journal of Emergency Medicine*, vol. 42, pp. 260.e3–260.e5, 2021.

[6] L. Gagliardi, C. Bertacca, C. Centenari et al., "Orchiepididymitis in a boy with COVID-19," *Pediatric Infectious Disease Journal*, vol. 39, no. 8, pp. e200–e202, 2020.

[7] M. Samsami, J. Z. Bagherpour, H. Tahmasbi, A. M. Tofigh, S. P. Shojaee, and H. Hatamabadi, "Review of unusual presentations of COVID-19," *Journal of Hearing Sciences and Otolaryngology*, vol. 6, no. 1, pp. 1–5, 2020.

[8] A. Mohammadi and S. M. K. Aghamir, "The hypothesis of the COVID-19 role in acute kidney injury: a literatures review," *Translational Research in Urology*, vol. 2, no. 3, pp. 74–78, 2020.

[9] A. Fakhr Yasseri and D. Taheri, "Urinary stone management during COVID-19 pandemic," *Translational Research in Urology*, vol. 2, no. 1, pp. 1–3, 2020.

[10] J. Kim, T. Thomsen, N. Sell, and A. J. Goldsmith, "Abdominal and testicular pain: an atypical presentation of COVID-19," *The American Journal of Emergency Medicine*, vol. 38, no. 7, pp. 1542.e1–1542.e3, 2020.

[11] M. Haydar, S. Baghdadi, M. Taleb, B. Al-Dali, H. Badr, and Y. Ghanem, "Orchiepididymitis in the context of multisystem inflammatory syndrome in a child with COVID-19 from Syria: a very rare presentation for SARS-Cov-19 in children," *Oxford Medical Case Reports*, vol. 2021, no. 7, article omab052, 2021.

[12] M. Creta, C. Sagnelli, G. Celentano et al., "SARS-CoV-2 infection affects the lower urinary tract and male genital system: a systematic review," *Journal of Medical Virology*, vol. 93, no. 5, pp. 3133–3142, 2021.

[13] H. Alkhatatbeh, D. Alzaghari, A. Alkhashman, M. Azab, G. M. A. Edwan, and M. Abufaraj, "Does severe acute respiratory syndrome coronavirus-2 (SARS-CoV-2) cause orchitis in patients with coronavirus disease 2019 (COVID-19)?," *Arab Journal of Urology*, vol. 18, no. 3, pp. 129–133, 2020.

[14] M. K. Aghamir, R. Hosseini, and F. Alizadeh, "A vacuum device for penile elongation: fact or fiction?," *BJU International*, vol. 97, no. 4, pp. 777-778, 2006.

[15] S. M. K. Aghamir, A. Salavati, R. Yousefie et al., "Does bone marrow-derived mesenchymal stem cell transfusion prevent antisperm antibody production after traumatic testis rupture?," *Urology*, vol. 84, no. 1, pp. 82–86, 2014.

[16] A. M. South, D. I. Diz, and M. C. Chappell, "COVID-19, ACE2, and the cardiovascular consequences," *American Journal of Physiology-Heart and Circulatory Physiology*, vol. 318, no. 5, pp. H1084–H1090, 2020.

[17] Y. Zhang, X. Geng, Y. Tan et al., "New understanding of the damage of SARS-CoV-2 infection outside the respiratory system," *Biomedicine & Pharmacotherapy*, vol. 127, article 110195, 2020.

[18] C. Fan, W. Lu, K. Li, Y. Ding, and J. Wang, "ACE2 expression in kidney and testis may cause kidney and testis infection in COVID-19 patients," *Frontiers in Medicine*, vol. 7, 2021.

[19] A. Di Vincenzo and M. Rossato, "COVID-19 and orchi-epididymitis," *The Pediatric Infectious Disease Journal*, vol. 39, no. 11, article e385, 2020.

[20] S. Aslan and U. Eryuruk, "Necrotizing orchitis due to COVİD-19," *Revista da Sociedade Brasileira de Medicina Tropical*, vol. 54, article e04082021, 2021.

[21] O. T. Olaniyan, A. Dare, G. E. Okotie et al., "Testis and blood-testis barrier in COVID-19 infestation: role of angiotensin-converting enzyme 2 in male infertility," *Journal of Basic and Clinical Physiology and Pharmacology*, vol. 31, no. 6, 2020.

13

The Intraoperative use of a Portable Cone-Beam Computed Tomography System for the Diagnosis of Intraperitoneal Bladder Perforation

Ankur Choksi,[1] **Benjamin Press**,[1] **Cayce Nawaf**,[1] **Shannon Longyear**,[2] **Marc Ferrante**,[2] **and Thomas V. Martin**[1]

[1]*Department of Urology, Yale University School of Medicine, New Haven, CT, USA*
[2]*Department of Radiology and Biomedical Imaging, Yale University School of Medicine, New Haven, CT, USA*

Correspondence should be addressed to Ankur Choksi; ankur.choksi@yale.edu and Thomas V. Martin; thomas.v.martin@yale.edu

Academic Editor: David Duchene

Background. Intraoperative imaging for endourologic procedures is generally limited to single-plane fluoroscopic X-ray. The O-arm™ is a mobile cone-bean CT scanner that may have applications in urologic surgeries. *Case Presentation.* We present a case of an 85-year-old male with radiation cystitis and recurrent gross hematuria who was identified to have a bladder perforation on cystoscopy during emergent clot evacuation. Single-view fluoroscopic evaluation was inconclusive as to whether an intraperitoneal bladder perforation occurred. A portable cone-beam CT scan was used to acquire a 3-D CT cystogram, which demonstrated intraperitoneal contrast extravasation, confirming the diagnosis of an intraperitoneal bladder perforation. *Conclusion.* We report the first use of a portable cone-beam CT scanner to perform an intraoperative CT cystogram to diagnose an intraperitoneal bladder perforation and guide surgical management.

1. Introduction

Cone-beam computed tomography (CBCT) is an increasingly available mobile imaging modality that can be used for intraoperative planning. The O-arm™ is a mobile imaging system that produces cone-beam X-rays in a rotating tube, capable of fitting around the surgical table, and can acquire 2-D fluoroscopic images and rapid 3-D volumetric reconstruction. The portability of a CBCT scanner, such as the O-arm™, allows for real-time intraoperative imaging and decision making, eliminating the need to transport the patient to a traditional CT scanner while the patient is under general anesthesia. Additional benefits of CBCT include lower radiation exposure to the patient compared to conventional CT, and superior spatial resolution and multidimensional image acquisitions when compared to fluoroscopy [1]. At our institution, the application of intraoperative CBCT is well established for neurosurgical, spinal, and orthopedic surgery. For urologic surgeries, intraoperative imaging is obtained through anterior-posterior plane 2-D fluoroscopic imaging.

For the diagnosis of bladder perforation, cystography with the use of water-soluble contrast is acquired either through fluoroscopy or CT imaging [2]. Cystography also allows for the determination as to whether the bladder perforation has occurred intraperitoneal or extraperitoneal, which would guide further management. If fluoroscopy is used, at least an anterior-posterior and lateral view must be acquired. For simple extraperitoneal bladder perforations, management may be limited to an indwelling urinary catheter. For intraperitoneal bladder perforations, tracking of the urine into the peritoneal cavity can cause ileus, peritonitis, sepsis, and abdominal compartment syndrome and is unlikely to heal with urinary drainage; hence, operative repair is warranted. For an intraoperative detection of bladder perforation visualized on rigid cystoscopy, a retrograde cystogram with single-plane fluoroscopy has limited utility due to the inability to obtain lateral plane views. Herein, we present the first reported utilization of a portable conical-beam CT scanner to perform an intraoperative CT cystogram to assist in the differentiation between an intraperitoneal and extraperitoneal bladder perforation visualized on cystoscopy.

2. Case Presentation

2.1. Clinical History. The patient is an 85-year-old male with a remote history of prostate cancer treated with an open radical prostatectomy and adjuvant radiation therapy who subsequently developed recurrent gross hematuria and clot retention secondary to radiation cystitis. He completed approximately forty sessions of hyperbaric oxygen therapies but continued to experience recurrent gross hematuria requiring multiple inpatient hospitalizations for continuous bladder irrigations and requiring transfusion of blood products. He was discharged from the hospital two weeks prior to his most recent admission with a urinary catheter after a prolonged hospital course during which he was treated for gross hematuria. His hospital course was also complicated by a small bowel obstruction managed nonoperatively and a *C. difficile* infection. On the night prior to this admission, he noticed poor drainage from his urinary catheter prompting his presentation to an outside Emergency Department where he was initiated on continuous bladder irrigation and transferred to our institution.

The following morning, the patient endorsed diffuse lower abdominal pain, had a marked increase in his leukocytosis, and had a poorly draining catheter with worsening gross hematuria. The patient was brought to the operating room emergently for a cystoscopy and clot evacuation. After clot was removed from the bladder and better visualization was obtained, a perforation was visualized at the dome of the bladder that extended towards the base of the bladder. In order to differentiate between an extraperitoneal and intraperitoneal bladder perforation, a fluoroscopic retrograde cystogram limited to the anterior-posterior view in lithotomy position was performed (Figure 1) using approximately 50 milliliters of iohexol (Omnipaque™) contrast dye; however, the image findings were equivocal.

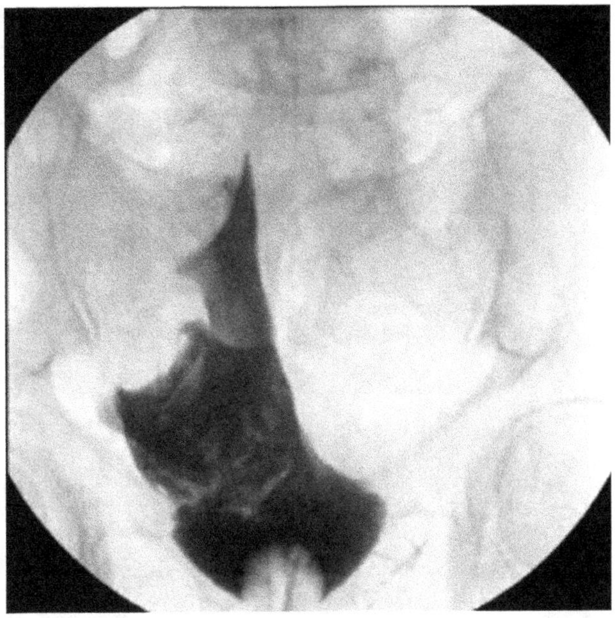

FIGURE 1: Intraoperative fluoroscopic cystography with images captured in the anterior-posterior view. Fluoroscopic images demonstrate the bladder perforation; however, with a single view, it is unclear whether the extravasation of contrast is intraperitoneal.

2.2. Technique. A portable cone-beam CT scanner (O-arm™, Medtronic, Minneapolis, MN) was brought into the operating room and positioned around the surgical table. An additional 50 milliliters of Omnipaque™ contrast was instilled by gravity drainage into the bladder. Two-dimensional fluoroscopic images and three-dimensional conical-beam computed tomography (CBCT) images of the abdomen and pelvis were obtained (Figure 2), to represent an intraoperative CT cystogram. Contrast extravasation was visualized in the peritoneal cavity. After the images were reviewed by radiology, it was confirmed that the patient had an intraperitoneal bladder perforation. The patient was repositioned and prepped and underwent an exploratory laparotomy and repair of his intraperitoneal bladder perforation. The total fluoroscopy radiation exposure from the O-arm™ was 9.23 mGy over an irradiation duration of 5.43 seconds. For the 3-D CBCT acquisition at 120 kVP, the CT dose index was 27.47 mGy with a dose-length product of 439.39 mGy∗cm.

3. Discussion

We described the first reported use of an intraoperative CBCT cystogram for the diagnosis of an intraperitoneal bladder perforation that was first identified during a cystoscopy for bladder clot evacuation. This patient was at an increased risk of morbidity from an abdominal exploratory laparotomy given his poor performance status, history of prior abdominal surgeries and pelvic radiation, and multiple prolonged hospitalizations over the past six months. The accurate and rapid diagnosis of an intraperitoneal bladder perforation was deemed necessary prior to proceeding with an exploratory laparotomy. In this case, the initial identification of the bladder perforation occurred cystoscopically while the patient was under general anesthesia; hence, obtaining a multiplanar fluoroscopic cystogram was challenging. The intraoperative acquisition of a CT cystogram using a portable CBCT scanner allowed for the rapid radiographic determination of an intraperitoneal bladder perforation without having to transport a patient under general anesthesia.

Conventional management of an intraperitoneal bladder perforation includes laparotomy with its own associated morbidity. With the advent of laparoscopic surgical techniques, the laparoscopic repair of an isolated intraperitoneal bladder has been described, with an associated shorter hospital stay, faster return to functionality, and decreased morbidity [3]. Although laparoscopic repair of bladder perforations is less frequent, a diagnostic laparoscopy can

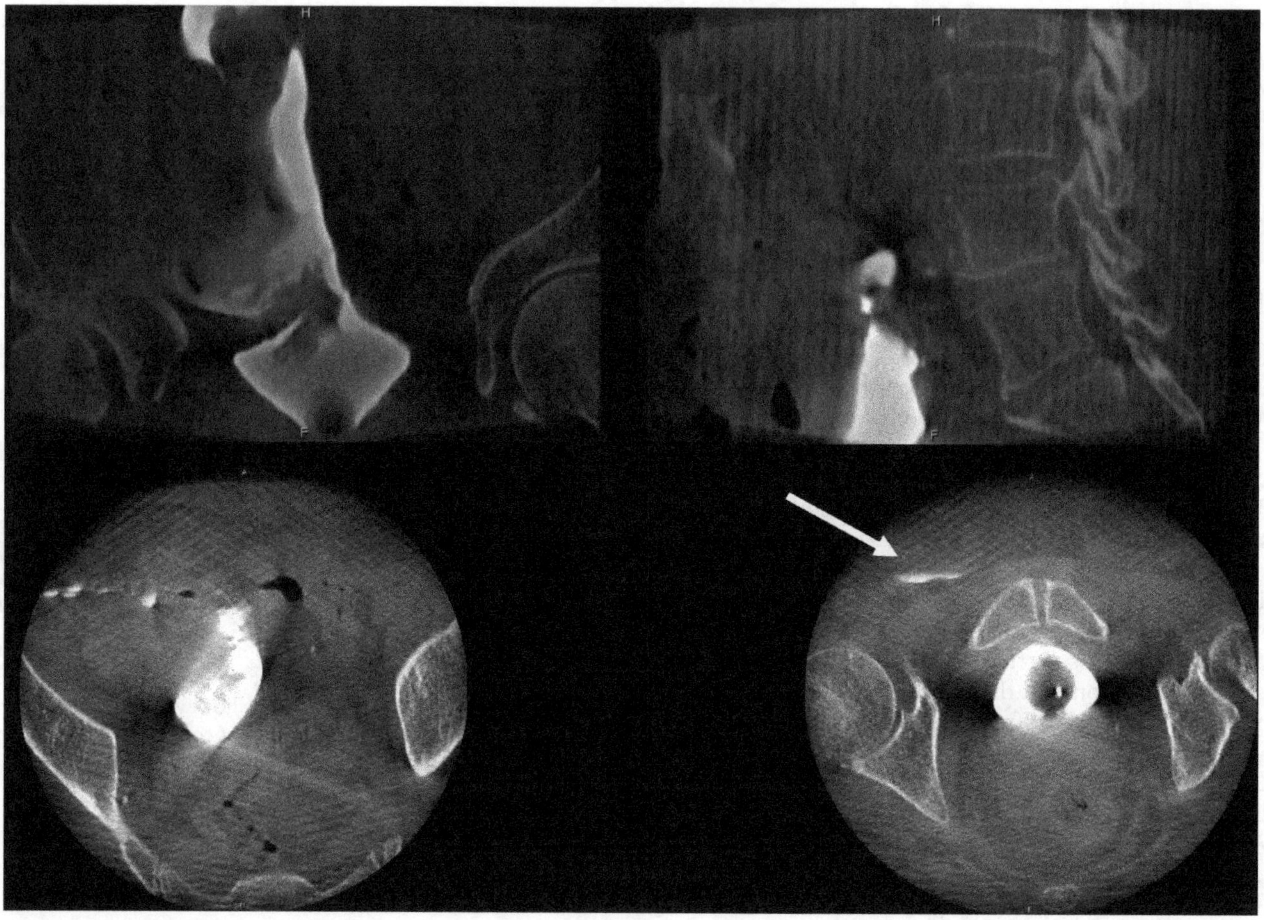

FIGURE 2: Intraoperative CT cystogram obtained using an O-arm™ surgical imaging system with three-dimensional volumetric reconstruction. Image acquisition in the coronal (top left), sagittal (top right), axial abdomen (bottom left), and axial pelvis (bottom right) planes was obtained. Contrast is visible in the intraperitoneal cavity and around the bowel, confirming the diagnosis of an intraperitoneal bladder perforation. Note the extravasation of contrast into a right inguinal hernia in the axial pelvis plane, also confirming an intraperitoneal bladder perforation.

replace the need to obtaining intraoperative cross-sectional imaging when a perforation is diagnosed cystoscopically. A laparoscopic approach would have been challenging in this patient given his prior history of pelvic radiation and abdominal surgeries.

The reported use of an intraoperative portable CBCT scanner in urologic surgeries is limited. Intraoperative CBCT scans were utilized by Zelefsky et al. to verify the positioning and dosimetry of prostate artery brachytherapy seeds [4]. The urologists were able to adjust the surgical plan and place additional seeds prior to anesthesia reversal based on the intraoperative CBCT scans obtained. The results were verified with a postoperative traditional CT scan, which demonstrated accurate correlation to the intraoperative CBCT scans. For patients with complex spinal anatomy and congenital malformations, intraoperative O-arm™ CBCT scans have been demonstrated by Hellström et al. to assist in surgical planning and navigate placement of an S3 stimulation electrode for sacral nerve stimulator lead implantation [5]. More recently, the use of a CBCT scan at the conclusion of a percutaneous nephrolithotomy was performed to evaluate for residual stone burden [6]. In a review of 19 cases, CBCT scans positively identified 9 patients with residual stone fragments that were removed by the urologist prior to anesthesia reversal. An eventual stone-free burden was confirmed with a postoperative noncontrast CT scan.

4. Conclusion

When an intraoperative bladder perforation is identified during cystoscopy, a single-view fluoroscopic cystogram may be inconclusive in differentiating between an intraperitoneal and extraperitoneal perforation. We describe the use of an O-arm™, a portable conical-beam CT scanner, to acquire an intraoperative CT cystogram to definitively diagnose an intraperitoneal bladder perforation and guide further management.

Consent

The patient provided informed consent for allowing the publishing of this information.

References

[1] E. Tabaraee, A. G. Gibson, D. G. Karahalios, E. A. Potts, J.-P. Mobasser, and S. Burch, "Intraoperative cone beam–

computed tomography with navigation (O-ARM) versus conventional fluoroscopy (C-ARM)," *Spine*, vol. 38, no. 22, pp. 1953–1958, 2013.

[2] D. P. N. Chan, H. H. Abujudeh, G. L. Cushing Jr., and R. A. Novelline, "CT cystography with multiplanar reformation for suspected bladder rupture: experience in 234 cases," *American Journal of Roentgenology*, vol. 187, no. 5, pp. 1296–1302, 2006.

[3] T. D. Marchand, R. H. Cuadra, and D. J. Ricchiuti, "Laparoscopic repair of a traumatic bladder rupture," *Journal of The Society of Laparoscopic & Robotic Surgeons*, vol. 16, no. 1, pp. 155–158, 2012.

[4] M. J. Zelefsky, M. Worman, G. N. Cohen et al., "Real-time intraoperative computed tomography assessment of quality of permanent interstitial seed implantation for prostate cancer," *Urology*, vol. 76, no. 5, pp. 1138–1142, 2010.

[5] P. A. Hellström, J. Katisko, P. Finnilä, and M. H. Vaarala, "Sacral nerve stimulation lead implantation using the o-arm," *BMC Urology*, vol. 13, no. 1, 2013.

[6] R. A. Kingma, M. J. H. Voskamp, B. H. J. Doornweerd, I. J. de Jong, and S. Roemeling, "Intraoperative cone beam computed tomography for detecting residual stones in percutaneous nephrolithotomy: a feasibility study," *Urolithiasis*, 2021.

14

A Mislocated Intrauterine Device Migrating to the Urinary Bladder: An Uncommon Complication Leading to Stone Formation

Mohamed Ali Nouioui, Tarek Taktak, Seif Mokadem, Houssem Mediouni, Ramzi Khiari, and Samir Ghozzi

Department of Urology, Military Hospital of First Instruction of Tunis, University of Tunis El Manar, Tunisia

Correspondence should be addressed to Mohamed Ali Nouioui; mednouiouimed@gmail.com

Academic Editor: Shiou-Sheng Chen

Intrauterine devices are a popular form of reversible contraception among women. Its administration can lead to some uncommon but serious complications such as perforation leading to its migration into adjacent organs. Like any foreign body, the presence of an IUD in the bladder can result in stone formation due to its lithogenic potential. We report a case of an IUD migrating from its normal position in the uterine cavity into the urinary bladder causing chronic low urinary tract symptoms in a 43-year-old female patient. The device was securely removed without complications using grasping forceps under cystoscopy, and no parietal defect was detected. A mislocated IUD is a rare complication that should be considered in female patients presenting with chronic urinary symptoms.

1. Introduction

Intrauterine devices (IUD) are a frequently used reversible form of contraception.

As any medical device, its administration can lead to complications such as perforation and extrauterine migration to adjacent organs.

The most common sites for IUD migration are the omentum, rectum, sigmoid colon, peritoneum, and bladder [1].

Here, we report a case of an IUD migrating from the uterus cavity into the urinary bladder.

2. Case Presentation

A 43-year-old female was referred to our outpatient department for a one-year history of chronic pelvic pain with lower urinary tract symptoms such as dysuria, urgency, and pollakiuria.

Her medical history was unremarkable other than the insertion of a Copper-T IUD four years ago by her gynaecologist and with no regular follow-up afterwards.

Physical pelvic examination was normal.

Urinalysis was indicative of leucocyturia, but urine culture was negative.

An abdominal ultrasonography revealed an echogenic intravesical lesion suggestive of urinary bladder calculus (Figure 1).

Plain abdominal radiography did not show any stone but demonstrated the IUD in the lower left quadrant of the abdomen (Figure 2).

A cystoscopy was done after written informed consent of the patient. It revealed a calcified T-shaped foreign object identified as the IUD, embedded into the muscular wall of the bladder.

No stones were found.

The IUD was extracted easily with gentle traction using endoscopic forceps.

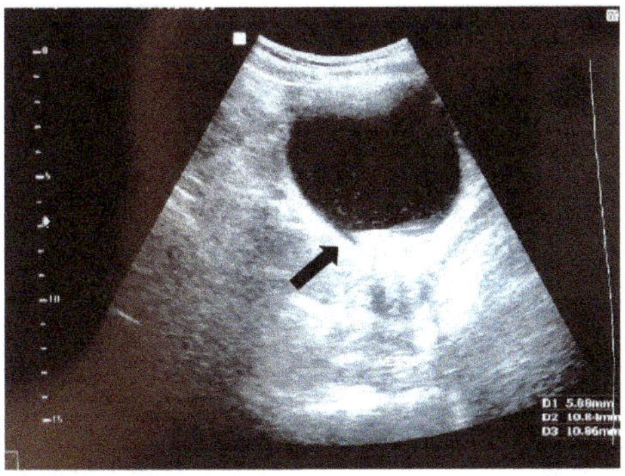

FIGURE 1: Pelvic US revealing an echogenic intravesical foreign object (arrow) initially suggestive of urinary bladder calculus.

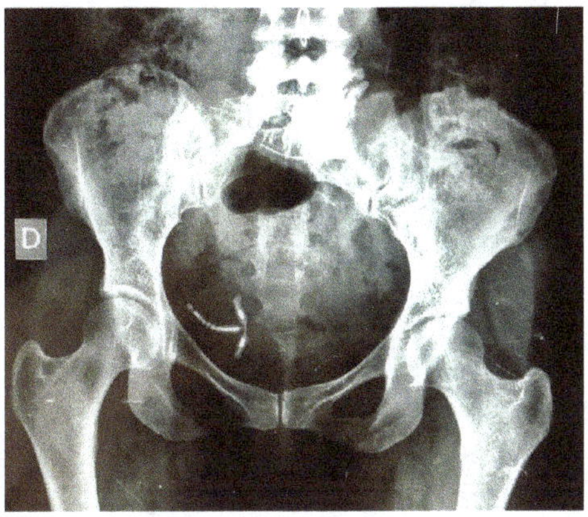

FIGURE 2: A mislocated IUD in the lower left quadrant of the abdomen showed on the plain abdominal X-ray.

After the removal of the foreign object, we did not find any fistula tract between the posterior wall of the bladder and the uterus.

One month following the procedure, the patient was reassessed and reported a significant improvement in lower urinary symptoms including no evidence of infections in the urine culture or persistence of fistula at the flexible cystoscopy.

3. Discussion

Intrauterine device is a regular form of mechanical contraception widely used. More than 150 million women use IUDs, mainly in emerging countries [2].

Its administration can be accompanied by several complications.

Perforation is one the most serious but rare complication secondary to the insertion of IUD, eventually leading to its migration from its normal position in the fundus either into the abdominal cavity or into other organs adjacent to the uterus.

The incidence of perforation is estimated as being between 1.9 and 3.6 per 1000 insertions [3].

The true incidence of perforation is most likely higher because of the frequently asymptomatic nature of the perforation, with over 30% of perforations recognized only when pregnancy [4].

The urinary bladder is one of the organs where the mislocated IUD can be embedded.

Table 1 shows five similar cases with different therapeutic approaches reported in literature.

Bladder stones (BS) are uncommon in women. Approximately, 5% of bladder stones occur in female patients [5].

Therefore, foreign bodies should be considered when assessing the presence of BS.

These foreign bodies such as IUD in this case, with their lithogenic potential, act as a nidus for stone formation in the urinary bladder [6].

Although perforation of the uterus by IUD is often a silent phenomenon, erosion of the bladder wall is usually symptomatic [7].

In this case, the patient presented with irritative low urinary tract symptoms, such as frequency and urgency, frequently associated with haematuria.

Recurrent urinary tract infections, chronic pelvic pain syndrome, and sexual complaints such as dyspareunia can be part of the clinical manifestations.

Typically, at pelvic examination, the retrieval string of the IUD should protrude approximately 2-3 cm through the external cervical os.

A missing string is a common and strong indication of displacement, uterine perforation, or expulsion.

Various imaging modalities can be used in the evaluation of IUDs and in establishing the etiological diagnosis of low urinary tract symptoms in female patients.

Abdominal ultrasonography (US) can easily help determine whether the IUD is correctly positioned.

IUD displacement and myometrial perforation can be fully investigated by performing US alone [8].

However, abdominal radiography can be helpful in demonstrating an extrauterine IUD.

In some cases, the IUD can be misdiagnosed for a bladder stone due to the calcium tone opacity acquired when intravesical.

Thus, diagnostic cystoscopy allows a direct visualisation of the bladder, allowing to identify the foreign body, its extraction using a mechanical forceps if possible, and the search for any vesicouterine fistula.

However, the management of migrated IUDs is controversial.

According to the World Health Organization (WHO) recommendation, any translocated IUD following uterine perforation within the abdomen should be removed whether symptomatic or asymptomatic irrespective of location [9].

An IUD that migrated to the bladder eventually leads to stone formation, making its removal necessary.

Three approaches to remove the device include the use of open cystolithotomy, transurethral grasping forceps, or minimally invasive laparoscopy [10].

Open and laparoscopic surgery should be considered for the removal of IUD with partial penetration due to the possibility of a vesicouterine fistula that needs repair [7].

In case of endoscopic approach, both the cystoscope and the transurethral nephroscope can be used.

Table 1: Review of intravesical migration of IUD cases reported in English language literature.

Author and year	Age	Time of IUD insertion	Clinical presentation	Urinalysis	Imaging performed	Radiological findings	Calculus formation	Peri-op findings	Treatment	Outcome and Follow-up
Niu et al., 2018	57	26 years ago	Chronic supra-pubic pain	Unremarkable	Plain abdominal X-ray US	Hyperechoic foreign body penetrating through the anterior uterine wall into the posterior supratrigonal bladder wall	On the tip of the penetrating IUD	Shifted IUD horizontal limb protruding through the anterior uterine wall into the bladder. Needle-like calculus on the IUD.	Endoscopic approach: Laser fragmentation of the calculus encapsulating the IUD. Removal of the IUD with forceps through the nephroscope. Placed in the uterine cavity, 2 weeks indwelling Foley catheter.	No subsequent evidence of residual perforation or fistula
Shin et al., 2011 [12]	38	11 years ago	Recurrent UTI dysuria, dyspareunia chronic pelvic pain	Leucocyturia	Plain abdominal Radiograph Pelvic CT	Stone opacity around the IUD 1.6 × 1.9 cm stone around the IUD located in the bladder	Yes	IUD deeply embedded into the muscular bladder wall. No vesico-uterin fistula	Laparoscopic approach: Removal of the IUD and the bladder stone via laparoscopic cystolithotomy	No leakage on cystography.
Yahsi et al., 2015 [13]	37	6 years ago	Supra-pubic pain Polyuria, urgency	Leucocyturia	Plain abdominal x-ray Pelvic US, CT	1,5 × 2 cm bladder stone on the IUD whose 1 cm tipn outside of the baldder.	Yes	Intravesical encrusted IUD entering the bladder lumen posteriorly.	Endoscopic approach: IUD stuck to the bladder. Removal with cystoscopic forceps failed. Laparoscopic approach.	Discharged after normal post-op cystography.
De Silva et al., 2017 [14]	48	15 years ago	Recurrent UTI Dysuria, hematuria	Proteus growth	Plain abdominal X-ray US	Intra-vesical large stone with three limbs and an imprint of a typical IUCD in the middle of the stone.	Yes	6 × 5 cm bladder stone with three limbs shaped to cover the IUCD found inside.	Open cystolithotomy.	Uncomplicated post-op period, asymptomatic afterwards, no further..
Gharbi M. et al., 2019 [15]	62	9 years ago	Intermittent pelvic pain	Pyuria, hematuria	Plain abdominal X-ray US	15-mm calcified pelvic mass overlying the copper-T echogenic intravesical lesion with distal acoustic shadow.	Yes	Large calculus at the end of the IUD wire penetrating the posterior wall of the bladder.	Endoscopic approach: Ballistic lithotripsy of the stone removal of the IUD after calculi fragmentation.	Uncomplicated post period.

Ballistic or laser lithotripsy should be used for the initial fragmentation of the calculi that formed around the IUD to facilitate its extraction.

In this case, cystoscopy was sufficient for the management of this mislocated IUD.

Although delicate surgical procedures are available nowadays, traditional noninvasive options such as herbal formulas have been reported for patients living in developing areas with known or unidentified mechanisms of actions, but an evidence based practice should be kept in mind [11].

4. Conclusion

IUD migrating to the urinary bladder is an uncommon complication that should be considered in female patients complaining of chronic low urinary tract symptoms.

Endoscopic approach of a mislocated IUD is considered a safe and effective minimally invasive approach.

References

[1] B. Kassab and P. Audra, "The migrating intrauterine device. Case report and review of the literature," *Contraception, Fertilite, Sexualite (1992)*, vol. 27, no. 10, pp. 696–700, 1999.

[2] C. d'Arcangues, "Worldwide use of intrauterine devices for contraception," *Contraception*, vol. 75, no. 6, pp. S2–S7, 2007.

[3] I. Chi, P. J. Feldblum, and S. M. Rogers, "IUD-related uterine perforation: an epidemiologic analysis of a rare event using an international dataset," *Contraceptive Delivery Systems*, vol. 5, no. 2, pp. 123–130, 1984.

[4] E. Caliskan, N. Oztürk, B. O. Dilbaz, and S. Dilbaz, "Analysis of risk factors associated with uterine perforation by intrauterine devices," *The European Journal of Contraception & Reproductive Health Care*, vol. 8, no. 3, pp. 150–155, 2003.

[5] K. Stav and P. L. Dwyer, "Urinary bladder stones in women," *Obstetrical & Gynecological Survey*, vol. 67, no. 11, pp. 715–725, 2012.

[6] r. H. Atakan, M. Kaplan, and E. Ertrk, "Intravesical migration of intrauterine device resulting in stone formation," *Urology*, vol. 60, no. 5, p. 911, 2002.

[7] A. S. El-Hefnawy, A. R. El-Nahas, Y. Osman, and M. A. Bazeed, "Urinary complications of migrated intrauterine contraceptive device," *International Urogynecology Journal and Pelvic Floor Dysfunction*, vol. 19, no. 2, pp. 241–245, 2008.

[8] H. E. Boortz, D. J. A. Margolis, N. Ragavendra, M. K. Patel, and B. M. Kadell, "Migration of intrauterine devices: radiologic findings and implications for patient care," *RadioGraphics*, vol. 32, no. 2, pp. 335–352, 2012.

[9] WHO Scientific Group on the Mechanism of Action Safety and Efficacy of Intrauterine Devices & World Health Organization, *Mechanism of action, safety and efficacy of intrauterine devices: report of a WHO Scientific Group*, vol. 753 of World Health Organization technical report series, , World Health Organization, 1987.

[10] J. M. Scovell, R. C. Chan, and C. P. Smith, "Transurethral use of a nephroscope significantly AIDS in the surgical management of an intrauterine device eroding into the bladder," *Female Pelvic Medicine & Reconstructive Surgery*, vol. 20, no. 6, pp. e8-11, 2014.

[11] A. Hosseinkhani, F. Tabatabaei, M. Mosaffa-Jahromi, and M. Pasalar, "Urinary bladder stone passing using a Persian herbal recipe," *Journal of Evidence-Based Integrative Medicine*, vol. 23, 2018.

[12] D. G. Shin, T. N. Kim, and W. Lee, "Intrauterine device embedded into the bladder wall with stone formation: laparoscopic removal is a minimally invasive alternative to open surgery," *International Urogynecology Journal*, vol. 23, no. 8, pp. 1129–1131, 2012.

[13] S. Yahsi, B. K. Aktas, G. Erbay, R. Salar, and C. S. Gokkaya, "Intravesical migration of intrauterine device mimicking bladder stone on radiologic imaging: a case report," *Indian Journal of Surgery*, vol. 77, Supplement 1, pp. 97–99, 2015.

[14] W. S. L. De Silva, K. A. S. U. A. Kodithuwakku, G. U. E. Aponsu, R. M. M. Rathnayake, and E. Rajasegaram, "A large bladder stone caused by the intravesical migration of an intrauterine contraceptive device: a case report," *Journal of Medical Case Reports*, vol. 11, no. 1, p. 293, 2017.

[15] M. Gharbi, M. Chakroun, K. Chaker, S. Mokadem, H. Ayed, and M. Chebil, "Intravesical migration of intrauterine device resulting in stone formation: about a case report," *Urology Case Reports*, vol. 23, pp. 65-66, 2019.

15

Septic Shock Immediately following Percutaneous Suprapubic Catheterization

Cale E. Leeson[1] **Brianna-Lee Beaudry,**[2] **and Geoffrey R. Wignall**[3]

[1]*Division of Urology, Department of Surgery, University of Ottawa, Ottawa, Ontario, Canada*
[2]*Faculty of Medicine, Northern Ontario School of Medicine, Thunder Bay, Ontario, Canada*
[3]*Division of Urology, Grey Bruce Health Services, Owen Sound, ON, Canada*

Correspondence should be addressed to Cale E. Leeson; clees033@uottawa.ca

Academic Editor: Tun-Chieh Chen

Suprapubic catheterization (SPC) is considered a safe and effective procedure for long-term bladder decompression. With proper technique and appropriate patient selection, significant complications of SPC are rare. Immediate postoperative septic shock (i.e., within the first 24 hours of surgery) is rarely reported. We report a case of an 83-year-old patient who developed septic shock within one hour of suprapubic catheterization for a chronic hypotonic bladder, highlighting the importance of early recognition of complications from SPC and prompt management to ensure positive outcomes.

1. Introduction

Suprapubic catheterization (SPC) is widely considered a relatively safe procedure for both emergent and long-term bladder decompression. It is a management option for patients with neurogenic lower urinary tract dysfunction [1]. Compared to urethral catheterization, SPC may improve independence, reduce episodes of bacteriuria and pain, avoid the risk of urethral erosion, facilitate engagement in sexual activity, and decrease the risk of epididymitis in males [1, 2]. With proper technique and patient selection, major complications of SPC, such as bowel injury, are rare [2]. Immediate postoperative septic shock is rarely reported in the literature, though may be reduced when preoperative prophylactic antibiotics are administered in select patients [3]. We report a case of septic shock immediately following an elective percutaneous SPC in a patient with a chronic decompensated bladder.

2. Case Report

An 83-year-old female presented to the operating room to undergo an elective suprapubic catheter placement for chronic urinary retention secondary to a hypotonic bladder. Past medical history included hypertension, aortic stenosis, atrial fibrillation, transient ischemic attack, peripheral vascular disease, five vaginal deliveries, and longstanding pelvic floor dysfunction. The patient weighed 53 kilograms. Preoperative cystoscopy revealed a grossly trabeculated bladder consistent with long-standing urinary retention. A trial of clean intermittent catheterization was found undesirable by the patient, and a urethral catheter was placed. After discussion regarding long-term options, the patient decided to proceed with SPC.

In the operating room, cefazolin 1 g was administered intravenously on induction of procedural sedation. The bladder was distended with approximately 500 mL of normal saline instilled through a urethral catheter and adequately palpated. A spinal needle was used to infiltrate the tract with 0.5% Marcaine without epinephrine. The spinal needle was then advanced into the bladder, and urine was aspirated. A trocar was passed, and an 18 French Foley catheter was advanced into the bladder. Hematuria was noted, and continuous bladder irrigation (CBI) was started through the urethral catheter. The patient was transferred to the post anesthesia care unit (PACU) in stable condition. Within one hour of surgery, nausea, vomiting, rigors, pyrexia (temperature 39°C), and significant hypertension (229/165 mmHg) became apparent. On examination, the patient was alert and the abdomen was moderately distended and firm. Intravenous labetalol was administered, and a stat computed-tomography (CT) scan of the abdomen and pelvis was ordered to rule out bowel injury. Marked hypotension (82/50 mmHg) was then noted, and blood cultures as well as intravenous crystalloid resuscitation were ordered. The CT scan showed no evidence of bowel puncture and confirmed appropriate placement of the suprapubic catheter tip within the bladder.

The patient was then transferred to the intensive care unit (ICU) for management of postoperative septicemia. Fluid resuscitation and empirical antibiotics were administered until blood cultures and sensitivities were available. Vasopressors were required overnight and discontinued on postoperative day one, as was the CBI and the urethral catheter. The suprapubic catheter was well positioned and draining clear, yellow urine. White blood cell counts peaked at 30.6×10^9/L. Blood cultures were positive for *Enterococcus faecalis* and *Proteus mirabilis*, for which the patient completed a seven-day course of piperacillin-tazobactam. *P. mirabilis* was sensitive to ampicillin, cefazolin, ciprofloxacin, gentamicin, and trimethoprim/sulfa, while *E. faecalis* showed sensitivity to ampicillin, gentamicin synergy, streptomycin synergy, and vancomycin.

The admission was further complicated by increased left ventricular afterload in the context of aortic stenosis, leading to poor coronary perfusion (postoperative troponin I peaking at 1917 ng/L) during the hypertensive episode in PACU. Coronary angiography was performed, and severe disease in the first obtuse marginal artery was treated with a drug-eluting stent. The patient was discharged in stable condition on postoperative day ten.

3. Discussion

Suprapubic catheters are indicated for chronic urinary retention in the elective setting [2]. Compared to urethral catheterization, SPC may reduce episodes of bacteriuria and pain and decrease the risk of epididymitis, prostatitis, and meatal erosion in males [1, 2, 4, 5]. Contraindications for SPC include patients presenting with carcinoma of the bladder or undiagnosed hematuria, sepsis of the abdominal wall, uncorrected bleeding disorders, or anticoagulation treatment or patients with a subcutaneous vascular graft in the suprapubic region [2]. Urologists should develop an individualized bladder management strategy for each patient [1].

SPC may be performed open or percutaneously, typically guided by ultrasound (US) or flexible cystoscopy [2]. The open technique is generally indicated for patients at high risk for bowel injury (previous lower abdominal surgery where the bladder has been mobilized or those in which the bladder cannot be distended sufficiently) [2]. US-guided SPC is recommended if the bladder cannot be sufficiently palpated, to avoid bowel injury [2]. The bladder should be adequately distended with at least 300 mL of irrigant to allow safe insertion, with larger volumes potentially increasing the margin of safety by providing a larger area of entry into the bladder [2]. In our case, the bladder was adequately distended and urine was aspirated to confirm placement. However, cystoscopy was not used to visualize for adequate distension, as the patient's urethral catheter was used to distend the bladder.

SPC is considered a relatively safe procedure for long-term bladder decompression. Complications include hematuria, catheter misplacement, surgical site infection, urinary tract infection, and bowel injury [2]. However, literature pertaining to immediate postoperative septic shock (i.e., within the first 24 hours) is limited. Two cases by Vaidyanathan et al. [6, 7] discuss fatal septicemia immediately following SPC for neurogenic bladder in patients with spinal cord injuries. They recommended that clinicians obtain a urine culture with appropriate antibiogram prior to cystostomy and avoid forcible distension of the bladder in patients with small bladder capacity or a colonized bladder from chronic indwelling urethral catheters [6, 7]. One study of 219 patients undergoing SPC found that 19% had complications at 30 days postoperatively, including 4.6% with septicemia secondary to a urinary tract infection (UTI) [3]. However, the study does not specify whether urosepsis occurred in the immediate postoperative period or whether septicemia secondary to UTI was merely associated with the presence of an indwelling suprapubic catheter. Bacteriuria will inevitably be present in any patient with an indwelling catheter and can result in symptomatic infection [2, 8]. Our patient developed sepsis within one hour of surgery. It is possible that the patient had a colonized bladder and low bladder volume, with rapid distension of the bladder during the procedure potentially contributing to the mechanism for the urosepsis. In a bladder with low compliance, acute distension can cause mucosal trauma facilitating entry of organisms present in the urine into the bloodstream, leading to bacteremia and, rarely, septicemia [7]. Acute distention of the bladder may also contribute to hematuria, such as in our case, from the overly stretched vesical mucosa [7]. Bladder distention has also been shown to significantly decrease coronary artery diameter at stenotic segments, leading to decreased coronary blood flow and increased coronary resistance [9]. This effect may have been compounded in our patient who had severe disease in the first obtuse marginal artery, contributing to the postoperative myocardial ischemia and subsequent rise in troponin.

As per current guidelines, our patient was managed for sepsis with adequate fluid resuscitation and vasopressors [10]. Microbiological cultures were obtained before promptly starting antimicrobial therapy [10]. Additionally, clinicians should have a low index of suspicion for bowel complications; thus, a rapid CT scan was ordered to rule out bowel injury [2]. Patients at high risk for infectious complications undergoing urologic procedures should receive preprocedural antibiotics [11]. Perioperative antimicrobial prophylaxis may reduce the risk of urosepsis following SPC [3]. Our patient had a chronic indwelling urethral catheter prior to undergoing SPC, increasing the risk for bladder colonization. Thus, cefazolin was administered intraoperatively, to which *P. mirabilis* was sensitive, though cefazolin may have been ineffective against *E. faecalis* based on postoperative culture and sensitivities. Despite this, our patient still developed septic shock, highlighting the importance of close monitoring following SPC in patients with chronic urethral catheterization for hypotonic bladder.

4. Conclusion

SPC is considered a safe and effective procedure for a decompensated bladder in appropriately selected patients. However, significant complications can arise. Preoperative urine cultures and antibiotic prophylaxis should be considered in patients who are high risk for bladder colonization, such as those with a chronic urethral urinary catheter. Our case highlights the importance of appropriate patient selection, risk factor identification, early recognition of complications from SPC, and prompt management to ensure positive outcomes.

References

[1] L. Campeau, S. Shamout, R. J. Baverstock et al., "Canadian Urological Association best practice report: catheter use," *Canadian Urological Association Journal*, vol. 14, no. 7, pp. E281–E289, 2020.

[2] S. Jane Hall, S. Harrison, C. Harding, S. Reid, and R. Parkinson, "British Association of Urological Surgeons suprapubic catheter practice guidelines - revised," *BJU International*, vol. 126, no. 4, pp. 416–422, 2020.

[3] R. S. Ahluwalia, N. Johal, C. Kouriefs, G. Kooiman, B. S. Montgomery, and R. O. Plail, "The surgical risk of suprapubic catheter insertion and long-term sequelae," *The Annals of The Royal College of Surgeons of England*, vol. 88, no. 2, pp. 210–213, 2006.

[4] A. Kavanagh, R. Baverstock, L. Campeau et al., "Canadian urological association guideline: diagnosis, management, and surveillance of neurogenic lower urinary tract dysfunction - Full text," *Canadian Urological Association Journal*, vol. 13, no. 6, pp. E157–E176, 2018.

[5] S. Saint and B. A. Lipsky, "Preventing catheter-related bacteriuria: should we? Can we? How?," *Archives of Internal Medicine*, vol. 159, no. 8, pp. 800–808, 1999.

[6] S. Vaidyanathan, B. M. Soni, T. Oo, P. L. Hughes, and G. Singh, "Fatal septicaemia following suprapubic cystostomy in a paraplegic patient: never do a cystostomy without prior urine culture and appropriate antibiogram!," *Case Reports in Medicine*, vol. 2010, Article ID 461514, 4 pages, 2010.

[7] S. Vaidyanathan, B. M. Soni, G. Singh, and P. L. Hughes, "Fatality due to septicemia and hemorrhage in a patient with spinal cord injury and ischemic heart disease with the need for long-term catheter drainage," *Advances in Therapy*, vol. 23, no. 2, pp. 354–358, 2006.

[8] P. A. Cadieux, G. R. Wignall, R. Carriveau, and J. D. Denstedt, "Implications of biofilm formation on urological devices," *AIP Conference Proceedings*, vol. 1049, pp. 147–163, 2008.

[9] T. M. Lee, S. F. Su, and C. H. Tsai, "Effects of distension of urinary bladder on coronary conduit and resistance vessels in hyperlipidemic patients," *Clinical Cardiology: An International Indexed and Peer-Reviewed Journal for Advances in the Treatment of Cardiovascular Disease*, vol. 25, no. 10, pp. 467–473, 2002.

[10] A. Rhodes, L. E. Evans, W. Alhazzani et al., "Surviving sepsis campaign: international guidelines for management of sepsis and septic shock: 2016," *Intensive Care Medicine*, vol. 43, no. 3, pp. 304–377, 2017.

[11] M. Mrkobrada, I. Ying, S. Mokrycke et al., "CUA guidelines on antibiotic prophylaxis for urologic procedures," *Canadian Urological Association Journal*, vol. 9, no. 1-2, pp. 13–22, 2015.

16

Pulmonary Embolism following Percutaneous Nephrolithotomy: An Uncommon and Life-Threatening Complication

Spyridon Papantidis,[1] **Antonios Katsimantas**,[1] **Dimitrios Oikonomidis**,[2] **and Nikolaos Ferakis**[1]

[1] *Urology Department, Korgialenio-Benakio Hellenic Red Cross Hospital, Athanasaki 1, 11526 Athens, Greece*
[2] *Second Cardiology Department, Korgialenio-Benakio Hellenic Red Cross Hospital, Athanasaki 1, 11526 Athens, Greece*

Correspondence should be addressed to Spyridon Paparidis; sppap86@yahoo.gr

Academic Editor: Apul Goel

High risk pulmonary embolism is a rare and life-threatening complication following percutaneous nephrolithotomy. We report the case of a previously healthy, 44-year-old male, who developed acute pulmonary embolism following right percutaneous nephrolithotomy. On the 1st postoperative day, the patient presented with hemodynamic instability, acute respiratory distress, hypoxia, and loss of consciousness. He was urgently intubated and placed on mechanical ventilation. Clinical findings set the suspicion of pulmonary embolism with shock. Chest computed tomography scan confirmed the diagnosis. The patient underwent urgent thrombolysis in the cardiac care unit. On the 2nd postoperative day, the patient was admitted to the intensive care unit due to hemodynamic instability and fever. The postoperative course was complicated by right renal bleeding on the 3rd postoperative day, which was managed through angiography and angioembolization of the lower segmental right renal artery, followed by recurrent respiratory and urinary tract infections. The patient was transferred back to the urology department on the 66th postoperative day and was discharged seven days later.

1. Introduction

Complications of percutaneous nephrolithotomy (PCNL), according to the literature, are minor ones such as extravasation (7,2%), renal hemorrhage (0,6-1,4%), blood transfusion (11,2-17,5%), and fever (21-32,1%), which can be managed conservatively or minimally invasively on early diagnosis, and major ones such as septicemia (0,3-4,7%), colonic injury (0,2-0,8%), and pleural injury (0-3,1%) [1]. Complication rates vary from 20 to 83% [2]. Death rates after PCNL range from 0,1 to 0,7% [2]. Pulmonary embolism (PE) and myocardial infraction occur in less than 3% of patients undergoing PCNL [2]. Our aim is to present an interesting and uncommon complication of PCNL.

2. Case Report

A 44-year- old Caucasian male, with body mass index: 29.3, was admitted to our department due to bilateral nephrolithiasis, in order to undergo right PCNL. Preoperative computed tomography (CT) scan demonstrated a 22 mm calculus in the right renal pelvis, causing pyelocaliceal obstruction and dilatation, and smaller calculi in the lower calyceal group of the ipsilateral kidney. Multiple calculi in the upper, median, and lower calyceal group of the left kidney were also present, with no signs of pyelocaliceal obstruction (Figure 1). The patient had no medical history and the preoperative urine culture was negative.

The patient underwent right PCNL in prone position under general anesthesia. Following placement of a 7Fr ureteral catheter in lithotomy position and injection of contrast agent, a single tract at the median calyceal group was created above the 12th rib under fluoroscopy. After tract dilation with a balloon dilator, a 30Fr Amplatz sheath was positioned inside the calyx of puncture. Following stone fragmentation with a pneumatic lithotripter, the stones were removed using grasping forceps and an 18Fr nephrostomy tube was inserted for postoperative drainage. There were no intraoperative complications and the patient was rendered stone-free on the right side.

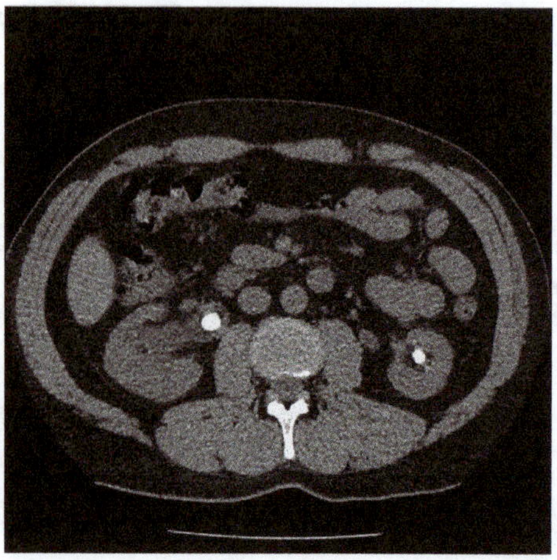

FIGURE 1: Preoperative CT scan. Bilateral nephrolithiasis.

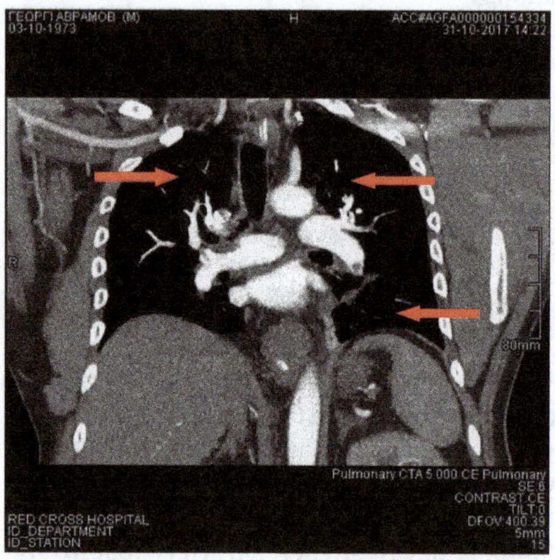

FIGURE 2: Chest CT angiography scan, depicting filling defects in subsegmental branches of the right pulmonary lobes, in segmental branch of the left lower pulmonary lobe, and in subsegmental branches of the left upper pulmonary lobe.

On the first postoperative day, the patient developed hemodynamic instability, acute respiratory distress, hypoxia, and loss of consciousness. His vital signs included blood pressure (BP) of 88/48 mmHg, heart rate of 110-120 bpm, and oxygen saturation of 50%, on room air. He was urgently intubated and placed on mechanical ventilation. Clinical findings set the suspicion of PE with shock. Chest CT scan demonstrated filling defects in subsegmental branches of the right pulmonary lobes, in segmental branch of the left lower pulmonary lobe, and in subsegmental branches of the left upper pulmonary lobe (Figure 2). Brain and abdominal CT scans were normal. These findings were indicative of high-risk PE with shock.

The patient underwent immediate thrombolysis, with recombinant tissue plasminogen activator (rt-PA) administration (100 mg Alteplase over 2 hours) in the cardiac care unit (CCU), and became hemodynamically stable. Subcutaneous enoxaparin sodium 12.000 iu twice daily (according to his body weight) and vasopressors were also administered. Subsequently, bedside echocardiography revealed both ventricles with normal size and function and normal values of pulmonary artery pressure. Hematuria through nephrostomy tube was present the first three hours after thrombolysis. Seven hours later, he developed hemodynamic instability and fever (38.6°C). Blood and urine cultures were obtained and Piperacillin/Tazobactam and Amikacin were administered empirically. Inotropic agents and blood transfusion were administered, and the patient was transferred to the intensive care unit (ICU).

During the first hours in the ICU, lower limbs venous ultrasonography was negative for deep vein thrombosis (DVT). On the 3rd postoperative day, an abdominal CT scan was performed due to continuous macroscopic hematuria through nephrostomy tube and a decrease in hemoglobin levels, despite blood transfusion. CT scan demonstrated a sizable right retroperitoneal hematoma and the patient underwent angiography and angioembolization of the lower segmental right renal artery. Moreover, the postoperative course was complicated by recurrent respiratory and urinary tract infections due to Acinetobacter Baumanii, Pseudomonas Aeruginosa, Klebsiella pneumoniae, and Klebsiella Oxytoca, which were isolated on sputum, blood, and urine cultures. Antibiotics were administered according to the sensitivity analysis.

The patient developed progressive recovery and was transferred back to the urology department on the 66th postoperative day and was discharged on the 73rd postoperative day. Apixaban 5 mg, twice/day, was orally administered for six months, following the instructions of cardiologists.

3. Discussion

PCNL is a well-established treatment option for patients with large, multiple, or inferior calyx renal stones [3–6]. Parameters that influence the complication rate are the surgeon's experience, the operative time, the stone's size and opacity, the number of punctures or tracts, and the presence of bacteria within the stone [3, 4, 6]. PE after PCNL is an uncommon complication. This is the first incident in our department since 2006, in our series exceeding 400 cases. Tae Seung Shin et al. reported one death from PE in their series of 698 patients who underwent PCNL [7], while Hentschel et al. reported one death in their series of 158 cases [8]. S.V Krishna Reddy et al. 2016 report that overall mortality of PCNL due to urosepsis, hemorrhage, or PE ranges from 0,5 to 1,1% in a series of 367 patients that underwent PCNL from a single surgeon [9]. According to the literature, rare cases of air embolism and stone fragment migration through venous system, causing pulmonary embolism, are reported [6, 10].

Acute pulmonary embolism represents the sudden obstruction of the pulmonary arterial vasculature which is usually caused by embolization of thrombus from the deep veins within the lower limbs and pelvis [11]. Although no predisposing factors are identified in approximately 20% of patients (idiopathic or unprovoked PE), most patients have either patient-related or setting-related attributable risk factors (secondary or provoked PE). Patient-related factors include advanced age, previous venous thromboembolism, active cancer, underlying coagulopathy (including factor V Leiden and prothrombin mutations), smoking, hormone replacement therapy, and oral contraceptive pill. Medical conditions associated with an increased risk of PE include heart failure, sepsis, stroke, respiratory failure, and inflammatory bowel disease. Setting-related risk factors include protracted immobility secondary to major general or orthopedic surgery, major fracture, air travel, pregnancy, chemotherapy, or the presence of a central venous line. Commonly, more than one risk factors are present [11], unlike our case, in which no risk factors were present.

PE may be classified as high risk, intermediate, or low risk. When patients with acute pulmonary embolism present with hypotension defined as a systolic blood pressure <90mmHg or drop of >40mmHg, not explained by another cause, this is referred to as high risk PE in the European Guidelines [12, 13]. Thrombolytic therapy should be administered unless contraindicated, as the 30-day mortality risk is greater than 15% in this population. Recent surgery comprises an absolute contraindication to thrombolysis. However, absolute contraindications to thrombolysis might become relative in a patient with immediately life-threatening high-risk PE [13]. American College of Chest Physicians guidelines suggest that recent surgery, excluding recent brain or spinal surgery or trauma, is a relative contraindication and that the bleeding risk reduces significantly 2 weeks after surgery. [12].

International literature reveals a paucity of data concerning the experience of thrombolysis following urologic surgical procedures. Cincin et al. report a case of high-risk PE treatment, through ultrasound assisted transcatheter thrombolysis using rt-PA and low-dose unfractionated heparin (LDUH), in a patient with recent radical prostatectomy: a suggested treatment in intermediate and high-risk patients, with high chance of bleeding due to recent urologic surgery [14]. A review of 126,891 cases with venous thromboembolic events (VTE) following urological procedures showed an incidence of VTE to 0,66% (PE 0,37%). For PCNL especially the incidence of VTE is 0,55%. Procedures in supine position seem to have higher rate of VTE compared to lithotomy position. Prolongation of thromboprophylaxis in high risk patients and deprivation of pharmaceutical thromboprophylaxis in low-risk procedures are suggested [15].

A review on VTE in urologic surgery indicates that low molecular weight heparin (LMWH) treatment for postoperative PE is preferred due to rapid approach of therapeutic levels, decreased recurrent bleeding, thrombosis, and mortality and more effective thrombus size reduction compared to LDUH, while LDUH is preferred in postoperative patients undergoing PE with shock and high risk of bleeding, and in cases of renal impairment. The duration of anticoagulant treatment in a first episode of postoperative PE with no identifiable risk factors is 6 to 12 months [16].

Patients undergoing stone surgery should be stratified into groups according to the risk of bleeding and VTE [17]. Thromboprophylaxis with subcutaneous LMWH until complete mobilization is recommended in high-risk patients performing lithotripsy procedures [18].

Although it is a rare complication after percutaneous nephrolithotomy, it requires high index of suspicion so as not to be missed as a diagnosis, especially in hemodynamically unstable patients with respiratory distress. Early diagnosis followed by proper therapeutic actions can be crucial for patients.

References

[1] M. S. Michel, L. Trojan, and J. J. Rassweiler, "Complications in percutaneous nephrolithotomy," *European Urology*, vol. 51, no. 4, pp. 899–906, 2007.

[2] E. Taylor, J. Miller, T. Chi, and M. L. Stoller, "Complications associated with percutaneous nephrolithotomy," *Translational Andrology and Urolog*, vol. 1, no. 4, pp. 223–228, 2012.

[3] H. Sekar, S. Krishnamoorthy, N. Kumaresan, and V. Ramanan, "Supracostal punctures for PCNL: Factors that predict safety, success and stone free rate in stag horn and non-stag horn stones: A single centre experience and review of literature," *Journal of Clinical and Diagnostic Research*, vol. 10, no. 9, pp. PC17–PC21, 2016.

[4] M. Osman, G. Wendt-Nordahl, K. Heger, M. S. Michel, P. Alken, and T. Knoll, "Percutaneous nephrolithotomy with ultrasonography-guided renal access: experience from over 300 cases," *BJU International*, vol. 96, no. 6, pp. 875–878, 2005.

[5] N. Ferakis, A. Katsimantas, G. Zervopoulos et al., "Nontraumatic acute elevation of pancreatic enzymes following percutaneous nephrolithotomy: A rare complication," *Case Reports in Urology*, vol. 2017, Article ID 7430328, 3 pages, 2017.

[6] C. Seitz, M. Desai, A. Häcker et al., "Incidence, prevention, and management of complications following percutaneous nephrolitholapaxy," *European Urology*, vol. 61, no. 1, pp. 146–158, 2012.

[7] T. S. Shin, H. J. Cho, S.-H. Hong, J. Y. Lee, S. W. Kim, and T.-K. Hwang, "Complications of percutaneous nephrolithotomy classified by the modified Clavien grading system: a single center's experience over 16 years," *Korean Journal of Urology*, vol. 52, no. 11, pp. 769–775, 2011.

[8] H. Hentschel and V. Janitzky, "Percutaneous nephrolithotomy - always effective and free of complications?" *Aktuelle Urologie*, vol. 38, no. 3, pp. 232–236, 2007.

[9] S. V. Krishna Reddy, B. S. Ahammad, and V. Sri, "Outcome and complications of percutaneous nephrolithotomy as primary versus secondary procedure for renal calculi," *International Brazilian Journal of Urology*, vol. 42, no. 2, pp. 262–269, 2016.

[10] M. H. Zahran, Y. Osman, and T. EL-Diasty, "Calcular pulmonary embolism," *International Urology and Nephrology*, vol. 46, no. 4, pp. 727–730, 2014.

[11] M. Narain and S. Price, "Massive pulmonary embolism," *Cardiology Clinics*, vol. 31, no. 4, pp. 503–518, 2013.

[12] L. A. Igneri and J. M. Hammer, "Systemic thrombolytic therapy for massive and submassive pulmonary embolism," *Journal of Pharmacy Practice*, 2018.

[13] S. V. Konstantinides, A. Torbicki, and G. Agnelli, "2014 ESC Guidelines on the diagnosis and management of acute pulmonary embolism: The task force for the diagnosis and management of acute pulmonary embolism of the European Society of Cardiology (ESC) endorsed by the European Respiratory

Society (ERS)," *European Heart Journal*, vol. 35, no. 43, pp. 3033–3073, 2014.

[14] A. Cincin, M. Bozbay, M. Oguz, A. Sahin, Y. Tanidir, and B. Mutlu, "Successful treatment of massive pulmonary embolism with catheter-directed thrombolysis in a patient with lymphocele: A rare cause of thromboembolism," *American Journal of Therapeutics*, vol. 23, no. 5, pp. e1257–e1262, 2016.

[15] J. Dyer, S. Wyke, and C. Lynch, "Hospital Episode Statistics data analysis of postoperative venous thromboembolus in patients undergoing urological surgery: a review of 126,891 cases," *The Annals of The Royal College of Surgeons of England*, vol. 95, no. 1, pp. 65–69, 2013.

[16] K. R. Rice, S. A. Brassell, and D. G. McLeod, "Venous thromboembolism in urologic surgery: Prophylaxis, diagnosis, and treatment," *Reviews in Urology*, vol. 12, no. 2/3, 2010.

[17] P. D. Violette, R. Cartwright, M. Briel, K. A. Tikkinen, and G. H. Guyatt, "Guideline of guidelines: thromboprophylaxis for urological surgery," *BJU International*, vol. 118, no. 3, pp. 351–358, 2016.

[18] A. Bourdoumis, T. Stasinou, S. Kachrilas, A. G. Papatsoris, N. Buchholz, and J. Masood, "Thromboprophylaxis and bleeding diathesis in minimally invasive stone surgery," *Nature Reviews Urology*, vol. 11, no. 1, pp. 51–58, 2014.

17

Exceptional Response of Metastatic Chromophobe Renal Cell Carcinoma to Vascular Endothelial Growth Factor (VEGF) Inhibitors: Should Increased VEGF-C Expression be used to Guide Treatment?

Jacob W. Bruinius,[1,2] **Karl J. Dykema,**[3] **Sabrina L. Noyes,**[1] **Bin Tean Teh,**[4] **and Brian R. Lane**[1,5]

[1]*Spectrum Health, Grand Rapids, MI, USA*
[2]*Helix Scribes Solutions, Grand Rapids, MI, USA*
[3]*Van Andel Research Institute, Grand Rapids, MI, USA*
[4]*National Cancer Centre Singapore, Singapore*
[5]*Michigan State University College of Human Medicine, Grand Rapids, MI, USA*

Correspondence should be addressed to Brian R. Lane; brian.lane@spectrumhealth.org

Academic Editor: Shiou-Sheng Chen

There is sparse literature demonstrating effective treatments for metastatic chromophobe renal cell carcinoma (ChRCC). The tyrosine kinase inhibitor (TKI) sunitinib selectively inhibits the VEGF pathway and it is a standard care for metastatic clear cell renal cell carcinoma (ccRCC), although data supporting its use in ChRCC is much more limited. A 56-year-old underwent palliative nephrectomy for locally-advanced ChRCC with sarcomatoid differentiation. Tumor gene expression profiling using Affymetrix HG-U133 Plus 2.0 GeneChip platform demonstrated significantly elevated VEGF-C expression compared to normal renal tissue (n = 12) and other types RCC (n = 158). Adjuvant sunitinib was used to treat his residual unresectable retroperitoneal lymph nodes. He demonstrated an exceptional response and underwent complete surgical resection four months later. He has been managed with TKIs for nearly nine years with only minimal disease progression. Additional studies exploring treatment options for patients with non-clear cell RCC are needed; in their absence, we would recommend TKIs for patients whose tumors bear a similar molecular profile.

1. Introduction

With 73,820 new cases estimated to be diagnosed in 2019, kidney cancer is one of the most frequently diagnosed forms of cancer in the United States [1]. Most of these (≥90%) were diagnosed as renal cell carcinoma (RCC), which includes a diverse classification of cancers originating from the epithelial cells of the renal tubule [2]. The three most common forms of RCC are clear cell (ccRCC), papillary, and chromophobe (ChRCC) which respectively account for 65%, 20%, and 5% of all reported cases of RCC [3]. ChRCC generally carries a more favorable prognosis compared to other histologic subtypes of RCC, with a five-year survival rate >90% [4]. Paradoxically, median progression-free survival (PFS) is reduced with metastatic ChRCC compared to metastatic clear cell RCC (ccRCC) [5]. Currently, there is limited data available to guide the medical management of metastatic nccRCC, as registration trials of targeted therapies have either excluded nccRCC in favor of the more common diagnosis of ccRCC, or enrolled nccRCC in numbers too small to make definitive recommendations [6]. There are no guideline-recommended systemic therapies for ChRCC at present, leaving treatment to physician discretion.

Elucidation of the molecular pathogenesis of RCC has led to the development of targeted therapies for patients who initially present with advanced disease or who experience recurrence after primary treatment [7]. Sunitinib is a small-molecule tyrosine kinase inhibitor (TKI) of vascular endothelial growth

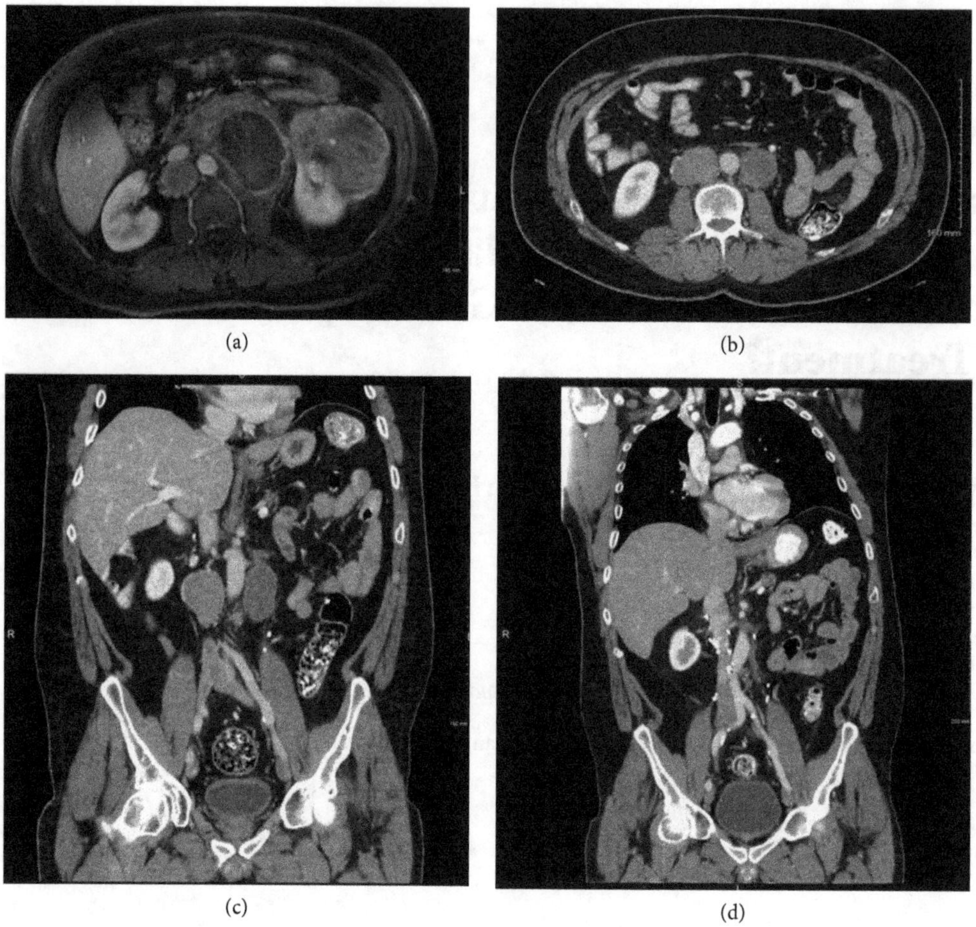

FIGURE 1: Magnetic resonance imaging (MRI) showing the large renal mass and metastatic lymph nodes. Dramatic reduction in tumor volume in an enlarged lymph node as demonstrated by MRI taken at initial presentation (a) vs. after 5 months of sunitinib (b) and (c). After retroperitoneal lymph node dissection, a complete response was obtained (d).

factor (VEGF), which drives tumor angiogenesis [8]. Other strategy approaches involve the inhibition of mammalian target of rapamycin (mTOR) or immunotherapy based on the programmed cell death protein 1 (PD-1). Each of these targeted therapeutic approaches offers increased efficacy when compared to the previous standard of care (high-dose interleukin-2) and boast a more tolerable toxicity profile [2].

Over the past 12 years several additional TKIs have also demonstrated activity in RCC including sorafenib, pazopanib, axitinib, and cabozantinib [7]. These have proven efficacious in prolonging PFS in patients with ccRCC, although a recent study was published which found that nccRCC patients treated with TKIs have worse clinical outcomes compared to matched ccRCC patients, with a median PFS of 11.8 months versus 6.5 months ($p = 0.018$) in ccRCC and nccRCC patients, respectively [9]. In this report, we describe the molecular profile of a patient who presented with advanced ChRCC and demonstrated an exceptional response to sunitinib with continued TKI therapy for nearly nine years.

2. Case Presentation

A 56-year-old man presented with complaints of generalized body aches, back pain, and bilateral flank pain. Noncontrast computed tomography (CT) imaging revealed a $13.3 \times 12.3 \times 10.4$ cm left renal mass and multiple enlarged retroperitoneal lymph nodes (LN), including $11.9 \times 10.1 \times 8.7$ cm necrotic para-aortic LN and $5.3 \times 4.4 \times 4.0$ cm interaortocaval LNs. Subsequent CT of the head, neck, and thorax were negative for metastases. Magnetic resonance imaging (MRI) revealed significant necrotic components in the tumor with no venous tumor thrombus (Figure 1(a)). Pathology from renal mass biopsy indicated an eosinophilic renal neoplasm in favor of non-clear cell RCC (nccRCC).

The patient underwent open left radical nephrectomy within two weeks of initial presentation. During surgery, the large necrotic LNs were densely adherent to the duodenum and small bowel mesentery and determined to be unresectable. Surgical pathology described a $16.0 \times 13.0 \times 12.5$ cm pT3a ChRCC with prominent sarcomatoid features (grade 4) and positive medial surgical margins. Immunohistochemistry revealed one component with plant-like tumor cells that were positive for CK7 and C-KIT and negative for CD10 and a spindle sarcomatoid tumor component positive for CD10 and vimentin.

Based on the histopathologic results, the patient was treated with a 4/2 schedule of sunitinib 50 mg once daily. After four cycles, the para-aortic LN had shrunk by 91% (Figures 1(b) and 1(c)). Complete retroperitoneal LN dissection 7 months after nephrectomy included, a grossly necrotic para-aortic LN

(6.0 × 4.0 × 3.8 cm) and golden, nonnecrotic interaortocaval LN (6.0 × 5.0 × 4.2 cm).

After LN dissection (Figure 1(d)) the patient achieved a continued response on sunitinib and continued therapy for another 23 months (28 months total). Side effects of systemic therapy were minimal, apart from fatigue noted after 16 months of treatment. An enlarged left mediastinal LN (1.5 cm) was noted 21 months after presentation and eventually grew to 2.1 cm over the next 8 months. After resection of this pathologically-confirmed metastatic ChRCC, sunitinib was discontinued and he started second-line therapy with axitinib (5 mg daily) which continued for 36 months without disease progression. He discontinued therapy for 2 months due to fatigue, but resumed TKI therapy with pazopanib (800 mg daily) when imaging revealed progression of a retro-aortic LN to 1.7 cm. He continued on pazopanib for 22 months with only minimal disease progression, before switching to cabozantinib (40 mg Mon–Fri), which was continued for 17 months. During this time, he received intensity modulated radiation therapy (4500 cGy) to the retro-aortic LN which had grown to 2.1 cm. Notably, the patient has achieved an ongoing prolonged response on systemic anti-VEGF therapy for nearly nine years.

3. Results

The patient's tumor underwent gene expression profiling using the Affymetrix HG-U133 Plus 2.0 GeneChip platform. This data was compared to normal renal tissue (n = 12) as well as multiple forms of RCC (n = 158) publicly available within the Gene Expression Omnibus database [10]. The data were read using Bioconductor [11] and processed using the Affymetrix [12] and MBNI custom CDF packages [13]. The whole gene expression matrix is attached as a Supplementary Table 1. To determine the molecular relationship between the patient and the other renal samples, a unrooted cluster tree was plotted based on 500 most variable genes from the dataset (Figure 2). The patient's tumor clustered with the other oncocytic neoplasms (ChRCC and oncocytoma), but was the most divergent of these tumors.

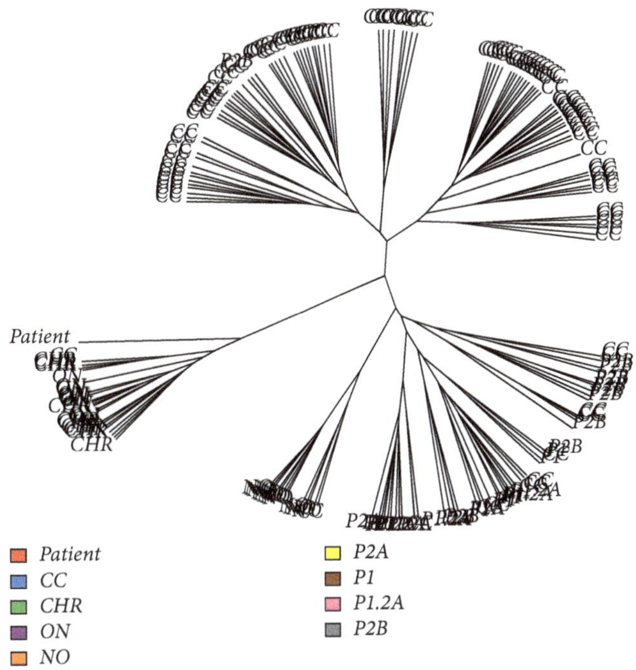

FIGURE 2: Unrooted cluster tree comparing the index tumor (*Patient*) to normal renal tissue (*NO*, n = 12), chromophobe RCC (*CHR*, n = 10), oncocytoma (*ON*, n = 14), clear cell RCC (*CC*, n = 102), papillary type 1 RCC (*P1*, n = 5), papillary mixed type 1/type 2a RCC (*P1.2A*, n = 4), papillary type 2a RCC (*P2A*, n = 4), and papillary type 2b RCC (*P2B*, n = 1) based on the 500 most variable genes.

Gene expression of VEGF-A, VEGF-B, and VEGF-C were determined for a range of renal epithelial neoplasms, including 102 ccRCC, 14 papillary RCC, 10 ChRCC, 14 oncocytoma, and 12 normal kidney controls. Normalized gene expression levels of VEGF-A were significantly elevated compared to all other subgroups (Figure 3). In contrast, VEGF-B and VEGF-C expression varied greatly in ccRCC, with a range of values overlapping that of the other renal epithelial neoplasms. The ChRCC and oncocytoma samples had similar expression of VEGF-A, VEGF-B, and VEGF-C, with greater variability of VEGF-C expression among the ChRCC samples.

Patient VEGF-C expression was significantly elevated (9.0) when compared to the 10 ChRCC tumor samples (median 6.9) and normal renal tissue (median 6.9). The 10 ChRCC samples had a wide range of VEGF-C expression (5.6–8.8) as did the 102 ccRCC samples (5.7–11.1), indicating wide heterogeneity of expression in these tumors. The patient's tumor also displayed increased VEGF-B expression (8.4) compared with normal renal tissue (median 6.7) although the range of expression among the 10 ChRCC overlapped the test patient (median 8.3, range 7.7–8.7). In contrast, VEGF-A expression (10.6) was similar to the levels seen in other ChRCC (median 9.7), oncocytoma (median 10.5), and normal renal tissue (median 10.1).

4. Discussion

To date there are limited clinical trial data [6] and few long-term responses documented for patients with metastatic ChRCC [14], none of which have included any molecular analysis of the responders. While ChRCC commonly involves extensive chromosomal losses (Y, 1, 2, 6, 10, 13, 17, and 21), it is generally regarded as a particularly indolent subtype of RCC [15]. This is intriguing, as excessive aneuploidy can compromise cellular proliferation, increasing the potential for cancer metastasis [16]. Comprehensive molecular profiling of 66 ChRCC tumors listed in The Cancer Genome Atlas (TCGA) database observed recurrent genomic structural arrangements involving the *TERT* promoter region and elevated *TERT* expression, as well as, diffusely increased mitochondrial function and mitochondrial DNA alterations [17]. Another comprehensive genomic analysis of nccRCC by Durinck et al. examined 49 ChRCC tumors and found *TP53*, *PTEN*, *FAAH2*, *PDHB*, *PDXDC1*, and *ZNF765* to be significantly mutated relative to normal tissue; this is in contrast to ccRCC, which is characterized by mutations in *VHL*, *TCEB1*, *PTEN*, *PBRM1*, *SETD2*, *BAP1*, *KDM5C*, *MTOR*, *PIK3CA*, and *TP53* relative

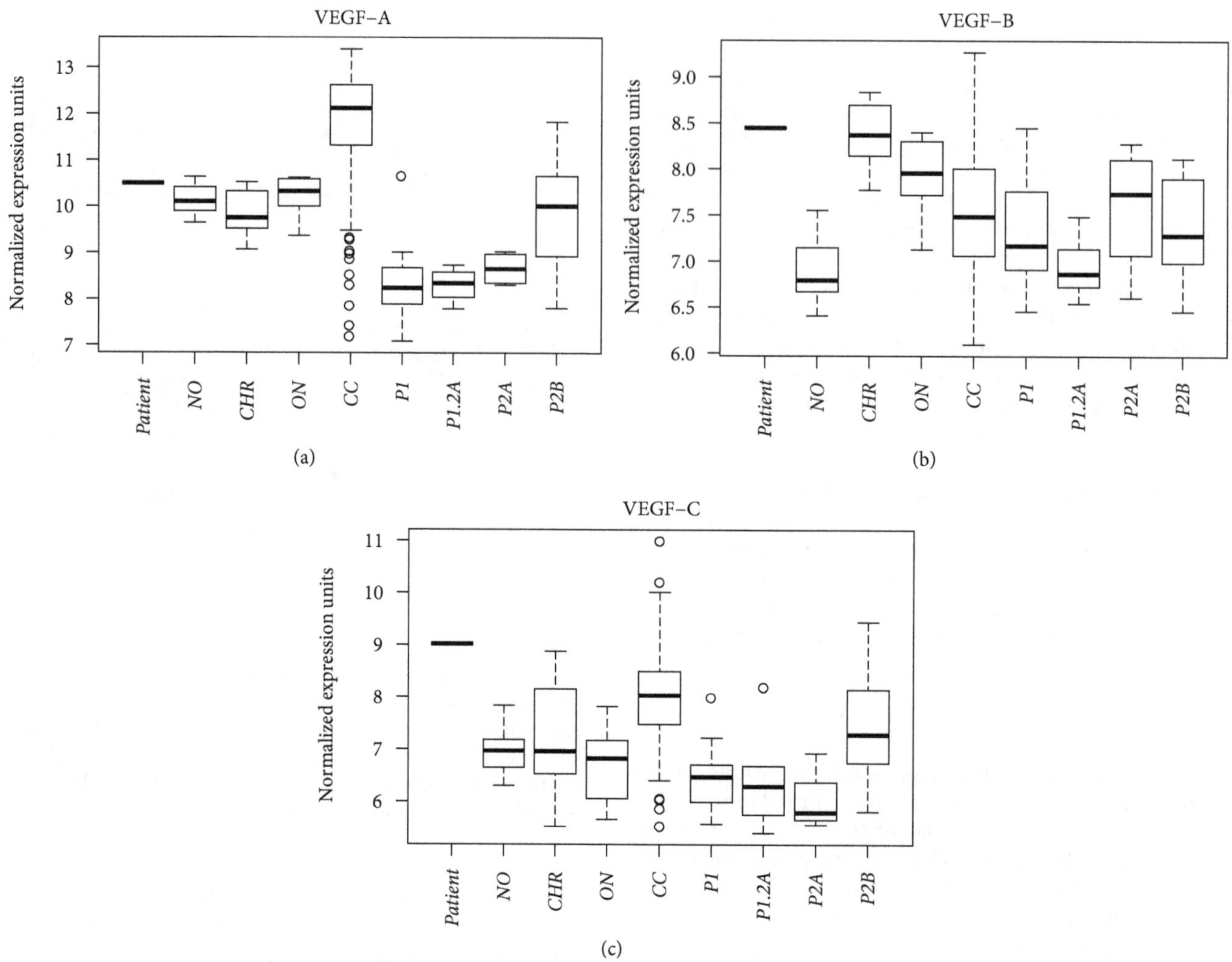

FIGURE 3: VEGF expression levels of the exceptional responder. Normalized gene expression levels of VEGF-A (a), VEGF-B (b), and VEGF-C (c) measured in the patient's tumor (*Patient*) compared to normal renal tissue (*NO*), chromophobe RCC (*CHR*), oncocytoma (*ON*), clear cell RCC (*CC*), papillary type 1 RCC (*P1*), papillary mixed type 1/type 2a RCC (*P1.2A*), papillary type 2a RCC (*P2A*), and papillary type 2b RCC (*P2B*).

to normal tissue [18]. The fundamental molecular differences between ccRCC and nccRCC, and ChRCC in particular, have profound clinical importance, particularly when these cancers require systemic therapy. Despite the lack of evidence and differences in tumor histology, most patients with metastatic nccRCC are treated with the same targeted therapies that are used for ccRCC. Choueiri et al. examined a cohort of 53 patients with nccRCC, including 12 with ChRCC. Of those, 3 (25%) achieved a response on TKI therapy and the median PFS for the entire group was 10.6 months. Phase II clinical trial data from RECORD-3 [19], ESPN [20], and ASPEN [21] have shown sunitinib to be slightly more efficacious than everolimus in treating metastatic nccRCC, although this effect is modest at best. Conclusions that can be drawn from these studies are limited as they do not indicate results according to the varying histology of each nccRCC subtype. A systematic review and meta-analysis examining systemic treatment options for patients with nccRCC concluded that VEGF-targeted therapies were slightly favored over mTOR inhibitors, although this did not reach the level of statistical significance [22]. A more recent cross-channel group study examining anti-angiogenic therapy vs. mTOR inhibitors for metastatic ChRCC came to a similar conclusion [23]. Immunotherapy has also recently emerged as another option to treat metastatic RCC, and clinical trials that compare TKI therapy vs. immunotherapy are currently underway, although these studies have only enrolled patients with ccRCC [24]. The role of immunotherapy in treating nccRCC, for now, remains an open question.

Certain genomic features have been identified which may assist in predicting clinical outcomes for patients with metastatic ChRCC. Casuscelli et al. examined genomic features specific to 35 metastatic ChRCC tumors and found that mutations to *TP53* and *PTEN,* and imbalanced chromosome duplication in ≥3 chromosomes, were associated with inferior clinical outcomes [25]. A recent report examining differentially expressed genes within the TCGA database found that two such genes, *SKA1* and *ERCC6L*, were associated with improved overall survival in patients with ChRCC [26]. While these data could certainly be used to guide further research into the genomic background of ChRCC, their immediate clinical utility is limited as they do not point towards any specific treatment option. The outcome of patients with ChRCC with sarcomatoid differentiation have poorer prognosis, as is the case for other RCC subtypes with sarcomatoid features [27]. Indeed, since variability of clinical outcomes are largely determined by tumor heterogeneity, the diverse genomic landscape of ChRCC (and nccRCC in general) better lends itself towards precision medicine, which can deliver tailored targeted therapies exploiting the specific subtype of cancer expressed in a given patient [28]. This is an emerging field and no predictive biomarkers are currently available to guide patients towards particular therapies [2].

Our data suggest VEGF-C could be utilized as a clinically viable biomarker to guide patients with ChRCC towards TKI therapy. While a major limitation of this study is that our data comes from a single patient, examinations of exceptional responders provide a unique opportunity to generate hypotheses which may prove useful in elucidating key molecular mechanisms behind disease processes. These so-called "N of 1" case reports have been previously used to uncover new cancer treatment options [29] and the nation's leading cancer research centers have been systematically collecting data on exceptional responders to guide future work on targeted therapies and drug discovery [30].

5. Conclusion

In this report, we report a patient diagnosed with ChRCC bearing increased expression of VEGF-C and VEGF-B who exhibited a prolonged response to sunitinib and has been stable on anti-VEGF therapies for nearly nine years. We feel that TKI's could be effective for other patients with ChRCC, particularly for patients whose tumors bear a similar molecular profile. Additional studies exploring potential treatment options for patients with nccRCC may help identify efficacious treatments for these uncommon cancers.

Acknowledgments

The corresponding author would like to thank the Betz Family Endowment for Cancer Research for their continued support. Funding was provided in part by the Spectrum Health Foundation (RG0813-1036). We would also like to acknowledge the Van Andel Research Institute where the gene expression profiling was done in Dr. B. T. Teh's laboratory at the time.

References

[1] R. L. Siegel, K. D. Miller, and A. Jemal, "Cancer statistics, 2019," *CA: A Cancer Journal for Clinicians*, vol. 69, no. 1, pp. 7–34, 2019.

[2] J. J. Hsieh, M. P. Purdue, S. Signoretti et al., "Renal cell carcinoma," *Nature Reviews Disease Primers*, vol. 3, 17009 pages, 2017.

[3] E. Jonasch, J. Gao, and W. K. Rathmell, "Renal cell carcinoma," *British Medical Journal*, vol. 349, pp. g4797–g4797, 2014.

[4] J. C. Cheville, C. M. Lohse, H. Zincke, A. L. Weaver, and M. L. Blute, "Comparisons of outcome and prognostic features among histologic subtypes of renal cell carcinoma," *The American Journal of Surgical Pathology*, vol. 27, no. 5, pp. 612–624, 2003.

[5] F. E. Vera-Badillo, A. J. Templeton, I. Duran et al., "Systemic therapy for non-clear cell renal cell carcinomas: a systematic review and meta-analysis," *European Urology*, vol. 67, no. 4, pp. 740–749, 2015.

[6] S. Agrawal, N. B. Haas, M. Bagheri et al., "Eligibility and radiologic assessment in adjuvant clinical trials in kidney cancer: report of a U.S. Food and Drug Administration and National Cancer Institute Public Workshop," *JAMA Oncology*, 2019.

[7] R. R. McKay, D. Bosse, and T. K. Choueiri, "Evolving systemic treatment landscape for patients with advanced renal cell carcinoma," *Journal of Clinical Oncology*, vol. 36, no. 36, pp. 3615–3623, 2018.

[8] R. J. Motzer, T. E. Hutson, P. Tomczak et al., "Sunitinib versus interferon alfa in metastatic renal-cell carcinoma," *New England Journal of Medicine*, vol. 356, no. 2, pp. 115–124, 2007.

[9] A. Poprach, K. Rumanova, R. Lakomy et al., "Tyrosine kinase inhibitors in the first-line treatment for metastatic nonclear cell renal carcinoma: a retrospective analysis of a national database," *In Urologic Oncology: Seminars and Original Investigations*, vol. 37, no. 4, 294-e1 pages, 2019.

[10] T. Barrett, S. E. Wilhite, P. Ledoux et al., "NCBI GEO: archive for functional genomics data sets—update," *Nucleic Acids Research*, vol. 41, no. D1, pp. D991–D995, 2012.

[11] R. C. Gentleman, V. J. Carey, D. M. Bates et al., "Bioconductor: open software development for computational biology and bioinformatics," *Genome Biology*, vol. 5, no. 10, R80 pages, 2004.

[12] L. Gautier, L. Cope, B. M. Bolstad, and R. A. Irizarry, "Affy–analysis of affymetrix GeneChip data at the probe level," *Bioinformatics*, vol. 20, no. 3, pp. 307–315, 2004.

[13] M. Dai, P. Wang, A. D. Boyd et al., "Evolving gene/transcript definitions significantly alter the interpretation of GeneChip data," *Nucleic Acids Research*, vol. 33, no. 20, e175 pages, 2005.

[14] J. M. Larkin, R. A. Fisher, L. M. Pickering et al., "Chromophobe renal cell carcinoma with prolonged response to sequential sunitinib and everolimus," *Journal of Clinical Oncology*, vol. 29, no. 9, pp. e241–e242, 2011.

[15] M. Brunelli, J. N. Eble, S. Zhang, G. Martignoni, B. Delahunt, and L. Cheng, "Eosinophilic and classic chromophobe renal cell carcinomas have similar frequent losses of multiple chromosomes from among chromosomes 1, 2, 6, 10, and 17, and this pattern of genetic abnormality is not present in renal oncocytoma," *Modern Pathology*, vol. 18, no. 2, pp. 161–169, 2005.

[16] S. Santaguida and A. Amon, "Short- and long-term effects of chromosome mis-segregation and aneuploidy," *Nature Reviews Molecular Cell Biology*, vol. 16, no. 8, pp. 473–485, 2015.

[17] C. F. Davis, C. J. Ricketts, M. Wang et al., "The somatic genomic landscape of chromophobe renal cell carcinoma," *Cancer Cell*, vol. 26, no. 3, pp. 319–330, 2014.

[18] S. Durinck, E. W. Stawiski, A. Pavia-Jimenez et al., "Spectrum of diverse genomic alterations define non-clear cell renal carcinoma subtypes," *Nature Genetics*, vol. 47, no. 1, pp. 13–21, 2015.

[19] R. J. Motzer, C. H. Barrios, T. M. Kim et al., "Phase II randomized trial comparing sequential first-line everolimus and second-line sunitinib versus first-line sunitinib and second-line everolimus in patients with metastatic renal cell carcinoma," *Journal of Clinical Oncology*, vol. 32, no. 25, pp. 2765–2772, 2014.

[20] N. M. Tannir, E. Jonasch, L. Albiges et al., "Everolimus versus sunitinib prospective evaluation in metastatic non-clear cell renal cell carcinoma (ESPN): a randomized multicenter Phase 2 trial," *European Urology*, vol. 69, no. 5, pp. 866–874, 2016.

[21] A. J. Armstrong, S. Halabi, T. Eisen et al., "Everolimus versus sunitinib for patients with metastatic non-clear cell renal cell carcinoma (ASPEN): a multicentre, open-label, randomised phase 2 trial," *The Lancet Oncology*, vol. 17, no. 3, pp. 378–388, 2016.

[22] S. Fernandez-Pello, F. Hofmann, R. Tahbaz et al., "A systematic review and meta-analysis comparing the effectiveness and adverse effects of different systemic treatments for non-clear cell renal cell carcinoma," *European Urology*, vol. 71, no. 3, pp. 426–436, 2017.

[23] E. Colomba, G. Le Teuff, T. Eisen et al., "Metastatic chromophobe renal cell carcinoma treated with targeted therapies: a renal cross channel group study," *European Journal of Cancer*, vol. 80, pp. 55–62, 2017.

[24] M. Santoni, F. Massari, V. Di Nunno et al., "Immunotherapy in renal cell carcinoma: latest evidence and clinical implications," *Drugs Context*, vol. 7, p. 212528, 2018.

[25] J. Casuscelli, N. Weinhold, G. Gundem et al., "Genomic landscape and evolution of metastatic chromophobe renal cell carcinoma," *JCI Insight*, vol. 2, no. 12, Article ID e92688, 2017.

[26] X. Yin, J. Wang, and J. Zhang, "Identification of biomarkers of chromophobe renal cell carcinoma by weighted gene co-expression network analysis," *Cancer Cell International*, vol. 18, no. 1, p. 206, 2018.

[27] B. Shuch, G. Bratslavsky, W. M. Linehan, and R. Srinivasan, "Sarcomatoid renal cell carcinoma: a comprehensive review of the biology and current treatment strategies," *The Oncologist*, vol. 17, no. 1, pp. 46–54, 2012.

[28] S. Signoretti, A. Flaifel, Y. B. Chen, and V. E. Reuter, "Renal cell carcinoma in the era of precision medicine: from molecular pathology to tissue-based biomarkers," *Journal of Clinical Oncology*, vol. 36, no. 36, pp. 3553–3559, 2018.

[29] I. M. Subbiah and V. Subbiah, "Exceptional responders: in search of the science behind the miracle cancer cures," *Future Oncology*, vol. 11, no. 1, pp. 1–4, 2015.

[30] C. Sheridan, "Cancer centers zero in on exceptional responders," *Nature Biotechnology*, vol. 32, no. 8, pp. 703–704, 2014.

18

Macrocystic Adult Penile Lymphangioma: A Rare Presentation

Jaisukh Kalathia, Kaushal Patel, and Santosh Agrawal

Department of Urology and Kidney Transplantation, Fortune Urology Clinic, India

Correspondence should be addressed to Jaisukh Kalathia; jaisukh2010@yahoo.com

Academic Editor: David Duchene

Adult penile lymphangioma (APL) is a rare multifactorial vascular malformation. Usually, it is asymptomatic and located on the coronal sulcus or shaft of the penis. It is benign in nature with rare chances of recurrence. APLs can be approached via various modalities from simple "watch and wait" to electrofulguration, laser ablation, and surgical excision. We report a rare variant of lymphangioma of the penis inculcating the shaft being excised surgically with favorable outcome along with brief review of literature.

1. Introduction

Lymphangioma is a benign condition which may occur due to abnormal development of the lymphatic system. Lymphangiomas are usually found in the head and neck region with rare exception of genital involvement. There are only few reported cases of penile lymphangioma in the literature. The congenital variant become more apparent over time as reported by Handa et al. [1], whereas the acquired variant could occur as a result of lymphatic vessel occlusion due to infections such as frequent cellulitis [2]. These lymphatic malformations are further classified as microcystic (lymphangioma circumscriptum), cavernous lymphangiomas, macrocystic (cystic hygromas), and the acquired lymphangiomas (lymphangiecatsis) [3]. The signs and symptoms vary depending on the size and location of the mass. They can disfigure the affected area and may potentially disrupt the function if left untreated.

2. Case Report

A-24-year-old unmarried male patient presented with a mass over dorsum of the penis for the past 10 years. It was painless and gradually increasing in size. As per the history, there were no predisposing factors. On examination, the mass was approximately of size 3 cm × 2 cm lying on the dorsal aspect at the midshaft of the penis. It was nontender, mobile, and firm in consistency with absent inguinal lymph nodes. The ultrasonography of the penis showed cystic mass involving midshaft of the penis.

A circumferential subcoronal incision was given to deglove the penis. The plane was developed below the external Colles fascia remaining above the Buck's fascia to avoid inadvertent injury to neurovascular bundles. On proximal dissection, the cystic mass was found severely adhered to midshaft. The two large feeding vessels were found at the ventral aspect of the mass which were dissected and ligated so as to remove the mass intact (Figure 1). The postoperative period was uneventful, and the patient was discharged on postoperative day one. In follow-up, the patient had normal erection, and the histopathological examination confirmed benign vascular lesion suggestive of lymphangioma (Figure 2).

3. Discussion

Lymphangiomas or "lymphatic malformations" were first described by Redenbacher et al. in 1828 [4]. These lymphatic malformations are relatively rare and not connected with the lymphatic system. They are ubiquitous because of the universal distribution of the lymphatic system but are commonly found in the head and neck. Lymphangioma are usually diagnosed during infancy or childhood. But, only few acquired cases can manifest in early and late adulthood with incidence slightly higher in males. The congenital lymphangioma may result from failure of fetal lymph vessel to involute or to join

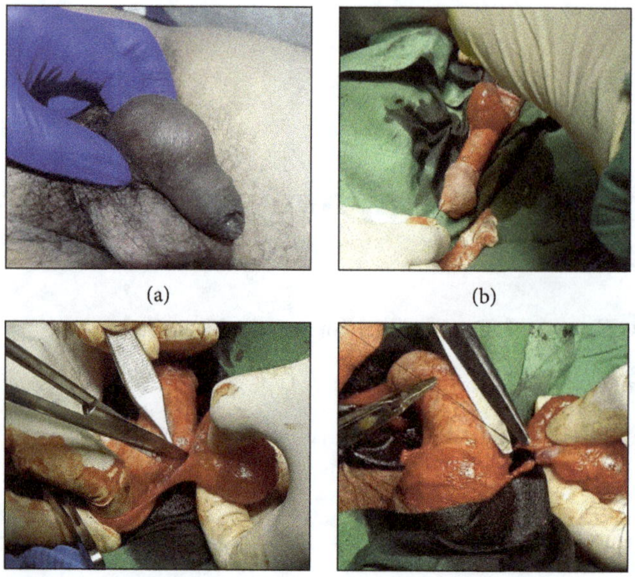

(a) (b) (c) (d)

Figure 1: (a) Cyst involving shaft of penis. (b) Degloving of penis. (c) Dissection of cyst. (d) Ligation of the two feeding vessels.

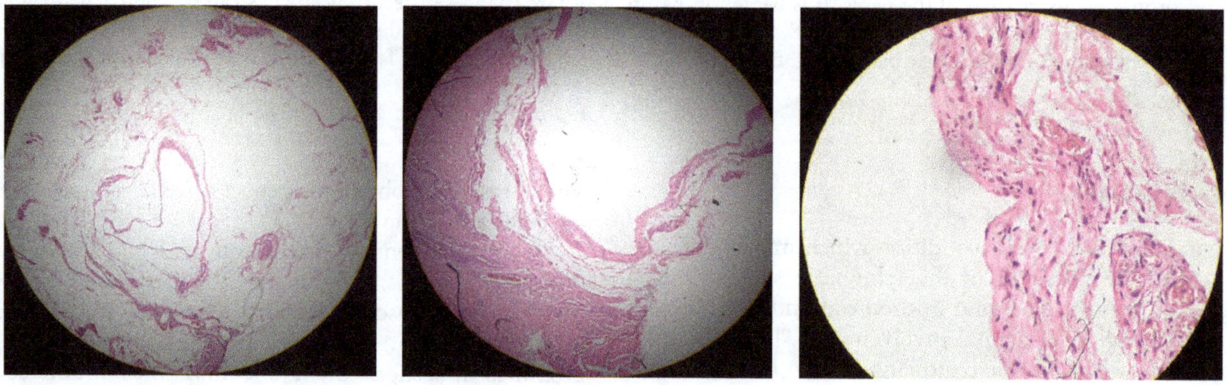

(a) (b) (c)

Figure 2: (a–c) Histopathological examination showing microcystic lymphatic malformation with irregular vascular channels and some containing slips of smooth muscle.

with the central lymphatic system. However, multiple etiology including trauma, infections, radiotherapy, pregnancy, scleroderma, severe phimosis, or STDs may result in acquired lymphangioma [5].

So far, less than 50 cases have been reported since Ferris and Holmes first described penile lymphangioma in 1944 [6]. The lymphangiomas are classified based on depth and size of lymph vessels: (1) lymphangioma circumscriptum (most superficial) composed of small thin-walled lymphatics, (2) cavernous lymphangioma composed of large lymphatics, and (3) cystic lymphangioma or cystic hygromas (deepest) with major lymphatic dilatation [7].

Penile lymphangiomas are commonly located on the coronal sulcus or shaft of penis.

The presentation is asymptomatic in majority of patients but those symptomatic can have sexual dysfunction. Given the benign nature of penile lymphangioma and rare likelihood of recurrence, these can be managed conservatively in those asymptomatic. However, acquired large lymphangiomas causing disfigurement of the penis or for the cosmetic purpose surgical excision should be adopted.

Various treatment modalities can be offered to treat lymphangiomas from simple "wait and watch" to electrofulguration, laser ablation, and surgical excision with favorable prognosis in each. However, during surgical excision, staged excision may be required depending on size [8]. In our case, the large lymphangioma was surgically excised intact to prevent further disfigurement of the penis.

4. Conclusion

APL is a benign tumor of lymphatic system which can be excised surgically with favorable outcome to prevent long-term sequelae of being permanently disfigured.

Consent

Informed consent was received from the participant.

Authors' Contributions

Kalathia Jaisukh is responsible for manuscript writing and project development. Patel Kaushal is responsible for data collection and manuscript writing. Santosh Agrawal is responsible for project development.

References

[1] N. Handa and P. Rao, "Penile lymphangioma circumscriptum-a rare case report," *Journal of Clinical & Experimental Dermatology Research*, vol. 7, no. 1, 2015.

[2] D. L. Swanson, "Genital lymphangioma with recurrent cellulitis in men," *International Journal of Dermatology*, vol. 45, no. 7, pp. 800–804, 2006.

[3] O. Enjorlas, "Vascular malformations," in *Dermatology*, J. Bolognia, J. Jorizzo, and J. Schaffer, Eds., pp. 1711–1723, Elsevier Limited, 2012.

[4] E. A. H. Redenbacher, *Dissertatio inauguralis medica de Ranula sub lingua, speciali cum casu congenito: Lindauer*, 1828.

[5] S. Adikari, M. Philippidou, and M. Samuel, "A rare case of acquired lymphangioma circumscriptum of the penis," *International Journal of STD & AIDS*, vol. 28, no. 2, pp. 205–207, 2016.

[6] D. O. Ferris and C. L. Holmes, "Extensive lymphangioma of scrotum, penis and adjacent areas: report of a case," *The Journal of Urology*, vol. 58, no. 6, pp. 453–457, 1947.

[7] F. M. Enzinger and S. W. Weiss, "Tumors of lymph vessels," in *Soft Tissue Tumors*, F. M. Enzinger and S. W. Weiss, Eds., pp. 679–699, Mosby-Year Book, St. Louis, 3rd edition, 1995, chapt 26.

[8] N. Feins, "Lymphatic disorders," in *Pediatric Surgery*, J. A. O'Neill Jr., M. I. Rowe, J. L. Grosfeld, E. W. Fonkalsrud, and A. G. Coran, Eds., pp. 1973–1981, Mosby, St. Louis, 5th edition, 1998.

19

Colon Cancer Metastasis to the Right Testis: Case Report and Review of Literature

Mizuki Kasahara, Tomo Shimizu, Hiroshi Aoki, Mizuho Okawa, Fumito Yamabe, Hideyuki Kobayashi, Koichi Nagao, Koichi Nakajima, and Yozo Mitsui

Department of Urology, Toho University Faculty of Medicine, 143-8540 Tokyo, Japan

Correspondence should be addressed to Mizuki Kasahara; mizuki.kasahara@med.toho-u.ac.jp

Academic Editor: Fumitaka Koga

Introduction. A metastatic testicular tumor is uncommon. We report here a case of testicular metastasis associated with recurrent colorectal cancer. *Case Presentation.* A 75-year-old male was presented with right scrotum pain one year after undergoing a right hemicolectomy combined with resection of the small intestine and omentum for ascending colon cancer (pT4N0M0). Magnetic resonance imaging of the pelvis showed a 7.3 × 5.4 × 4.5 cm mass consisting of a cystic solid tumor. A right inguinal orchiectomy was performed and right testicular pain improved after surgery. Pathology results showed that the tumor was a metastatic adenocarcinoma. The patient subsequently died two months later due to progression of the colon cancer. *Conclusion.* Although colorectal cancer metastasis to the testis is very uncommon, it should be kept in mind in clinical situations, especially for older males with a testicular mass or discomfort.

1. Introduction

A metastatic carcinoma to the testis is rare, accounting for only 0.8-2.3% of all testicular tumors [1, 2], with the most common primary site of the prostate gland, accounting for approximately 40% of all reported cases [3]. Here, details are presented regarding the treatment of a patient with a painful right testicular tumor found to be a metastasis from ascending colon cancer surgically treated one year prior. A right inguinal orchiectomy was performed for providing a pathological diagnosis and reducing pain.

2. Case Presentation

A 75-year-old male was referred to our hospital for right scrotal pain that was initially noted three weeks prior. One year before referral, the patient had undergone a right hemicolectomy combined with resection of the small intestine and omentum for ascending colon cancer (pT4N0M0) and subsequently received adjuvant chemotherapy with oxaliplatin for three cycles. Following that treatment, he did not visit the treating hospital regularly for follow-up examinations. Our physical examination findings revealed right scrotal swelling as well as tenderness. Scrotal ultrasonography showed a liquid component in the scrotum, while neoplastic lesions, normal testicle components, or the epididymis were not clearly visualized (Figure 1). A scrotal puncture was performed followed by a physical examination, during which palpation revealed a mass above the testis to the epididymis along with remaining scrotal tenderness. Magnetic resonance imaging (MRI) of the pelvis was then performed for reevaluation, which showed a 7.3 × 5.4 × 4.5 cm cystic solid tumor in the right scrotum, suspected to be a seminoma or malignant lymphoma (Figure 2, T2-weighted image). Laboratory results revealed normal or slightly elevated levels of prostate-specific antigen, alpha-fetoprotein, carbohydrate antigen 19-9, soluble inteleukin-2 receptor, beta-human gonadotrophin, and lactate dehydrogenase, while those of carcinoembryonic antigen (1,174 ng/mL) and cancer antigen 125 (56 U/mL) were markedly elevated. In addition, computed tomography (CT) findings indicated the presence of multiple metastatic tumors in the lungs, liver, lymph nodes,

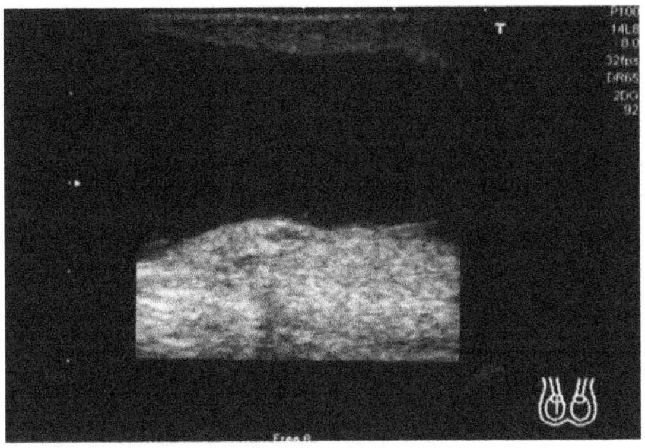

FIGURE 1: Scrotal ultrasonography image showing liquid component. Neoplastic lesions, normal testicle components, and the epididymis were not clearly visible.

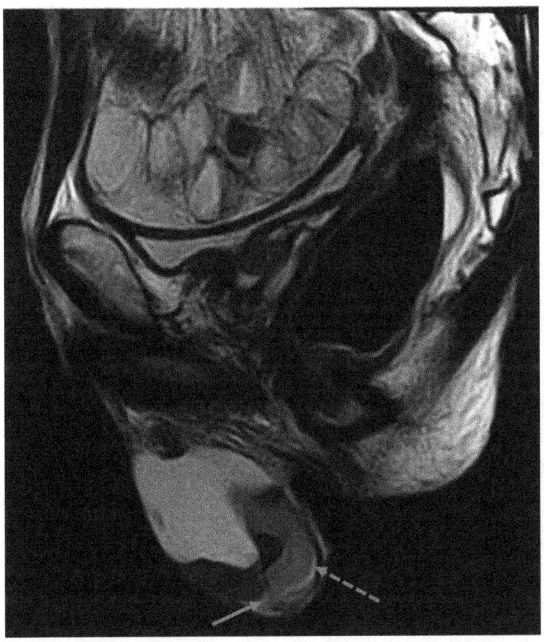

FIGURE 2: MRI T2-weighted image of the pelvis showing a 7.3 × 5.4 × 4.5 cm testicular mass consisting of a cystic solid tumor (arrow) as well as normal testicle components (dashed line arrow).

skin, and abdominal cavity. Based on the imaging and laboratory results, it was considered that colorectal cancer had recurred and metastasized throughout the body.

The patient was subsequently admitted to our hospital for pain control and anorexia. Right scrotal pain did not improve after administering a narcotic preparation for systemic pain, thus a right orchiectomy via an inguinal approach was performed for pain relief and diagnosis, during which a part of the scrotal wall was resected to treat adhesions. As shown in Figure 3, an ill-defined white solid mass was found above the right testis (3.0 cm) and another in the epididymis (1.3 cm). Histopathological results also showed an adenocarcinoma with moderate differentiation, which was identical to the primary colon cancer (Figure 4). In addition, cancer cells were found disseminated on the serosal surface of the peritoneal sheath of the spermatic cord and extended to the dartos fascia at the bottom of the scrotum. Based on these findings, the mass in the right testis was diagnosed as a metastatic tumor from primary colon cancer. Right scrotal pain improved after surgery, though the patient died two months later due to cancer progression.

3. Discussion

Metastasis of a carcinoma to the testis is rare and accounts for only 0.8-2.3% of all testicular tumors. The diagnosis is most often incidental in an autopsy examination [1, 2, 4]. Occurrence has been noted in males from 29 to 90 years old; the prostate is the most common primary site, followed by the lung, melanoma, and the kidney [4]. A previous study estimated that metastatic testicular tumors from digestive organs comprised 17.5% of all such tumors, among which colorectal cancer is the most likely to metastasize to a testicular cancer, though fewer than 80 cases have been reported thus far [5, 6].

Most patients with a metastatic testicular tumor from colon cancer are presented with testicular swelling or a hydrocele, with or without pain, and the mass is not solid [1, 7]. Thus, careful diagnostic testing is necessary, as this disease can be confused with a benign or inflammatory condition. Diagnosis of metastasis of carcinoma to the testis is generally confirmed based on microscopy results, though other important factors including patient age, history of present or prior malignancy, and results obtained with imaging modalities such as ultrasonography, CT, or MRI can assist with the final determination. In the present case, important information regarding the scrotum was easily obtained with minimally invasive ultrasonography, while MRI results provided evidence of the testicular tumor in greater details. CT imaging is also useful for assessing the spread of cancer cells to systemic organs, while increased gastrointestinal tumor markers in the present case was an important finding strongly suggesting colon cancer recurrence/metastasis. Thus, a multidisciplinary approach based on patient history, blood sampling data, and use of various imaging modalities can contribute to the diagnosis of a metastatic testicular tumor.

Although details regarding the mechanism of testicular metastasis of colon cancer remain largely unknown, several candidate theories have been suggested [7, 8], including arterial embolization, retrograde venous or lymphatic spread, and direct spread. Interestingly, it was recently proposed that microscopic channels of communication may be present between the peritoneum and testes, because most cases are presented with a testicular hydrocele [4], indicating that cancer cells may invade and extend from the original or a disseminated lesion through microscopic sized channels between the peritoneum and testes. The present findings also support this hypothesis from the perspective of hydrocele presence, though additional investigations are needed to clarify the precise mechanisms of metastatic carcinoma development in the testis.

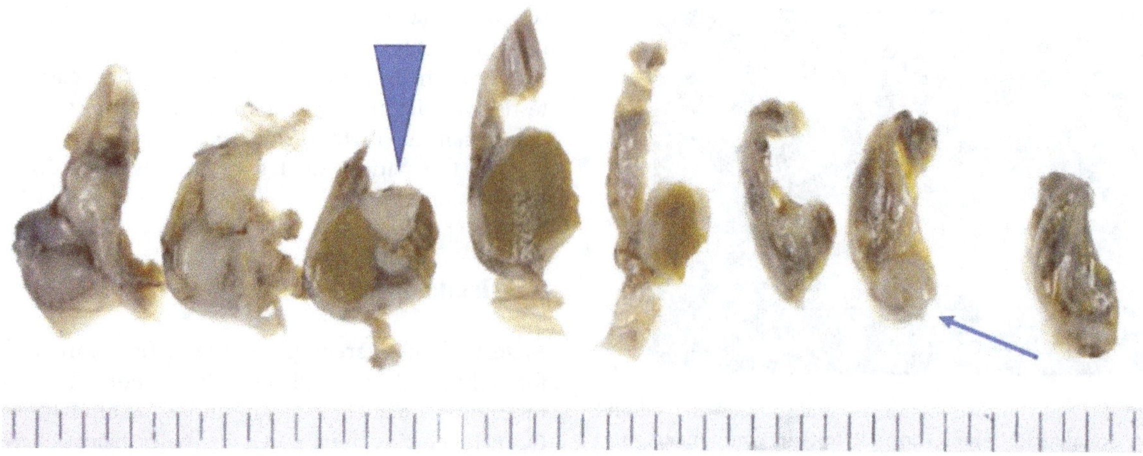

Figure 3: Macroscopic views of the resected specimen showing ill-defined white solid mass found above the testis (arrow) and in the epididymis (arrowhead).

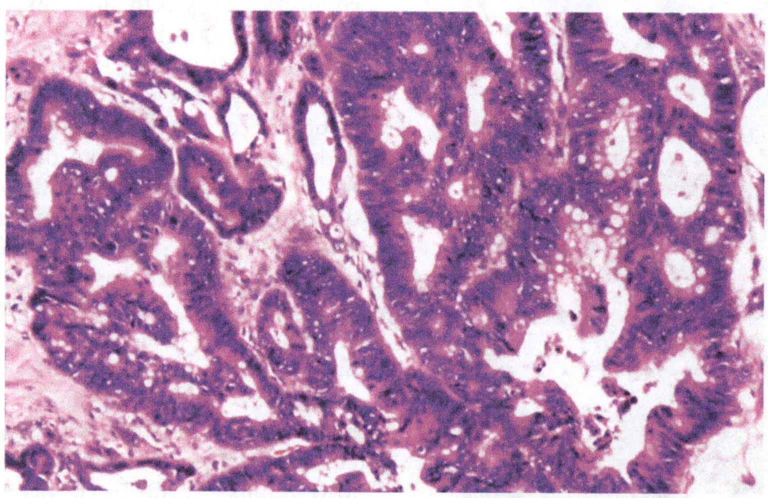

Figure 4: Histological findings of resected testis showed an adenocarcinoma with moderate differentiation, identical to the primary colon cancer (H&E stain, ×200).

Resection performed for liver or lung metastasis from primary colon cancer can improve prognosis in some cases [9, 10]. However, the significance of surgical treatment for testicular metastasis from colon cancer is unclear, since that is regarded as a late manifestation of a systemic spread of cancer cells. Indeed, in most cases with an initial presentation of colon cancer as testicular metastasis, an average survival was found to be 6-12 months regardless of treatment [1]. However, if the site is symptomatic, as in the present case, we think that a surgical approach should be considered for improving patient's quality of life.

In summary, we experienced a rare case of right testicular metastasis from colon cancer, for which the patient was treated with inguinal orchiectomy. Although metastasis to the testis is rare, awareness of the possibility is important for clinicians, especially when an older male is presented with a testicular mass or discomfort. Moreover, surgical treatment should be considered for relief of symptoms.

Additional Points

Keynote Message. We encountered a rare case of right metastatic testicular tumor from the ascending colon cancer in a patient who was presented with pain in that area. Local treatment for testicular metastasis does not typically prolong survival, because the condition is generally a late manifestation of systemic spreading of cancer cells. However, surgical removal of a metastatic testis is reasonable for improving quality of life such as relief of pain as well as providing findings for a definitive diagnosis.

References

[1] W. Charles, G. Joseph, B. Hunis, and L. Rankin, "Metastatic colon cancer to the testicle presenting as testicular hydrocele," *Journal of Clinical Oncology*, vol. 23, no. 22, pp. 5256-5257, 2005.

[2] T. Kiriyama and S. Yoshida, "The review of testicular tumor from Japanese pathological department," *Hinyokikakiyo*, vol. 29, pp. 155–168, 1983.

[3] T. M. Ulbright and R. H. Young, "Metastatic carcinoma to the testis: a clinicopathologic analysis of 26 nonincidental cases with emphasis on deceptive features," *The American Journal of Surgical Pathology*, vol. 32, no. 11, pp. 1683–1693, 2008.

[4] H. A. Omar, M. Mohiuddin, and A. Sharif, "Colon cancer presenting as a testicular metastasis," *Translational Gastroenterology and Hepatology*, vol. 1, p. 89, 2016.

[5] R. B. Meacham, J. A. Mata, R. Espada, T. M. Wheeleer, C. W. Schum, and P. T. Scardino, "Testicular metastasis as the first manifestation of colon carcinoma," *The Journal of Urology*, vol. 140, no. 3, pp. 621-622, 1988.

[6] A. Gabsi, A. Mnif, O. Adouni, F. Mghirbi, A. Mokrani, and A. Mezlini, "Testicular metastasis of colorectal carcinoma: a new observation," *Urology Case Reports*, vol. 35, article 101544, 2021.

[7] H. A. Hatoum, G. S. Abi Saad, Z. K. Otrock, K. A. Barada, and A. I. Shamseddine, "Metastasis of colorectal carcinoma to the testes: clinical presentation and possible pathways," *International Journal of Clinical Oncology*, vol. 16, no. 3, pp. 203–209, 2011.

[8] E. B. Price Jr. and F. K. Mostofi, "Secondary carcinoma of the testis," *Cancer*, vol. 10, no. 3, pp. 592–595, 1957.

[9] H. Shimada, K. Tanaka, I. Endou, and Y. Ichikawa, "Treatment for colorectal liver metastases: a review," *Langenbeck's Archives of Surgery*, vol. 394, no. 6, pp. 973–983, 2009.

[10] M. Riquet, C. Foucault, A. Cazes et al., "Pulmonary resection for metastases of colorectal adenocarcinoma," *The Annals of Thoracic Surgery*, vol. 89, no. 2, pp. 375–380, 2010.

20

Doubling of Decipher Biopsy Genomic Score is Related to Disease Reclassification on Subsequent Surveillance Biopsy but not Adverse Features on Radical Prostatectomy

Kamyar Ghabili,[1] Nathan Paulson,[2] Jamil S. Syed,[1] Cayce B. Nawaf,[1] Ghazal Khajir,[1] Darryl T. Martin,[1] John Onofrey,[3] Michael S. Leapman,[1] Angelique Levi,[2] Jeffrey C. Weinreb,[3] Peter A. Humphrey,[2] and Preston C. Sprenkle[1]

[1]Department of Urology, Yale University School of Medicine, New Haven, CT, USA
[2]Department of Pathology, Yale University School of Medicine, New Haven, CT, USA
[3]Department of Radiology and Biomedical Imaging, Yale University School of Medicine, New Haven, CT, USA

Correspondence should be addressed to Preston C. Sprenkle; preston.sprenkle@yale.edu

Academic Editor: Fumitaka Koga

The utility of serial Decipher biopsy scores in a true active surveillance population is still unknown. In a man on active surveillance for low-risk prostate cancer, a doubling of the Decipher biopsy score within genomic low-risk category from first to the second biopsy related to biopsy reclassification to Gleason grade group 4 on the third biopsy. However, the final pathology at radical prostatectomy showed Gleason grade group 2 with an organ-confined disease. This case suggests that the genomic risk category of Decipher biopsy scores during active surveillance may be more informative than either the interval genomic score change or the biopsy Gleason grade group.

1. Introduction

Active surveillance (AS) is a management option to defer immediate treatment for eligible patients with low-risk prostate cancer while monitoring disease progression [1]. However, distinguishing indolent versus aggressive tumor in patients on AS is challenging [2, 3]. Therefore, apart from repeat biopsies and prostate-specific antigen (PSA) measurements during surveillance, various serum, imaging, and genomic biomarkers are being used for better risk stratification of those patients [4].

The Decipher biopsy test is a genomic classifier that has been independently associated with metastasis, prostate-cancer-specific mortality, and adverse pathology at radical prostatectomy (RP) [2]. Nonetheless, the prognostic merit of the Decipher biopsy test in the true AS population and how the Decipher score changes over time on serial surveillance biopsies is still immature [4]. Here, we present a patient on AS for low-risk prostate cancer whose Decipher biopsy score doubling was related to disease reclassification on subsequent biopsy but not adverse features on radical prostatectomy.

2. Case Presentation

The patient is a Scandinavian male presented in 2016 at age 73 due to an elevated serum PSA of 6.3 ng/mL. His urologic history was notable for benign prostatic hyperplasia since 2014 managed with tamsulosin. He denied any family history of prostate cancer or any prior prostate biopsy. On digital rectal examination, no nodule/induration was palpable (clinical T1c). Following a negative multiparametric magnetic resonance imaging (mpMRI) with a prostate volume of 79 mL (PSA density = 0.08), he underwent 12-core transrectal ultrasound- (TRUS-) guided biopsy which showed Gleason grade group (GG) 1 prostate adenocarcinoma involving 80% and 5% of two cores. The Decipher prostate biopsy score (GenomeDx

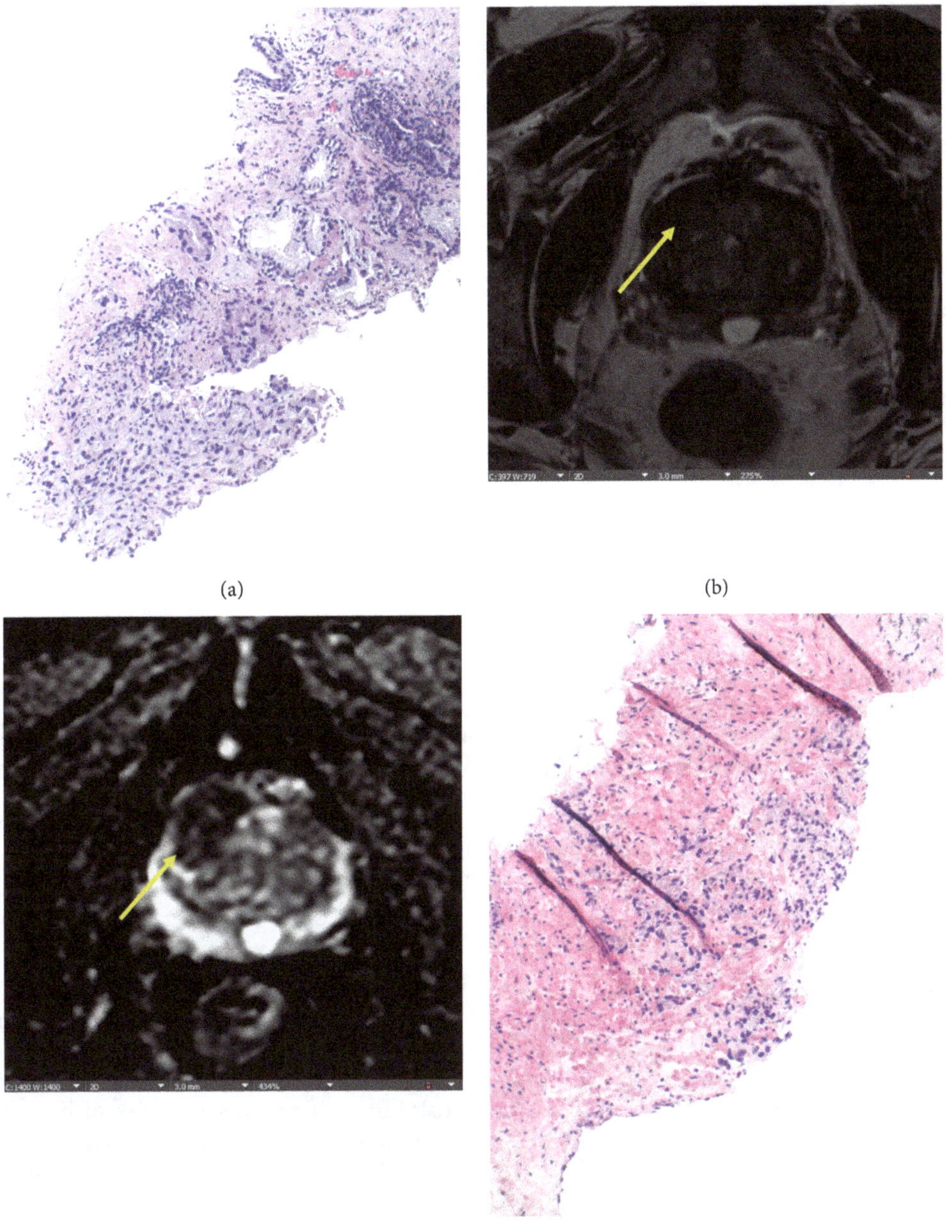

(a) (b)

(c) (d)

Figure 1: Continued.

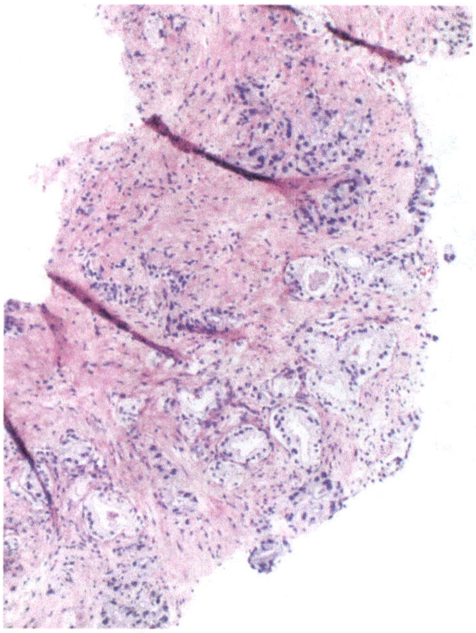

(e)

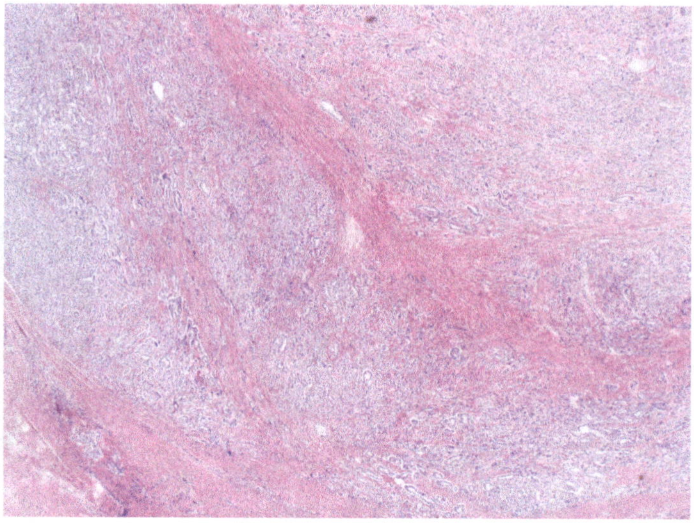

(f)

FIGURE 1: (a) A focus of Gleason GG2 prostatic adenocarcinoma on a targeted core in the 2nd biopsy; (b) T2-weighted image shows lenticular homogeneous moderately hypointense lesion (arrow) measuring 1.5 cm located in right anterior transitional zone in midgland, representative of Prostate Imaging Reporting and Data System category 5; (c) apparent diffusion coefficient map shows marked focal hypointensity (arrow); (d) a single focus of Gleason GG4 prostatic adenocarcinoma on a systematic core in the 3rd biopsy; (e) infiltrative growth of Gleason GG3 prostatic adenocarcinoma on a systematic core in the 3rd biopsy. Gleason pattern 3 is comprised of well-formed glands with relatively clear cytoplasm, small nuclei, and inconspicuous nucleoli. Gleason pattern 4 is made up of smaller, poorly formed glands with amphophilic cytoplasm, larger nuclei, and variably prominent nucleoli; (f) a radical prostatectomy specimen showing two distinct patterns of prostatic adenocarcinoma (the majority of Gleason pattern 3 and small population of pattern 4).

TABLE 1: Biomarker measures during active surveillance.

	First biopsy (7/2016)	Second biopsy (8/2017)	Third biopsy (12/2018)
PSA (ng/mL)	6.3	5.7	9.1
% free PSA	—	—	13.2
PHI	—	—	47.3
Biopsy	x	x	x
Decipher score	0.15	0.36	—
Prostate volume (mL)	79	91	90
PSA density (ng/mL/mL)	0.08	0.06	0.10

Biosciences, San Diego, CA) was 0.15 which was within genomic low risk and conveyed a 10% risk of high-grade disease at RP. After counseling with his provider for the diagnosed NCCN low-risk prostate cancer, the patient elected to undergo monitoring on AS.

His surveillance mpMRI one year from diagnosis illustrated a 91 mL prostate (PSA density = 0.06) with a 1.5 cm lesion in the right midgland to apex transition zone with Prostate Imaging Reporting and Data System (PI-RADS) score 5 but without extracapsular extension. A right-sided bulge was also palpable on his rectal exam (cT2a). Subsequent mpMRI/TRUS fusion biopsy revealed adenocarcinoma with Gleason GG2 (10% pattern 4) in 75% of a targeted core (Figure 1(a)) and Gleason GG1 in three other targeted cores with the highest involvement of 55%. The Decipher test performed on the biopsy specimen of the core with Gleason GG2 resulted in a score of 0.36 (genomic low risk but with an increased risk of high-grade disease at RP to 17.6%). At this time, the patient elected to stay on AS.

Follow-up serum biomarker, biopsy genomic, and prostate imaging data are listed in Table 1. A repeat mpMRI in 2018 demonstrated a stable 1.5 cm PI-RADS 5 lesion within the transition zone (Figures 1(b) and 1(c)). A simultaneous serum testing revealed a PSA of 9.1 ng/mL with 13% free PSA and prostate health index (PHI) of 47.3. The patient underwent a surveillance mpMRI/TRUS fusion biopsy which showed extensive cancer in 8 of total 17 cores. Five of 12 systematic cores were positive with the maximum Gleason GG4 (one core, Figure 1(d)), followed by Gleason GG3 (one core, Figure 1(e)), and Gleason GG2 (two cores). Three targeted biopsy cores showed Gleason GG1 disease. Preoperative whole body ^{99m}Tc-methylene diphosphonate bone scan demonstrated no uptake suspicious for osseous metastasis. The patient underwent robotic-assisted laparoscopic radical prostatectomy and bilateral pelvic lymph node dissection with pathology demonstrating Gleason GG2 acinar adenocarcinoma involving 20% of the gland (Figure 1(f)), positive perineural invasion, negative surgical margins, lymphovascular invasion, extracapsular extension, and 36 negative nodes (pT2 pN0).

3. Discussion

This case illustrated that a doubling of the Decipher score (yet within the genomic low-risk category) or Gleason GG4 on preoperative biopsy was not associated with any adverse features such as primary Gleason pattern 4 and/or pT3 in the final pathology. This suggests that the genomic risk category of Decipher biopsy scores during AS may be more informative than either interval genomic score change or biopsy Gleason GG. To the best of our knowledge, this case represents the first in which the relationship between changes of Decipher biopsy score over time and Gleason GG upgrade on biopsy and RP is reported. Nevertheless, studies of a larger cohort of patients on AS with serial Decipher biopsy scores are required before any conclusions can be made in terms of clinical decision-making.

In the present case, we observed a significant elevation in Decipher biopsy score on serial biopsies. By contrast, Cedars and colleagues found a relatively stable Oncotype DX Genomic Prostate Score (GPS) over time during AS. Given that GPS at baseline, but not follow-up, was associated with an upgrade at second biopsy, they concluded that serial genomic testing might be of limited utility in the AS [5]. The present case highlighted the need for a similar study with the Decipher biopsy score as our observation was in favor of a potential association between elevation of the Decipher score and biopsy grade reclassification in the AS setting.

Several other biomarkers are also used during AS to predict biopsy progression which triggers for intervention. Although postdiagnostic PSA-based tests (PSA density, % free PSA, and PHI) have been shown to predict later progression, the prognostic utility of PSA kinetics as well as mpMRI in the AS population is debatable [6]. The present case challenges the benefits of PSA density in the surveillance setting, given that his highest PSA density value was 0.10. We were unable to interpret the values of % free PSA and PHI due to unavailable baseline data.

4. Conclusion

This case report demonstrates how serial genomic assessments during AS can provide valuable data regarding the final pathology. It is anticipated that combining biopsy genomic risk category assessment with other biomarkers such as PHI during AS would improve patient risk stratification and offer further evidence for rational management approaches in the setting of biopsy grade reclassification.

References

[1] W. Hsiang, K. Ghabili, J. S. Syed et al., "Outcomes of serial multiparametric magnetic resonance imaging and subsequent biopsy in men with low-risk prostate cancer managed with active surveillance," *European Urology Focus*, vol. 7, no. 1, pp. 47–54, 2021.

[2] M. S. Leapman and P. R. Carroll, "New genetic markers for prostate cancer," *The Urologic Clinics of North America*, vol. 43, no. 1, pp. 7–15, 2016.

[3] D. T. Martin, K. Ghabili, A. Levi, P. A. Humphrey, and P. C. Sprenkle, "Prostate cancer genomic classifier relates more strongly to Gleason grade group than prostate imaging reporting and data system score in multiparametric prostate magnetic resonance imaging-ultrasound fusion targeted biopsies," *Urology*, vol. 125, pp. 64–72, 2019.

[4] S. Loeb and J. J. Tosoian, "Biomarkers in active surveillance," *Transl Androl Urol.*, vol. 7, no. 1, pp. 155–159, 2018.

[5] B. E. Cedars, S. L. Washington, J. E. Cowan et al., "Stability of a 17-gene genomic prostate score in serial testing of men on active surveillance for early stage prostate cancer," *The Journal of Urology*, vol. 202, no. 4, pp. 696–701, 2019.

[6] S. Loeb, S. M. Bruinsma, J. Nicholson et al., "Active surveillance for prostate cancer: a systematic review of clinicopathologic variables and biomarkers for risk stratification," *European Urology*, vol. 67, no. 4, pp. 619–626, 2015.

21

Reconstruction of a Scrotum by Combining Two Skin Flaps in a Ball Shape

Kazuya Kashiyama[1,2] **Motoi Nakano**[1,2] **Akihito Higashi**[1,2] **Shoko Ashizuka**[1,2] **Yuki Moriuchi**[2] **Atsuhiko Iwao**[2] **and Katsumi Tanaka**[2]

[1]*Department of Plastic and Reconstructive Surgery, Nagasaki Harbor Medical Center, Nagasaki, Japan*
[2]*Department of Plastic and Reconstructive Surgery, Nagasaki University Hospital, Nagasaki, Japan*

Correspondence should be addressed to Kazuya Kashiyama; tempnauts.2061@gmail.com

Academic Editor: Fumitaka Koga

Background. The scrotum functions to maintain spermatogenesis and hormonal production of Leydig cells by preventing the testicles from rising in temperature and protecting them from the outside world. The scrotum, along with the penis, is also an organ that symbolizes masculinity. Therefore, deformity or loss of the scrotum can be a major psychological problem. Various scrotal reconstruction techniques have been reported. In these papers, there is some discussion about the type of skin flap, but little discussion about the method of suturing the skin flap. We devised a way to reconstruct a scrotum to a natural size by suturing two skin flaps together to form a ball shape. *Case Presentation.* Case 1 was a patient with a missing scrotum due to Fournier's gangrene. Total resection of the scrotum, including the bilateral testes, was performed to save his life. Reconstructive surgery was performed 11 days after the initial surgery. Reconstruction was performed using bilateral gluteal fold flaps. Case 2 was a patient with a congenital defect of the scrotum. The testis on the right side exhibited cryptorchidism, and the scrotum was missing, and the testis on the left side was encased in a hypoplastic scrotum. Reconstruction was performed using an internal pudendal artery perforator flap. *Conclusion.* There are two types of scrotal defects: those with testes present and those with testes missing. This method can be used for both types of scrotal defects, and we were able to create a scrotum that satisfied each patient.

1. Background

The scrotum functions to maintain spermatogenesis and hormonal production of Leydig cells by preventing the testicles from rising in temperature and protecting them from the outside world [1]. The scrotum, along with the penis, is also an organ that symbolizes masculinity. Therefore, deformity or loss of the scrotum can be a major psychological problem. Congenital anomalies, trauma, malignancy, and infections such as Fournier's gangrene can cause scrotal defects [2, 3]. In recent years, scrotum reconstruction has become a very important issue in terms of gender-affirming surgery. Various scrotal reconstruction techniques have been reported [2, 4–6]. In these papers, there is some discussion about the type of skin flap, but little discussion about the method of suturing the skin flap. We devised a way to reconstruct a scrotum with a natural size by suturing two skin flaps together to form a ball shape.

2. Case Presentation

2.1. Case 1. The patient was a 66-year-old Japanese man who had type 2 diabetes. During treatment for epididymitis, the patient developed Fournier's gangrene and was rushed to our hospital. On the same day, a scrotal resection, including the testes, was performed by a urologist (Figure 1). The patient was then referred to the plastic surgery department for scrotal reconstruction. Reconstruction of the scrotum was performed 11 days after the initial surgery. The operation was performed with the patient in the lithotomy posi-

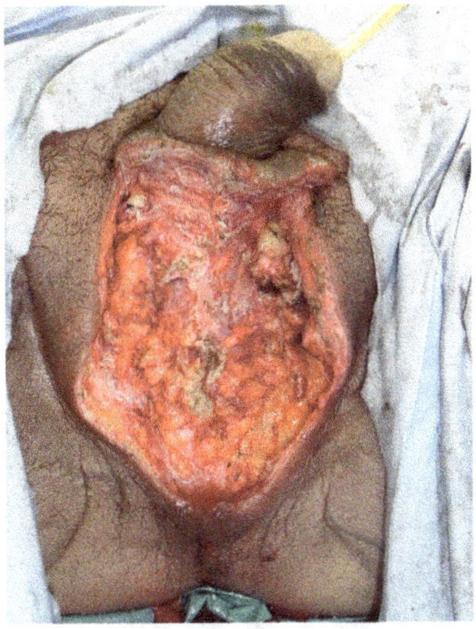

FIGURE 1: Case 1, primary surgery. Bilateral scrotum and testes were resected.

tion under general anesthesia. Reconstruction was performed using bilateral gluteal fold flaps (Figure 2(a)). The flap was rotated by more than 180 degrees towards the defect in a tension-free manner (Figure 2(b)). Two gluteal fold flaps were combined in a ball shape and sutured together to reconstruct the scrotum (Figures 2(c) and 2(d)). Immediately after the surgery, the patient complained that the reconstructed scrotum was too large and interfered with walking. However, during follow-up, the reconstructed scrotum gradually shrank. Eight months after surgery, there were no problems with the shape or size of the scrotum, and the patient was satisfied with the results (Figures 3(a)–3(c)).

2.2. Case 2. The patient was a two-year-Japanese boy who had popliteal pterygium syndrome. The testis on the right side exhibited cryptorchidism, and the scrotum was missing (Figure 4(a)). The testis on the left side was encased in a hypoplastic scrotum. The penis was located slightly to the right of the midline. Reconstruction was performed using an internal pudendal artery perforator flap. Two flaps were combined in a ball shape and sutured together to reconstruct the scrotum. Bilateral testes were wrapped and fixed in the inner envelope space of the two skin flaps (Figures 4(b)–4(e)). At 11 years postoperatively, the testes are still in the reconstructed scrotum. The scrotum is a suitable size and hangs down in the standing position, and the patient was satisfied with the results (Figure 5).

3. Discussion and Conclusions

Because the skin of the scrotum is extremely elastic, direct suturing is often possible in cases of partial defects [2]. However, if the defect is large or if there are cosmetic concerns, some form of reconstructive surgery should be considered.

There are two possible forms of total loss of the scrotum. The first is the total loss of the scrotum including the testes. The other is a total loss of the scrotum with the testes and spermatic cord remaining. Malignant tumors and infections may require removal of the scrotum, including the testes and spermatic cord. Total loss of the scrotum due to trauma is often caused by clothing being caught in machinery. In such cases, the testicles and spermatic cord are spared from damage due to the epididymis reflex at the time of injury, and degloving injury often occurs between the internal and external spermatic fascia [7–10].

When considering scrotal reconstruction, two issues need to be considered. One is a cosmetic issue, and the other is a functional issue of testicular protection. Several scrotum reconstruction methods have been reported, including skin grafts, fasciocutaneous flaps, and free flaps, all of which have advantages and disadvantages [1, 11–14].

Skin grafting is a simple method that can be used with or without remaining testes or the spermatic cord and is very useful in terms of testicular cooling because they are covered with a very thin skin [15, 16]. However, reconstruction with skin grafts does not look good [17]. It has also been reported that the presence of the testicles under thin skin prevents patients from leading a normal sex life for fear of hurting them [18, 19]. Therefore, reconstruction with more soft tissue such as a skin flap is preferred if possible [2, 11].

Several types of scrotum reconstruction with skin flaps have been reported, such as gluteal fold island flaps [2], pudendal thigh flaps [20], and gracilis myocutaneous flaps [2, 21–26]. The problem with reconstructing the scrotum with a skin flap is that the flap is bulky due to excessive soft tissue [4]. Therefore, a moderate size and thickness skin flap is needed to create an appropriately sized scrotum. We also have to take into account that the flap shrinks postoperatively due to elasticity [27], and the reconstructed scrotum may be deformed due to contraction of the skin flap.

In cases where the testes or spermatic cord remains, a skin flap large enough to contain the testes or spermatic cord is required. Since the scrotal region is symmetrical, it is often reconstructed using two skin flaps from the left and right sides [2, 4–6, 28, 29]. In this study, we tried to find a way to suture the skin flap so that it would morphologically resemble the scrotum and be able to contain a large space.

In case 1, we used a gluteal fold flap. Although there has been a report of scrotal reconstruction using bilateral gluteal fold flaps in the past, in the reported cases, the two flaps were sutured symmetrically at the midline [2]. We devised a new method for suturing the skin flaps. When suturing, the apex of one skin flap was fixed around the middle of the other skin flap to make a ball with the two skin valves and this was sutured. A baseball ball is made by using two sheets of skin-flap-like cloth, and the same thing was done with skin flaps to create a scrotum. Unlike combining two longitudinal flaps in this method, the force of contraction of the flap works in the direction of tightening the other flap, resulting in an overall reduction in the size of the valve while maintaining its shape. Therefore, the postoperative form is maintained.

In case 2, we used an internal pudendal artery perforator flap [30]. Skin flaps were created from the left and right sides in order to adequately cover the testes on both sides. Eleven years after the surgery, hair growth was observed in the scrotum reconstructed by the skin flap. In prepubertal patients,

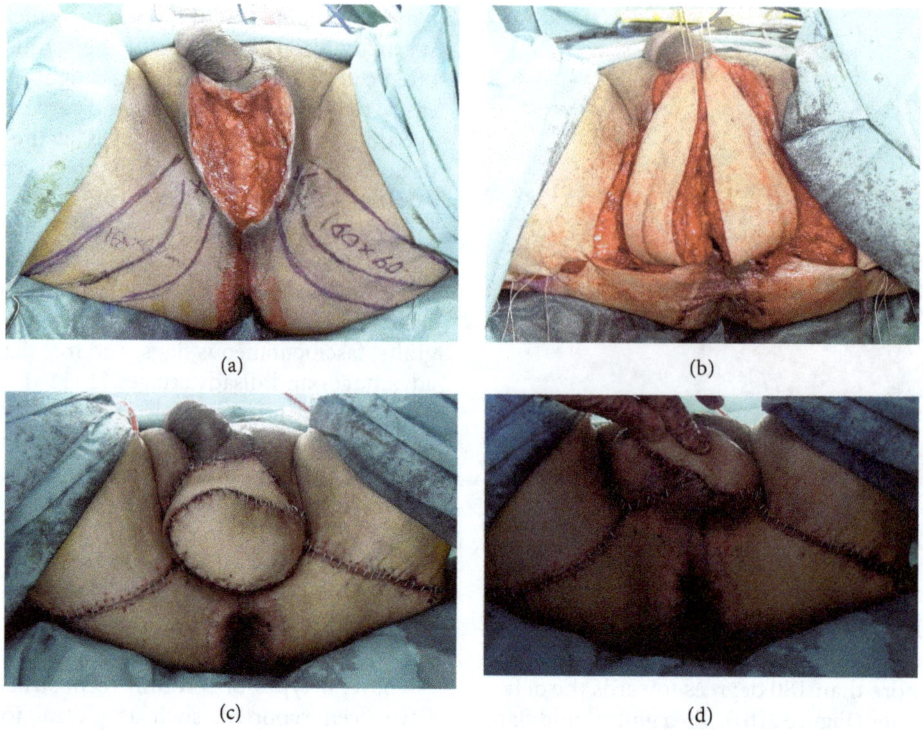

FIGURE 2: Case 1, reconstruction of a scrotum. (a) Skin flap design. X indicates a perforator. (b) Skin flaps were elevated. (c) Immediately postsurgery anterior view of the scrotum. (d) Immediately postsurgery posterior view of the scrotum.

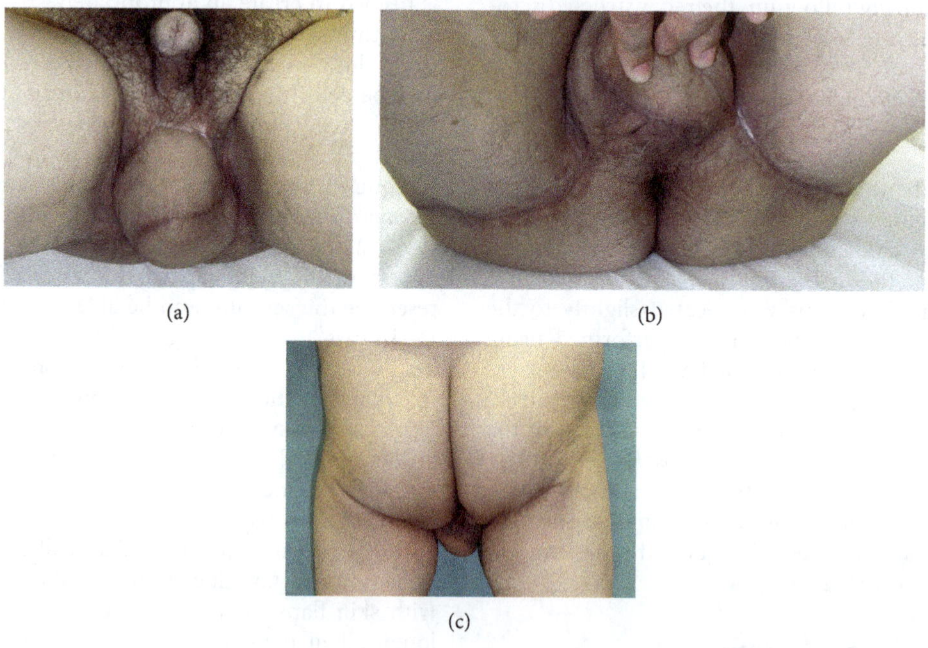

FIGURE 3: Case 1, eight months after reconstruction surgery. (a) Anterior view of the scrotum. (b) Posterior view of the scrotum. (c) Standing view.

careful consideration should be given to the choice of flap harvest site.

If the testes remain, it is necessary to obtain sufficient space to contain them. A single adult testis weighs about 15 g, is 5 cm long, 3 cm wide, and 1.5-2 cm thick, with a volume of about 20 cc [31–33]. There is some discussion about the type of skin flap used in the literature, but little discussion about the method of suturing the skin flap. It is thought that if the skin flap is sutured in a ball-like combination, it is possible to obtain an appropriate internal space rather than if the same size skin valves were sutured vertically. In addition, unlike combining two longitudinal skin flaps, when skin flaps are

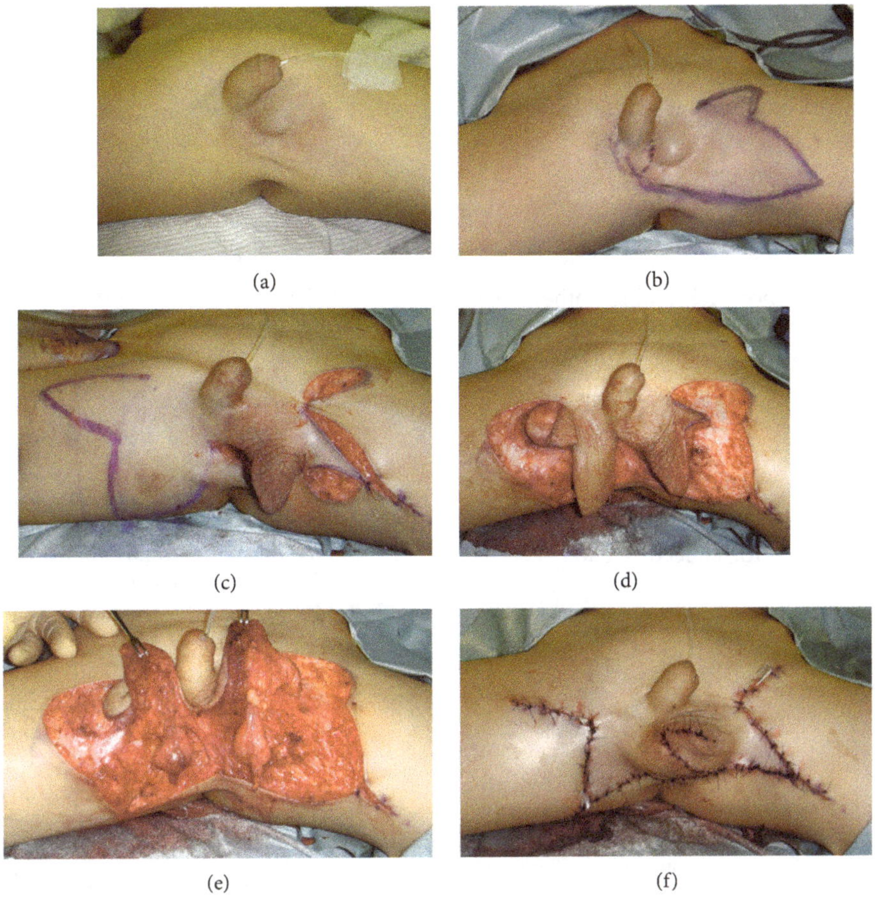

FIGURE 4: Case 2. (a) Presurgery. (b) Skin flap design of the left side. (c) Skin flap design of the right side. (d) Skin flaps were elevated. (e) Testes are present. (f) Immediately postsurgery.

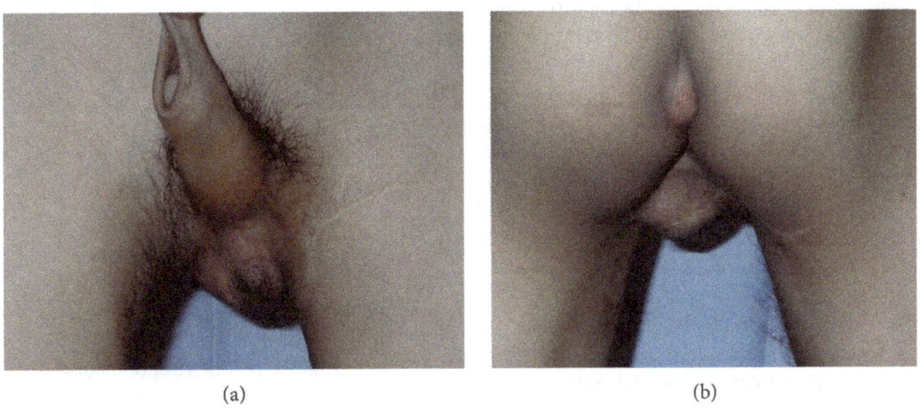

FIGURE 5: Case 2, eleven years after reconstruction surgery. (a) Anterior view of the scrotum. (b) Posterior view of the scrotum.

combined using this method, the force of contraction of the skin flaps works in the direction of tightening each other, resulting in an overall reduction in the size of the skin flaps while maintaining their shape. Therefore, the postoperative morphology can be maintained. The problem is that the concept of creating an appropriate space inside by combining skin flaps may create a dead space. Therefore, adequate drainage should be performed when suturing the skin flap using this approach.

Ethical Approval

The study was approved by our institutional research ethics board (No. 21101931).

Consent

Written informed consent was obtained from each patient and a parent of patient 2 for publication of this case report and accompanying images and other personal or clinical details.

Authors' Contributions

KK conceived and wrote the report. KK and the others were involved in treating the patient. KK participated in critically in editing the manuscript. All authors declare that they contributed to this article, and that they have read and approved the final manuscript.

Acknowledgments

We thank Miss Yukiko Kusano for collecting data.

References

[1] J. W. McAninch, "Management of genital skin loss," *The Urologic Clinics of North America*, vol. 16, no. 2, pp. 387–397, 1989.

[2] S. E. Han, E. J. Kim, H. H. Sung, and J. K. Pyon, "Aesthetic penoscrotal resurfacing: creating propeller flaps from gluteal folds," *European Urology*, vol. 73, no. 4, pp. 610–617, 2018.

[3] N. Quatan and R. S. Kirby, "Improving outcomes in Fournier's gangrene," *BJU International*, vol. 93, no. 6, pp. 691-692, 2004.

[4] N. Mopuri, E. F. O'Connor, and F. C. Iwuagwu, "Scrotal reconstruction with modified pudendal thigh flaps," *Journal of Plastic, Reconstructive & Aesthetic Surgery*, vol. 69, no. 2, pp. 278–283, 2016.

[5] A. Daigeler, B. Behr, B. D. Mikhail, M. Lehnhardt, and C. Wallner, "Bilateral pedicled gracilis flap for scrotal reconstruction," *Journal of Plastic, Reconstructive & Aesthetic Surgery*, vol. 69, no. 9, pp. e195–e196, 2016.

[6] J. Yang, S. H. Ko, S. J. Oh, and S. W. Jung, "Reconstruction of a perineoscrotal defect using bilateral medial thigh fasciocutaneous flaps," *Archives of Plastic Surgery*, vol. 40, no. 1, pp. 72–74, 2013.

[7] H. Baxter, M. Hoffman, E. Smith, and K. Stern, "Complete AVULSION of skin of penis and SCROTUM; SURGICAL endocrinological and psychological treatment," *Plastic and Reconstructive Surgery*, vol. 4, no. 6, pp. 508–521, 1949.

[8] J. M. Bruner, "Traumatic avulsion of skin of the male external genitalia; coverage with local remnants of genital skin," *Plastic and Reconstructive Surgery (1946)*, vol. 6, no. 4, pp. 334–338, 1950.

[9] M. Gonzalez-Ulloa, "Severe avulsion of the scrotum in a bullfighter: reconstructive procedure," *British Journal of Plastic Surgery*, vol. 16, pp. 154–159, 1963.

[10] E. S. Brintnall, D. A. Culp, R. H. Flocks et al., "Injuries to the male genitalia," *Plastic and Reconstructive Surgery (1946)*, vol. 18, no. 5, pp. 344–353, 1956.

[11] H. Hsu, C. M. Lin, T. B. Sun, L. F. Cheng, and S. H. Chien, "Unilateral gracilis myofasciocutaneous advancement flap for single stage reconstruction of scrotal and perineal defects," *Journal of Plastic, Reconstructive & Aesthetic Surgery*, vol. 60, no. 9, pp. 1055–1059, 2007.

[12] P. J. Nisar and H. J. Scott, "Myocutaneous flap reconstruction of the pelvis after abdominoperineal excision," *Colorectal Disease*, vol. 11, no. 8, pp. 806–816, 2009.

[13] T. N. Wang, T. Whetzel, S. J. Mathes, and L. O. Vasconez, "A fasciocutaneous flap for vaginal and perineal reconstruction," *Plastic and Reconstructive Surgery*, vol. 80, no. 1, pp. 95–103, 1987.

[14] C. T. Westfall and H. B. Keller, "Scrotal reconstruction utilizing bilateral gracilis myocutaneous flaps," *Plastic and Reconstructive Surgery*, vol. 68, no. 6, pp. 945–947, 1981.

[15] P. Maguiña, T. L. Palmieri, and D. G. Greenhalgh, "Split thickness skin grafting for recreation of the scrotum following Fournier's gangrene," *Burns*, vol. 29, no. 8, pp. 857–862, 2003.

[16] B. K. Tan, M. Z. Rasheed, and W. T. Wu, "Scrotal reconstruction by testicular apposition and wrap-around skin grafting," *Journal of Plastic, Reconstructive & Aesthetic Surgery*, vol. 64, no. 7, pp. 944–948, 2011.

[17] H. Boukind, M. Ezzoubi, N. Chafiki et al., "Scrotal reconstruction after necrotizing cellulitis of the perineum and external genital organs. Apropos of 21 cases," *Annales d'Urologie*, vol. 29, no. 5, pp. 308–312, 1995.

[18] R. M. Campbell, "Dermatome grafting of the totally denuded testes," *Plastic and Reconstructive Surgery (1946)*, vol. 19, no. 6, pp. 509–513, 1957.

[19] R. M. Campbell, "Follow-up clinic: dermatome grafting of the totally denuded testes," *Plastic and Reconstructive Surgery*, vol. 50, no. 3, p. 280, 1972.

[20] D. Maharaj, V. Naraynsingh, A. Perry, and M. Ramdass, "The scrotal reconstruction using the "Singapore sling"," *Plastic and Reconstructive Surgery*, vol. 110, no. 1, pp. 203–205, 2002.

[21] D. W. Banks, D. P. O'Brien 3rd, J. R. Amerson, and T. R. Hester Jr., "Gracilis musculocutaneous flap scrotal reconstruction after Fournier gangrene," *Urology*, vol. 28, no. 4, pp. 275-276, 1986.

[22] I. Hashimoto, H. Nakanishi, H. Nagae, H. Harada, and H. Sedo, "The gluteal-fold flap for vulvar and buttock reconstruction: anatomic study and adjustment of flap volume," *Plastic and Reconstructive Surgery*, vol. 108, no. 7, pp. 1998–2005, 2001.

[23] I. Hashimoto, G. Murakami, H. Nakanishi et al., "First cutaneous branch of the internal pudendal artery: an anatomical basis for the so-called gluteal fold flap," *Okajimas Folia Anatomica Japonica*, vol. 78, no. 1, pp. 23–30, 2001.

[24] P. K. Lee, M. S. Choi, S. T. Ahn, D. Y. Oh, J. W. Rhie, and K. T. Han, "Gluteal fold V-Y advancement flap for vulvar and vaginal reconstruction: a new flap," *Plastic and Reconstructive Surgery*, vol. 118, no. 2, pp. 401–406, 2006.

[25] R. Ragoowansi, N. Yii, and N. Niranjan, "Immediate vulvar and vaginal reconstruction using the gluteal-fold flap: long-term results," *British Journal of Plastic Surgery*, vol. 57, no. 5, pp. 406–410, 2004.

[26] J. T. Wee and V. T. Joseph, "A new technique of vaginal reconstruction using neurovascular pudendal-thigh flaps: a preliminary report," *Plastic and Reconstructive Surgery*, vol. 83, no. 4, pp. 701–709, 1989.

[27] R. W. Ng, J. Y. Chan, V. Mok, M. S. Leung, A. P. Yuen, and W. I. Wei, "Clinical implications of anterolateral thigh flap shrinkage," *Laryngoscope*, vol. 118, no. 4, pp. 585–588, 2008.

[28] S. H. Lee, D. K. Rah, and W. J. Lee, "Penoscrotal reconstruction with gracilis muscle flap and internal pudendal artery perforator flap transposition," *Urology*, vol. 79, no. 6, pp. 1390–1394, 2012.

[29] D. F. Mello and A. Helene Júnior, "Scrotal reconstruction with superomedial fasciocutaneous thigh flap," *Revista do Colégio Brasileiro de Cirurgiões*, vol. 45, no. 1, article e1389, 2018.

[30] I. Hashimoto, Y. Abe, and H. Nakanishi, "The internal pudendal artery perforator flap: free-style pedicle perforator flaps for vulva, vagina, and buttock reconstruction," *Plastic and Reconstructive Surgery*, vol. 133, no. 4, pp. 924–933, 2014.

[31] L. Johnson, C. S. Petty, and W. B. Neaves, "Influence of age on sperm production and testicular weights in men," *Journal of Reproduction and Fertility*, vol. 70, no. 1, pp. 211–218, 1984.

[32] T. Tasaka, S. Hiraga, M. Kitamura et al., "First report on studies of normal testicular weight and size in the Japanese," *Nihon Hinyokika Gakkai Zasshi*, vol. 77, no. 9, pp. 1506–1510, 1986.

[33] H. Takihara, J. Sakatoku, M. Fujii, T. Nasu, M. J. Cosentino, and A. T. Cockett, "Significance of testicular size measurement in andrology. I. A new orchiometer and its clinical application," *Fertility and Sterility*, vol. 39, no. 6, pp. 836–840, 1983.

22

Bladder Leiomyoma with Synchronous Solitary Fibrous Tumor of the Pleura

Charalampos Mavridis,[1] George Georgiadis,[1] Eleni D. Lagoudaki,[2] Iordanis Skamagkas,[1] Ioannis Heretis,[1] Anastasios V. Koutsopoulos,[2] and Charalampos Mamoulakis[1]

[1]*Department of Urology, University General Hospital of Heraklion, University of Crete, Medical School, Heraklion, Crete, Greece*
[2]*Department of Pathology, University General Hospital of Heraklion, University of Crete, Medical School, Heraklion, Crete, Greece*

Correspondence should be addressed to Charalampos Mamoulakis; mamoulak@uoc.gr

Academic Editor: Mehraj Sheikh

Bladder leiomyomas (BLs) are extremely rare benign tumors of mesenchymal origin. The exact pathophysiological mechanisms that lead to their appearance remain unclear including hormonal disorders, chromosomal abnormalities, and fetal remnants in the bladder. They usually remain asymptomatic for a long period of time. Solitary fibrous tumors (SFTs) are also rare neoplasms of mesenchymal origin with malignant potential usually affecting the pleura. The pathogenesis of SFTs remains unclear. We report the case of a 28-year-old male presenting with SFT of the pleura and synchronous BL. The patient presented with persistent cough as a sole symptom. Computed tomography (CT) of the thorax revealed a pleural mass, which was surgically removed and proved to be a SFT. At an early follow-up, abdominal CT scan revealed a bladder wall mass that proved to be a BL. This is the first report of BL with synchronous SFT of the pleura. Synchronous BLs and SFTs may be incidental, but the coexistence of two mesenchymal tumors at different sites, in a young patient, may raise the suspicion of a new clinical syndrome that warrants further investigation.

1. Introduction

Bladder leiomyomas (BLs) are very rare benign tumors of mesenchymal origin (<0.5%, <250 cases have been published) [1]. The exact pathophysiological mechanisms that lead to their appearance remain unclear. Several theories have been proposed for the interpretation of their development such as hormonal disorders, vestigial remnants in the bladder, perivascular inflammation-metaplasia of bladder structures, chromosomal abnormalities, and bladder wall infection or inflammation [2]. They are usually asymptomatic (80%) [1], manifesting rarely with hematuria and urge or obstructive urination depending on the localization (endovesical: 63%, extravesical: 30%, and intramural: 7%) [2, 3]. Solitary fibrous tumors (SFTs) are also very rare tumors of mesenchymal origin, usually affecting the pleura. Less than 800 cases have been published globally, accounting for 5% of chest tumors [4]. Extrapleural SFTs are commonly located at the visceral skull and the retroperitoneum [5]. The presence of SFTs in the genitourinary system is extremely rare (14 cases of prostate SFTs [6] and <50 cases of renal SFTs [7] have been published). The pathogenesis of SFTs has not been elucidated, and they usually remain asymptomatic [5]. The aim of this report is to present a unique case of pleural SFT with synchronous BL.

2. Case Presentation

A 28-year-old male visited the outpatient pulmonary clinic of our hospital due to persistent cough during the last six months. Medical history and physical examination did not reveal any pathology. Computed tomography (CT) scan of the thorax showed a tumor ($6.8 \times 5.5 \times 4.5$ cm) of the left pleura (Figures 1 and 2). The mass was surgically removed and proved to be a pleural tumor with varying cellularity composed of uniform spindle cells with fibroblastic morphology and rare mitotic activity (0-1 MF/10 HPF) arranged in a "patternless pattern" or forming short ill-defined

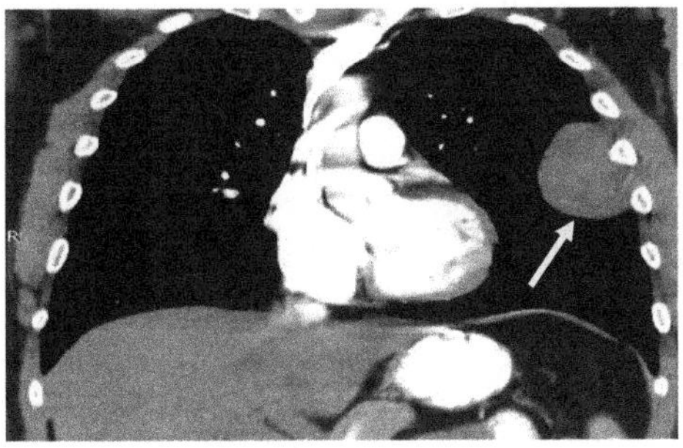

FIGURE 1: Solitary fibrous tumor of the left pleura (grey arrow). Computed tomography, thorax. Coronal view.

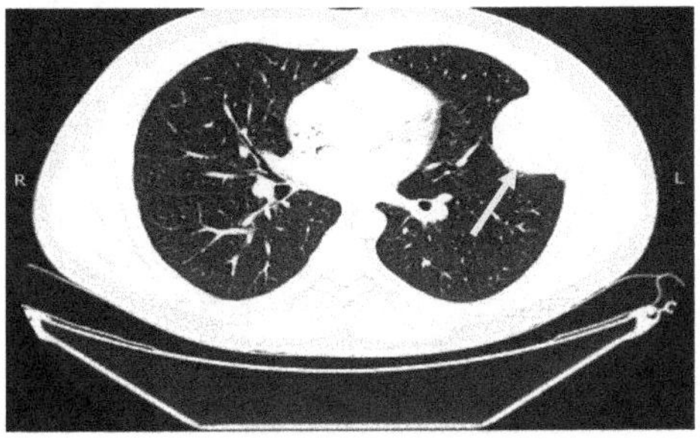

FIGURE 2: Solitary fibrous tumor of the left pleura (grey arrow). Computed tomography, thorax. Horizontal view.

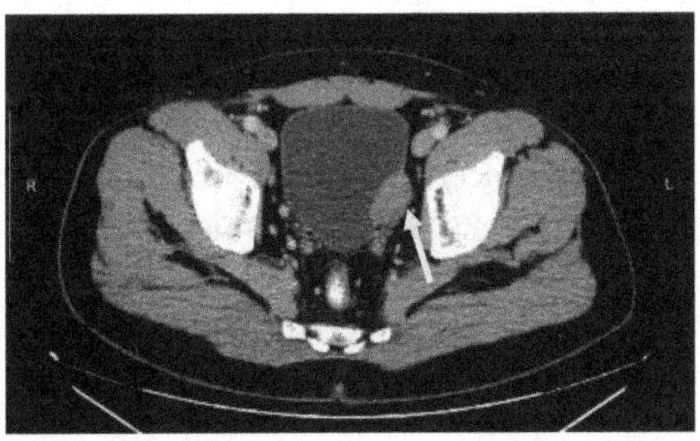

FIGURE 3: Bladder leiomyoma (grey arrow). Computed tomography, low abdomen. Horizontal view.

fascicles in an extensively collagenized and regionally myxoid stroma. Immunohistochemically, tumor cells expressed CD34, vimentin, and Bcl-2, showing no expression of smooth muscle actin (SMA), EMA, Cam 5.2, desmin, and calretinin. These findings were compatible with a SFT of the pleura [6]. At the time of diagnosis, imaging of the lower abdomen was not performed. During a routine follow-up at 6 months postoperatively, CT scan of the abdomen showed a mass at the left bladder wall, 3.7 cm in diameter (Figures 3 and 4). The patient was admitted to our Department of Urology for further evaluation.

The medical history was negative for any urological abnormalities or diseases. The patient did not report any symptoms from the genitourinary system, and the physical examination did not indicate any pathology. Flexible cystoscopy (IMAGE1 S™; Karl Storz, Tuttlingen, Germany) [8, 9] and bladder washout cytology were normal. The patient was submitted to open retropubic surgical exploration for mass

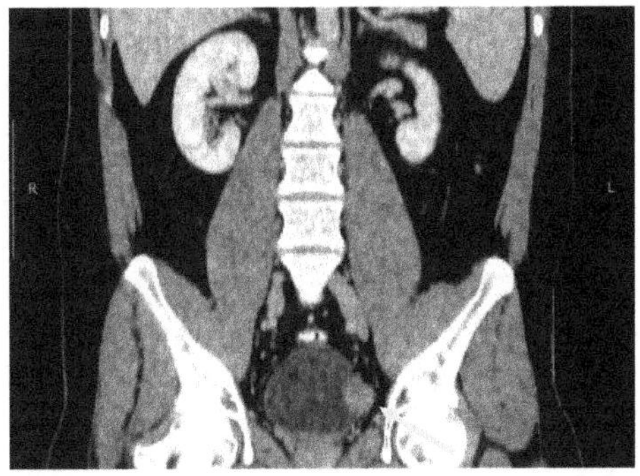

FIGURE 4: Bladder leiomyoma (grey arrow). Computed tomography, abdomen. Coronal view.

TABLE 1: Immunohistochemical markers in solitary fibrous tumors (SFTs) of the pleura and bladder leiomyomas (BL) [11, 18].

IHC tumor marker	SFTs of pleura	BL
STAT-6	+ (>95%)	−
CD34	+ (90-100%)	−
Bcl-2	+ (94.3-100%)	Mostly −
Vimentin	+ (100%)	+
Calretinin	− (0-13% +)	−
Desmin	− (0% +)	+
SMA	− (0% +)	+

removal. The histological examination revealed a benign neoplasm (3.3 × 2.7 × 2.2 cm) composed of dense intersecting fascicles of slender tapered smooth muscle cells, without mitotic activity, nuclear atypia, or areas of necrosis, arranged in a collagenous stroma containing vessels with mural hyalinization. Immunohistochemically, tumor cells expressed muscle antigens such as SMA and desmin, while they were negative for S-100 protein and CD34, [6]. Based on these findings, the diagnosis of BL was set. To the best of our knowledge, this is the first report of a patient presenting with SFT of the pleura and synchronous BL [10].

3. Discussion

The first reference for SFTs was made in 1870, and the first complete description of pleural SFTs in 1931 [11]. They are tumors of mesenchymal origin. Differential diagnosis includes various benign and malignant tumors, such as nerve sheath tumors, type A thymomas, sarcomatoid mesothelioma, and synovial sarcoma. Final diagnosis is based on the histopathological findings, corroborated by the immunohistochemical expression profile of the tumor cells. Immunohistochemical markers and their correspondent rate of expression in pleural SFTs are shown in Table 1; with the most specific being STAT6, which is positive in >95% of the cases. Even though the vast majority of lesions are CD34-positive, this is a nonspecific finding. Furthermore, Bcl-2 and CD99-positive staining is nonspecific and not helpful. SFTs are usually benign, although in 10-15% of the cases they may be

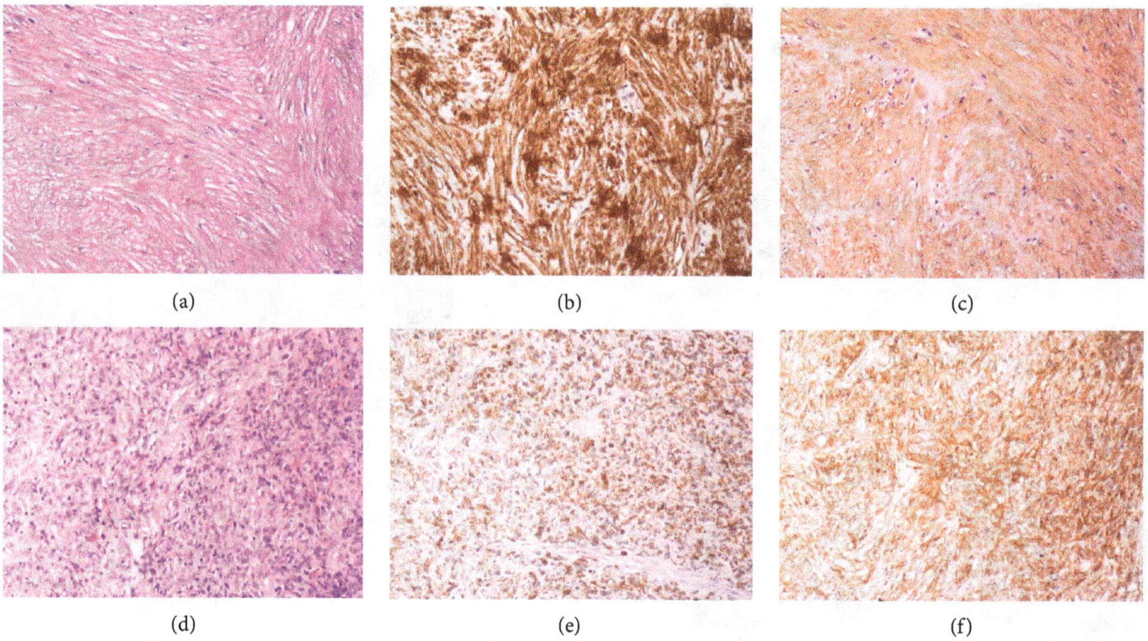

Figure 5: (a–c) Representative images of leiomyoma arising from the muscular wall of urinary bladder stained for H&E (a), desmin (b), and SMA (c), magnification ×200. (d–f) Representative images of pleural solitary fibrous tumor stained for H&E (d), Bcl-2 (e), and CD34 (c), magnification ×200.

metastatic or recurrent [12]. According to the World Health Organization, SFTs are classified as intermediate-rare metastatic tumors [5]. The main features of potential malignancy include tumor size (>15 cm), patient age (>55 years), and the presence of mitotic activity > 4/10 high fields of view (×400 magnification) [6]. None of these features was documented in our case, supporting a benign nature of the tumor.

BLs are tumors of mesenchymal origin, predominately found in women (76%) [13]. Most patients exhibit symptoms such as obstructive urinary symptoms, including acute urine retention, hematuria, and renal colic, while they may also be asymptomatic [13]. In the present case, BL was an incidental finding. Although patient's SFT of the pleura had no malignant characteristics, the possibility of metastasis had to be ruled out. Cystoscopy and negative cytological examination of bladder washout excluded the presence of an endovesical tumor. Imaging methods such as ultrasound, CT, and magnetic resonance imaging cannot differentiate mesenchymal tumors, and surgical removal of the mass is necessary for definite histopathological diagnosis [14]. The surgical methods that have been applied include laparoscopically assisted, robotically assisted, open, transurethral, and transvaginal excision [15] depending on the tumor location. In this case, the tumor was excluded by an open method since endovesical pathology had been excluded. The final diagnosis (extravesical BL) was based on the histopathological characteristics and the immunohistochemical characterization of the tumor cells. Table 1 and Figure 5 present the immunohistochemical markers and features of SFTs/BLs.

According to Moertel's classification for multiple primary cancers and multicentric cancers, multiple primary cancers are grouped into three groups [16]: group I (multiple primary cancers occurring in organs of the same histology), group II (multiple primary tumors originating from different tissues), and group III (cancers from different tissues/organs concurrently existing with group I cancers, and they form multiple primary cancers of three or more cancers). Group IA includes cancers that occur in the same tissue and organ, group IB includes cancers that are from the same tissue and different organs, and group IC includes cancers that occur in bilateral organs. Multiple primary cancers diagnosed simultaneously or within 6 months are termed as synchronous, while those developing at more than a 6-month interval are termed as metachronous [16]. Based on these classifications and definitions, our case is included in group II, and the tumors are considered synchronous.

The presence of multiple primary tumors may be incidental. Nevertheless, multiple primary tumors can be the result of inherited genetic/immunological defects [17]. To the best of our knowledge, synchronous BLs/SFTs are not related to any known syndrome. Nevertheless, coexistence of two mesenchymal tumors at different sites, in a young patient, may raise the suspicion of a new clinical syndrome that warrants further investigation.

4. Conclusion

BLs are very rare benign tumors that possibly coexist with SFTs in extremely rare cases. Surgical exception is the treatment of choice and confirms the diagnosis. Synchronous BL/SFT is not related to any known syndrome and may be incidental. Nevertheless, coexistence of two mesenchymal tumors at different sites, in a young patient, may raise the suspicion of a new clinical syndrome that warrants further investigation.

Acknowledgments

The authors would like to thank Mrs. D. Pantartzi, Scientific Secretary of the Clinical Trial Office of the Department of Urology, University of Crete, Medical School, Heraklion, Crete, Greece, for the administrative and technical support. The authors would like to thank the Special Research Account of the University of Crete for supporting the publication of this study (ELKE No. 3550).

References

[1] J. E. Mendes, A. V. Ferreira, S. A. Coelho, and C. Gil, "Bladder leiomyoma," *Urology Annals*, vol. 9, no. 3, pp. 275–277, 2017.

[2] N. Khater and G. Sakr, "Bladder leiomyoma: presentation, evaluation and treatment," *Arab Journal of Urology*, vol. 11, no. 1, pp. 54–61, 2013.

[3] J. L. Cornella, T. R. Larson, R. A. Lee, J. F. Magrina, and D. Kammerer-Doak, "Leiomyoma of the female urethra and bladder: report of twenty-three patients and review of the literature," *American Journal of Obstetrics and Gynecology*, vol. 176, no. 6, pp. 1278–1285, 1997.

[4] J. M. Ali, A. Ali, M. Van Leuven, and W. R. Bartosik, "Giant solitary fibrous tumour of the pleura an unpredictable entity: case series and literature review," *Annals of the Royal College of Surgeons of England*, vol. 99, no. 6, pp. e165–e171, 2017.

[5] A. Ronchi, I. Cozzolino, F. Zito Marino et al., "Extrapleural solitary fibrous tumor: a distinct entity from pleural solitary fibrous tumor. An update on clinical, molecular and diagnostic features," *Annals of Diagnostic Pathology*, vol. 34, pp. 142–150, 2018.

[6] A. Ronchi, E. La Mantia, V. Gigantino et al., "A rare case of malignant solitary fibrous tumor in prostate with review of the literature," *Diagnostic Pathology*, vol. 12, no. 1, p. 50, 2017.

[7] A. K. Lalwani, S. M. Faiq, and J. Ahuja, "Solitary fibrous tumor of kidney," *Journal of the College of Physicians and Surgeons–Pakistan*, vol. 28, no. 7, pp. 564-565, 2018.

[8] C. Mamoulakis, *The role of image enhancement systems in the management of patients with non-muscle invasive bladder cancer*, ISRCTN Registry, 2016.

[9] C. Mamoulakis, *The contribution of endoscopic image enhancement systems in the management of superficial bladder cancer*, ISRCTN Registry, 2016.

[10] A. Jena, R. Patnayak, A. Y. Lakshmi, B. Manilal, and M. K. Reddy, "Multiple primary cancers: an enigma," *South Asian Journal of Cancer*, vol. 5, no. 1, pp. 29–32, 2016.

[11] B. Geramizadeh, M. Marzban, and A. Churg, "Role of immunohistochemistry in the diagnosis of solitary fibrous tumor, a review," *Iranian Journal of Pathology*, vol. 11, no. 3, pp. 195–203, 2016.

[12] F. Khanchel, M. Driss, K. Mrad, and K. B. Romdhane, "Malignant solitary fibrous tumor in the extremity: cytopathologic findings," *Journal of Cytology*, vol. 29, no. 2, pp. 139–141, 2012.

[13] S. K. Jain, R. Tanwar, and A. Mitra, "Bladder leiomyoma presenting with LUTS and coexisting bladder and uterine leiomyomata: a review of two cases," *Reviews in Urology*, vol. 16, no. 1, pp. 50–54, 2014.

[14] B. Dodia, A. Mahajan, D. Amlani, and S. Bathe, "Leiomyoma of urinary bladder in middle-aged female," *Journal of Obstetrics and Gynaecology of India*, vol. 67, no. 2, pp. 147–149, 2017.

[15] L. He, S. Li, C. Zheng, and C. Wang, "Rare symptomatic bladder leiomyoma: case report and literature review," *The Journal of International Medical Research*, vol. 46, no. 4, pp. 1678–1684, 2018.

[16] C. G. Moertel, "Multiple primary malignant neoplasms: historical perspectives," *Cancer*, vol. 40, 4 Suppl, pp. 1786–1792, 1977.

[17] J. S. Lee, W. Moon, S. J. Park et al., "Triple synchronous primary cancers of rectum, thyroid, and uterine cervix detected during the workup for hematochezia," *Internal Medicine*, vol. 49, no. 16, pp. 1745–1747, 2010.

[18] S. Lott, A. Lopez-Beltran, G. T. Maclennan, R. Montironi, and L. Cheng, "Soft tissue tumors of the urinary bladder, part I: myofibroblastic proliferations, benign neoplasms, and tumors of uncertain malignant potential," *Human Pathology*, vol. 38, no. 6, pp. 807–823, 2007.

23

Extensive Prostatic Abscess in an Elderly Patient Requiring Multidisciplinary Drainage

John Michael Nesemann [1], **Kathy Huen,** [2] **and Jonathan Bergman** [3]

[1] *University of California Los Angeles, David Geffen School of Medicine, Los Angeles, USA*
[2] *Department of Urology, University of California Los Angeles David Geffen School of Medicine, Los Angeles, USA*
[3] *Olive-View UCLA Medical Center, Veterans Association Greater Los Angeles, David Geffen School of Medicine, Los Angeles, USA*

Correspondence should be addressed to John Michael Nesemann; jnesemann@mednet.ucla.edu

Academic Editor: Yankai Xia

Background. Prostatic abscess is rare and mainly affects immunocompromised individuals, classically presenting with both systemic and lower urinary tract symptoms. Our case is unique as the patient presented with an exceptionally long duration of symptoms prior to seeing a health-care provider, had no systemic symptoms, and was managed via a multidisciplinary approach. *Case Presentation.* We present a case of a 70-year-old man with type-two diabetes who endured two months of lower urinary tract symptoms and constipation without systemic symptoms prior to seeking medical attention. He had a positive urinalysis and culture and was initially thought to have a urinary tract infection; however, computed tomography scan revealed a large, complex, and multiloculated prostatic abscess. Multidisciplinary drainage of the abscess was performed by interventional radiology and urology. A postoperative Foley catheter was left in place, and the patient recovered without complications. *Discussion.* Prostatic abscess is uncommon and presents almost exclusively in patients with immunocompromising conditions such as diabetes. Prior to the advent of antibiotics, the major causes were gonorrheal and *Staphylococcus aureus* infections, but with the advent of antibiotics, microbial culprits have shifted to gram-negative organisms. Patients typically present with lower urinary tract symptoms, perineal or lower back pain, and systemic symptoms. Management often consists of intravenous antibiotics and surgical drainage either by transrectal ultrasound-guided needle aspiration, or transurethral deroofing of the prostate. Our case highlights the following: (a) the importance of a high index of suspicion for a prostatic abscess in an immunocompromised patient with persistent leukocytosis and perineal pain after treatment with antibiotics and (b) the potential for an early multidisciplinary approach to draining extensive, loculated prostatic abscesses.

1. Background

Prostatic abscess is a rare entity, described in 0.5-2.5% of patients presenting with inflammatory prostatitis [1]. Its incidence has declined in current clinical practice and is thought to be due to the introduction of broad spectrum antibiotics and the decreased incidence of gonococcal urethritis [2]. Because of its wide range of nonspecific presenting symptoms, it is commonly misdiagnosed as acute bacterial prostatitis or urogenital chronic pelvic pain syndrome, which are far more common [3]. While classically thought of as a sequela of untreated primary urinary tract infection, it is now a marker of men with immune compromise or chronic medical conditions such as diabetes mellitus (DM), human immunodeficiency virus (HIV), hepatic cirrhosis, renal dialysis, chronic indwelling catheters, genitourinary instrumentation, among others [4]. Prostatic abscess is thought to arise from acute or chronic bacterial prostatitis or to develop de novo from retrograde flow of contaminated urine during micturition or from hematogenous seeding. The microbial profile of prostatic abscess has changed drastically since the preantibiotic era, with a majority of cases now being gram-negative in origin and a rising number involving multidrug-resistant organisms [5]. We describe a case of bacterial prostatic abscess in a diabetic patient who waited an exceptionally long time, i.e., two months, prior to seeking medical attention and lacked systemic symptoms. We emphasize the high index of suspicion necessary to diagnose prostatic abscess and review proposed management guidelines, highlighting the potential for an early multidisciplinary approach to the treatment of extensive prostatic abscesses.

2. Case Presentation

A 70-year old man with a history of uncontrolled diabetes (hemoglobin A1c of 16.6%), diabetic foot ulcers for the past three years, and hypertension presented to the emergency room with a two month history of frequency, urgency, nocturia, and constipation requiring manual disimpaction. He denied a history of prostatitis or benign prostatic hyperplasia (BPH); however, he reported a resolved perirectal abscess one year prior to presentation. His lower urinary tract symptoms (LUTSs) had started with difficulty voiding and progressed over two months to frequency and nocturia ten to twelve times per night. He had started wearing a diaper at night and noticed drops of blood in the diaper over the past week but was unsure of the source. Three days prior to presentation, he developed perineal pain radiating to his urethra and rated it as 10/10. His family stated he had been ignoring his symptoms, but he was brought into the emergency department by his wife when she noticed the blood in his diaper. He denied any prior bleeding, fevers, chills, vomiting, or abdominal or flank pain.

On admission, he was afebrile with a heart rate of 95 and a blood pressure of 93/50. His hypotension improved with fluid resuscitation. Physical exam was remarkable for suprapubic tenderness on palpation and an enlarged and mildly tender prostate on digital rectal exam; however, there was no prostatic fluctuance or purulent urethral discharge. A 16 French Foley catheter was placed, and the initial 800 cc of urine was bloody but quickly cleared with irrigation.

Labs were remarkable for leukocytosis of 17.6/mm3, hyperkalemia of 7 mEq/L, bicarbonate of 18 mEq/L, anion gap of 18 mEq/L, creatinine of 1.46 mg/dL, BUN of 36 mg/dL, and a glucose of 883 mg/dL. His urinalysis showed glucose >1000 mg/d, positive ketones, >182 white blood cells/hpf(WBC), negative nitrite, 3+ red blood cells/hpf (RBC), and positive bacteria. Urine culture grew penicillin-resistant, methicillin-sensitive *Staphylococcus aureus* (MSSA), but blood cultures remained negative throughout the hospital stay. He was admitted to the hospital for management of his electrolyte abnormalities. The patient's negative blood cultures made invasive *S. aureus* less likely. As his urine culture grew *S. aureus*, it was suspected he had an isolated urinary tract infection (UTI) and he was started on IV ceftriaxone 1 gram every 24 hours for treatment.

The patient's pain and leukocytosis persisted after three days of hospitalization. After discussion with the primary medical team, it was decided there was a wide differential as to the cause of his urinary retention and leukocytosis and an intravenous contrast enhanced pelvic computed tomography (CT) scan was ordered to obtain more information. It demonstrated a complex multiloculated rim-enhancing fluid collection in the pelvis, predominantly centered within the prostate but extending to the right seminal vesicle, right pelvic sidewall, and the perianal region consistent with a prostatic abscess (Figure 1). The abscess measured 7.8 cm × 6.6 cm. Transesophageal echocardiogram revealed no cardiac vegetations. As his urine culture showed sensitivity to methicillin, he was started on 2 grams of cephazolin every 8 hours. After discussion with radiology, it was felt that the patient would benefit from multidisciplinary treatment due to the multiloculated and extensive nature of his abscess. Thus, a combined approach was pursued where interventional radiology (IR) performed a CT-guided percutaneous drainage of the posterior fluid collection, yielding approximately 10 mL of purulent fluid.

Our patient then underwent transurethral deroofing (TUD) of the abscess for which he was placed in the low lithotomy position after a time-out and initiation of anesthesia. He was given 1 g of vancomycin preoperatively and prepped and draped in a sterile fashion. After dilation, a 26-French rigid resectoscope was inserted. The prostate was noted to be about 2 cm in size and no frank pus was noted. The location of the abscess was determined using preoperative CT imaging. Upon identification of the ureteral orifice, we began to shave away thin layers of the prostate from both the right and left lateral walls. Once pus began to escape into the urethral cavity, several thin layers of the prostate were sequentially shaved away to allow for further evacuation of the abscess cavity (Video 1). Throughout this process, the bladder neck and anterior prostate were spared. A total of 70 mL of pus was removed. A final, vigorous digital rectal exam was performed to expel any residual pus. The infected urine was sent for culture, and the prostate chips were also irrigated out.

An 18-French 3-way Foley catheter was left in place after the procedure. Both wound and urine cultures grew penicillin-resistant, methicillin-sensitive *S. aureus*. He was transferred to the intensive care unit (ICU) postoperatively due to his risk of sepsis. His cefazolin regimen was continued, and his leukocytosis resolved. The patient did not experience any adverse events immediately following the intervention and reported tolerating the procedure well.

He was discharged home where he completed a four-week course of IV cefazolin. He returned to clinic 13 days later, where he was unable to pass a void trial. He passed a repeat void trial 16 days later, and the Foley catheter was removed. Almost a month and a half after the transurethral unroofing of his prostatic abscess, he presented to the emergency department for hyperkalemia and was found to have a post-void residual (PVR) of 400 cc. A Foley was placed and a repeat CT of the abdomen and pelvis showed no hydronephrosis and "near resolution of the previously demonstrated multi-loculated prostatic abscess" (Figure 2). His hyperkalemia resolved, and he was discharged from the medicine service with a Foley two days later. He passed a subsequent void trial, and on telephone follow-up, the patient reported he had no further adverse events and was happy with the outcome of his intervention.

3. Discussion and Conclusion

Prostatic abscess is an uncommon disease due to the widespread and early use of antibiotics in most individuals

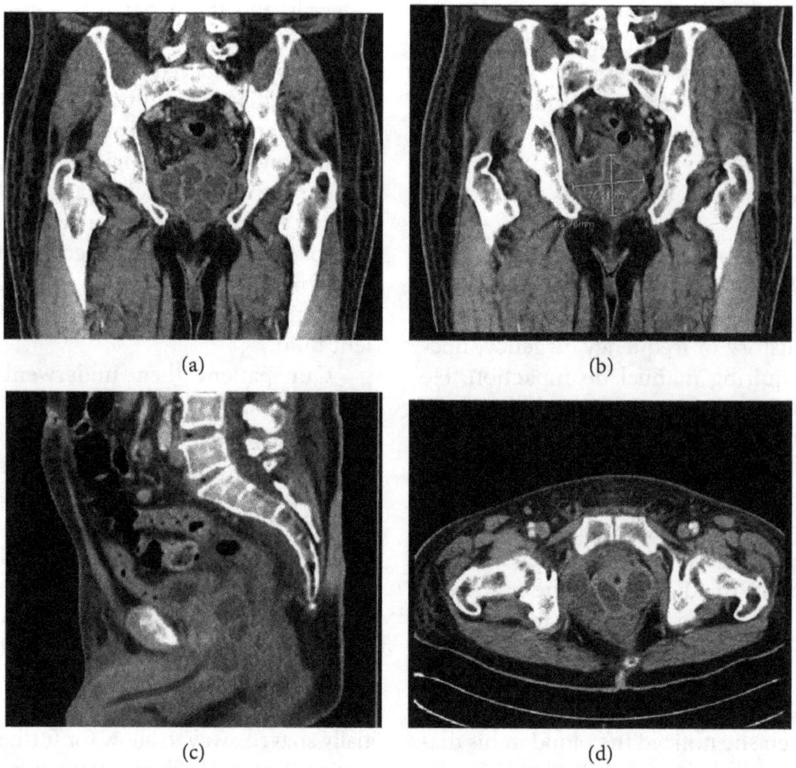

FIGURE 1: CT of the pelvis with contrast showing the multiloculated prostatic abscess in: (a) coronal view, (b) coronal section with measurements, (c) sagittal view showing involvement of the right perirectal/perianal region, and (d) axial view showing invasion of the right pelvic sidewall/obturator muscle.

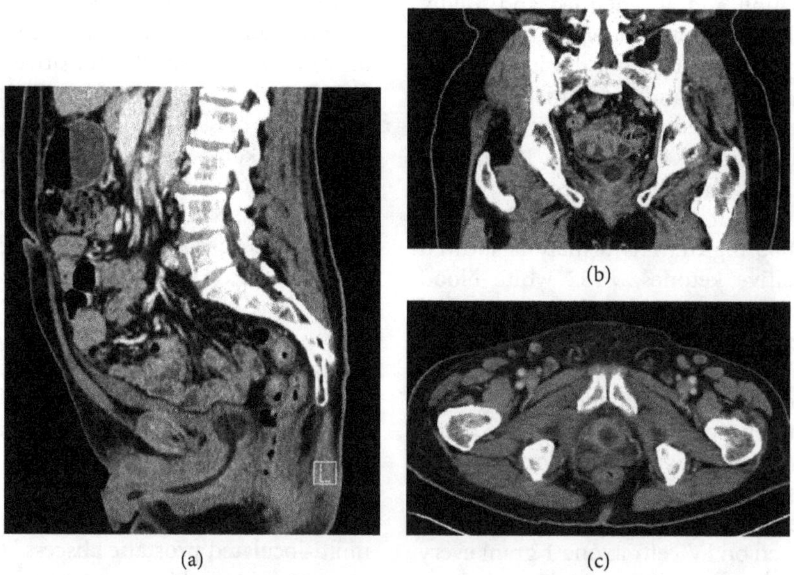

FIGURE 2: CT of the pelvis: (a) sagittal, (b) coronal, and (c) axial views of the prostate showing near resolution of the abscess with minimal residual fluid seen in the left posterior aspect at the base of the prostate.

presenting with lower urinary tract symptoms. It most commonly presents in patients with chronic medical conditions such as diabetes (the most common), cirrhosis, renal dialysis, and chronic indwelling catheters [6]. Other risk factors include HIV or other immunocompromising conditions and recent urogenital instrumentation or surgery. Prostatic abscess spreads hematogenously in approximately one quarter of patients, as may be the case with this patient's diabetic foot ulcers, but urinary tract infections and acute bacterial prostatitis are additional etiologies [2].

Prior to the advent of antibiotics, prostatic abscesses were a common complication of gonorrheal infection in otherwise healthy men, with *Staphylococcus aureus* being the other common causative organism [7]. The introduction of antibiotics shifted the microbial culprits to mostly gram-negative organisms, which have been detected in 60-90% of prostatic abscess cultures [8, 9]. Of the gram-negatives, the most common is *Escherichia coli* with 75% of isolates susceptible to first-line antibiotics in the 1990s but only 22% in the 2000s [5]. Recently, there have been increasing numbers of case reports detailing incidences of both methicillin-sensitive and resistant *S. aureus*, with 33 cases reported in the literature as of 2014 [10]. Other reported bacterial pathogens include *Klebsiella pneumoniae*, *Pseudomonas aeruginosa*, *Enterococcus* species, *Streptococcus* species, and *Burkholderia pseudomallei* [2, 5].

Prostatic abscess classically occurs in middle-aged men who present with hesitancy, weakened stream, dysuria, fever, perineal discomfort or low back pain, and leukocytosis. Urinary retention occurs in up to one-third of patients [2]. This case is atypical in that the patient had an exceptionally long duration of symptoms prior to presenting for care. Moreover, he denied systemic symptoms, which are the only presenting symptom in up to one-third of patients [2], and was afebrile, which according to Weinberger et al.'s [8] report, fever occurs in up to 72% of cases. A tender prostate is typically present on physical exam, but a normal digital rectal exam has been reported in 23% of patients [9]. While fluctuance is pathognomonic, its incidence varies from 16 to 88% [4, 8]. As symptoms are variable, diagnosing the condition requires a high index of suspicion in any patients with risk factors who present with lower urinary tract symptoms and signs of infection. When clinically suspected based on systemic and lower urinary tract symptoms in a patient with DM or other immunosuppressive conditions, the workup for prostatic abscess includes imaging with computed tomography or transrectal ultrasonography, and blood and urine cultures.

There is no clear consensus on treatment, but management typically consists of a combination of oral or parenteral antibiotics with surgical drainage via either transrectal ultrasound- (TRUS-) guided drainage or transurethral deroofing, depending on the size and location of the abscess [4, 11, 12]. As Collado et al. [9] reported symptoms of sepsis in 19% of their patients, it can be assumed that prostatic abscesses are high risk for sepsis and should be considered for inpatient management. These patients should be given parenteral antibiotics, with possible options including third-generation cephalosporins or aminoglycosides with ampicillin. Stable patients with a small abscess (<1 cm) may be tried on conservative therapy with serial imaging to ensure resolution; however, most individuals require surgical drainage [11, 13].

The most common surgical drainage option is TRUS-guided needle aspiration, which can be carried out at the bedside and allows for diagnosis and treatment in a single procedure. It has a low rate of infectious complications but serious, and sometimes fatal, episodes of sepsis have been reported [5]. It is also preferred for hemodynamically unstable patients as the anesthesia required for operating on these patients carries a high risk of further deterioration. However, the greatest limitation of this mode of treatment is abscess recurrence or incomplete treatment, which ranges from 16 to 22% [14, 15]. Some experts advocate transurethral deroofing (TUD) of the prostate for large, multiloculated abscesses (as in this patient) as up to one-third of prostatic abscess patients will eventually need transurethral resection of the prostate [5]. This is especially true if the prostate is very large (>80 g), there are residual abscesses, and if the patient suffers from symptomatic benign prostatic hyperplasia [12]. TUD is associated with lower rates of recurrence, as low as 7% in one study [12], and significant shorter hospital length when compared to needle aspiration [14]. A 2017 study of 44 patients with large (>2 cm) or multiple abscesses or abscesses not responding to antibiotic therapy compared patients who had received TRUS-guided needle aspiration with those who had received TUD and found that 96% of patients responded to transurethral deroofing while only 84.1% responded to TRUS-guided needle aspiration ($p < 0.23$) [16]. They also found that six patients in the TRUS group had abscess recurrence while only one in the transurethral deroofing group suffered recurrence ($p < 0.03$). TUD of the prostate carries the same risks as transurethral resection of the prostate, such as retrograde ejaculation, urethral stricture, and incontinence.

In the case of our patient, it was decided to pursue a multidisciplinary approach to management combining TUD of the abscess with a posterior needle aspiration. As our patient had a large (>2 cm), multiloculated abscess, we chose to pursue TUD as this is often recommended for large abscesses [12], and has been associated with lower rates of recurrence and shorter hospital stays [12, 14, 16]. Since the abscess extended out from the prostate to the right seminal vesicle, right pelvic sidewall, and the perianal region, it was decided a TUD of the abscess alone would not adequately drain all of the abscess cavities. Thus, a needle aspiration of the posterior fluid collection was also performed by IR. We believed this would give the patient the best chance at recovering from this serious condition.

The prostate deroofing procedure has been described by other authors [16, 17], and we have described our version in the case presentation. Our procedure is most similar to that described by Goyal et al. [17] as we spared the bladder neck and anterior prostate, although our deroofing was more focused as we did not resect other portions of the prostate once adequate drainage had been achieved. There is no mention of digital rectal exam during surgery in order to expel abscess contents, but we believe this maneuver was helpful.

Many of the case reports in the literature describe attempting TRUS-guided drainage, and if there is no improvement, proceeding to TUD of the prostate [18–21]. Here, we report a description of a multidisciplinary approach to draining an extensive and loculated prostate abscess. We believe this approach may be useful for abscess drainage as it has the potential to access multiple areas of loculated abscesses and thus theoretically provide greater drainage compared to a single approach. While this case report presents a new management possibility, the evidence is limited due to the single patient experience reported and lack of control group for comparison. However, further study could elucidate the potential benefits of this approach to the drainage of extensive prostate abscesses.

This case illustrates the importance of a high index of suspicion for a prostatic abscess if there is persistent leukocytosis and perineal pain in an immunocompromised patient with a urinary tract infection after treatment with intravenous antibiotics. Finally, the TUD- and IR-guided percutaneous drainage performed in quick succession for this patient highlights the potential for an early multidisciplinary approach to draining extensive, loculated prostatic abscesses.

Abbreviations

LUTS: Lower urinary tract symptoms
DM: Diabetes mellitus
HIV: Human immunodeficiency virus
WBC: White blood cells
RBC: Red blood cells
MSSA: Methicillin-sensitive Staphylococcus aureus
UTI: Urinary tract infection
IV: Intra-venous
CT: Computed tomography
ICU: Intensive care unit
PVR: Post void residual
TRUS: Trans-rectal ultrasound
TUD: Trans-urethral deroofing
IR: Interventional radiology.

Ethical Approval

All interventions were part of standard healthcare practices; thus, ethical approval was neither required nor sought.

Consent

Informed consent was obtained from the patient for publication of this case report and any accompanying images. A copy of the consent is available for review by the editor of this journal.

Disclosure

The content is solely the responsibility of the authors and does not necessarily represent the official views of the NIH or UCGHI. This institution is providing financial means for the corresponding author to conduct research for a year but had no role in the design, collection, analysis, and interpretation of data.

Authors' Contributions

JN gathered and interpreted the patient's clinical course in drafting the report. KH conceived the work, gathered the patient's clinical data, and substantially reviewed the drafted work. JB played a major role in the conception of the work and made significant contributions to the drafted work. All authors have read and approved the manuscript.

Acknowledgments

This project was supported by the National Eye Institute and the Fogarty International Center of the National Institutes of Health (NIH) under award number D43TW009343 as well as the University of California Global Health Institute (UCGHI) in the form of a Fogarty grant to John Nesemann.

Supplementary Materials

Video 1: This video demonstrates shaving away thin layers of the prostate. Prior to the start of the video the urethral orifice was identified and we began to shave away thin layers of the prostate from the lateral walls. As shown in the video, once pus began to escape into the urethral cavity several more layers of the prostate were sequentially shaved away to allow for further evacuation of the abscess cavity. Throughout this process the bladder neck and anterior prostate were spared. *(Supplementary materials)*

References

[1] J. E. Langer and F. Cornud, "Inflammatory disorders of the prostate and the distal genital tract," *Radiologic Clinics of North America*, vol. 44, no. 5, pp. 665–677, 2006, vii.

[2] A. L. Ackerman, P. S. Parameshwar, and J. T. Anger, "Diagnosis and treatment of patients with prostatic abscess in the post-antibiotic era," *International Journal of Urology*, vol. 25, no. 2, pp. 103–110, 2018.

[3] J. C. Nickel, J. Downey, D. Hunter, and J. Clark, "Prevalence of prostatitis-like symptoms in a population based study using the National Institutes of Health chronic prostatitis symptom index," *The Journal of Urology*, vol. 165, no. 3, pp. 842–845, 2001.

[4] E. A. Granados, G. Riley, J. Salvador, and J. Vicente, "Prostatic abscess: diagnosis and treatment," *The Journal of Urology*, vol. 148, no. 1, pp. 80–82, 1992.

[5] S. K. Bhagat, N. S. Kekre, G. Gopalakrishnan, V. Balaji, and M. S. Mathews, "Changing profile of prostatic abscess," *International Braz J Urol*, vol. 34, no. 2, pp. 164–170, 2008.

[6] A. Naboush, A. A. Yassine, M. Yasmin, and N. Mobarakai, "Community-acquired methicillin-resistant Staphylococcus aureus prostatic abscess presenting as acute urinary retention: a case report and review of the literature," *Case Reports in Infectious Diseases*, vol. 2013, 5 pages, 2013.

[7] J. C. Sargent and R. Irwin, "Prostatic abscess: a clinical study of 42 cases," *The American Journal of Surgery.*, vol. 11, no. 2, pp. 334–337, 1931.

[8] M. Weinberger, S. Cytron, C. Servadio, C. Block, J. B. Rosenfeld, and S. D. Pitlik, "Prostatic abscess in the antibiotic era," *Reviews of Infectious Diseases*, vol. 10, no. 2, pp. 239–249, 1988.

[9] A. Collado, J. Palou, J. Garcia-Penit, J. Salvador, P. de la Torre, and J. Vicente, "Ultrasound-guided needle aspiration in prostatic abscess," *Urology*, vol. 53, no. 3, pp. 548–552, 1999.

[10] T. Jana, J. D. Machicado, G. E. Davogustto, and J. J. Pan, "Methicillin-resistant Staphylococcus aureus prostatic abscess in a liver transplant recipient," *Case Reports in Transplantation*, vol. 2014, 7 pages, 2014.

[11] H. Abdelmoteleb, F. Rashed, and A. Hawary, "Management of prostate abscess in the absence of guidelines," *International Braz J Urol*, vol. 43, no. 5, pp. 835–840, 2017.

[12] A. M. Elshal, A. Abdelhalim, T. S. Barakat, A. A. Shaaban, A. Nabeeh, and E.-H. Ibrahiem, "Prostatic abscess: objective assessment of the treatment approach in the absence of guidelines," *Arab Journal of Urology*, vol. 12, no. 4, pp. 262–268, 2019.

[13] M. Ludwig, I. Schroeder-Printzen, H. G. Schiefer, and W. Weidner, "Diagnosis and therapeutic management of 18 patients with prostatic abscess," *Urology*, vol. 53, no. 2, pp. 340–345, 1999.

[14] K. Jang, D. H. Lee, S. H. Lee, and B. H. Chung, "Treatment of prostatic abscess: case collection and comparison of treatment methods," *Korean Journal of Urology*, vol. 53, no. 12, pp. 860–864, 2012.

[15] C. Gogus, E. Ozden, R. Karaboga, and C. Yagci, "The value of transrectal ultrasound guided needle aspiration in treatment of prostatic abscess," *European Journal of Radiology*, vol. 52, no. 1, pp. 94–98, 2004.

[16] B. Purkait, M. Kumar, A. K. Sokhal, A. Bansal, S. N. Sankhwar, and V. Bhaskar, "Outcome analysis of transrectal ultrasonography guided aspiration versus transurethral resection of prostatic abscess: 10 years' experience from a tertiary care hospital," *Arab Journal of Urology*, vol. 15, no. 3, pp. 254–259, 2019.

[17] N. K. Goyal, A. Goel, S. Sankhwar, and D. Dalela, "Transurethral resection of prostate abscess: is it different from conventional transurethral resection for benign prostatic hyperplasia?," *ISRN Urology*, vol. 2013, 5 pages, 2013.

[18] J. Docekal, J. Hall, B. Reese, J. Jones, and T. Ferguson, "A rare presentation of community acquired methicillin resistant Staphylococcus aureus," *Case Reports in Infectious Diseases*, vol. 2013, 3 pages, 2013.

[19] D. E. Carroll, I. Marr, G. K. L. Huang, D. C. Holt, S. Y. C. Tong, and C. S. Boutlis, "Staphylococcus aureus prostatic abscess: a clinical case report and a review of the literature," *BMC Infectious Diseases*, vol. 17, no. 1, p. 509, 2017.

[20] S. C. Park, J. W. Lee, and J. S. Rim, "Prostatic abscess caused by community-acquired methicillin-resistant Staphylococcus aureus," *International Journal of Urology*, vol. 18, no. 7, pp. 536–538, 2011.

[21] D. J. Lachant, M. Apostolakos, and A. Pietropaoli, "Methicillin resistant Staphylococcus aureus prostatic abscess with bacteremia," *Case Reports in Infectious Diseases*, vol. 2013, 5 pages, 2013.

Male Perineal Carcinoma: Experience in 4 Cases and Literature Review

Agustín Fraile Poblador,[1] Manuel Hevia Palacios,[1] Manuel Rodríguez Vegas,[2] Alberto Artiles Medina,[1] Enrique Sanz Mayayo,[1] Silvia García Barreras,[1] Guillermo Fernández Conejo,[1] Rafael Rodríguez Patrón,[1] Varona Crespo Constatino,[3] Ana Saiz González,[3] and Javier Burgos Revilla[1]

[1]*Urology Department, IRYCIS (Institute of Biosanitary Research of the Ramon y Cajal Hospital), Crta Colmenar Viejo, Km 9, 100, 28034 Madrid, Spain*

[2]*Plastic Surgery Department, IRYCIS (Institute of Biosanitary Research of the Ramon y Cajal Hospital), Crta Colmenar Viejo, Km 9, 100, 28034 Madrid, Spain*

[3]*Anatomic Pathology Department, IRYCIS (Institute of Biosanitary Research of the Ramon y Cajal Hospital), Crta Colmenar Viejo, Km 9, 100, 28034 Madrid, Spain*

Correspondence should be addressed to Agustín Fraile Poblador; agustinfraile78@hotmail.com and Manuel Hevia Palacios; manuel.hevia.palacios@gmail.com

Academic Editor: Claudio Simeone

Perineal carcinoma of unknown origin is a rare and aggressive disease, so an early diagnosis and adequate treatment are essential to prevent its progression. We report the first series of cases of perineal carcinoma of unknown origin: (I) a 62-year-old male patient being followed up for a urethral stricture treated with periodic dilations with subsequent development of perineal abscesses and perineal carcinoma; (II) a 67-year-old male patient who consults for urinary discomfort associated with a perineal abscess. Recurrence of the abscess in the first month revealed the presence of an underlying perineal carcinoma; (III) a 78-year-old male patient that underwent urethroplasty with graft with subsequent regimen of periodical dilations. Recurrent formation of perianal abscesses revealed the presence of an underlying perineal carcinoma; and (IV) a 78-year-old male patient with history of in situ penile carcinoma treated by glans resurfacing. He consulted for penile pain, and imaging tests revealed a perineal abscess adjacent to the left corpus cavernosum. The core needle biopsy revealed a squamous cell carcinoma. Penile exploration and negative glans biopsy ruled out possible recurrence of penile carcinoma. The form of presentation of the disease has been very similar in all patients, demonstrating the presence of perineal abscess in all cases. Two patients had inguinal lymph node disease at diagnosis. All patients were treated by surgery, and three of them required adjuvant systemic treatment. Surgery combined with systemic treatment is probably the best option if the patient's conditions allow it.

1. Introduction

Carcinomas of unknown primary (CUP) origin represent 3-5% of all malignant tumors. Squamous cell CUP accounts for 5-10% of CUP, and the involvement of the male pelvis is extremely rare [1]. Perineal carcinoma can be derived, as in our case, from a process of inflammation and chronic infection in a patient with a urological history. Inflammatory process sustains the proliferation and survival of malignant transformed cells, can promote angiogenesis and metastatic processes, can negatively regulate the antitumoral adaptive and innate immune responses, and may alter the efficacy of therapeutic agents [2]. Initial presenting symptoms include buttock pain, rectal urgency, constipation, diarrhea, and urinary frequency [1]. The uniqueness of this series of cases is supported by the lack of published case reports.

Surgical intervention remains the leading form of therapy; however, approaches are case specific, depending on the location of the tumor and the degree of invasiveness [3].

2. Case Presentation

2.1. Case 1. A 62-year-old male patient with a history of bulbar urethral stricture was treated with periodic dilations for three years. In this context, the patient develops a urethrocutaneous fistula that was treated conservatively with a suprapubic and a bladder catheter.

A combined cystography is performed through the suprapubic catheter and the bladder catheter, which reveals an extravasation of urine is observed at the level of the bulbar urethra compatible with urethral fistula. The endoscopic examination revealed a devitalized penile and bulbar urethra without finding a fistulous orifice. Conservative treatment fails, and the patient presents perineal abscesses that require treatment up to four times, two of them with percutaneous drainage and the other two by open surgery. The microbiological examination revealed the presence of gram +, gram -, and anaerobic bacteria. The patient was treated with piepracillin/tazobactan associated with IV metronidazole. During the follow-up, three months later, the patient underwent several CT scans in which anfractuous collection located in the root of the penis was observed, with approximate measurements of 66 × 25 mm, unchanged from previous studies. There are no images to suggest the presence of tumor tissue. Three months later and after the failure of conservative management, the case is discussed in the clinical session together with the other members of the urology department, and it is decided to perform a Wallace-type urinary diversion and a Friedrich of the perineal wound. The patient presented a good evolution after the intervention, and the pathological result of the debridement of the perineal wound was a well-differentiated perineal carcinoma that widely affects the margins of the analyzed tissue. An extension study was carried out with PET-CT after administration of 18-FDG in which a voluminous heterogeneous perineal mass was observed, with a significant increase in metabolism, affecting both the corpora cavernosa and spongiosum body, and involves the left ischiopubic branch as well as the anal canal. The prostatic apex is affected by contiguity.

Bilateral inguinal lymphadenopathies of up to 11 mm are observed with increased metabolic activity. The case was presented in the multidisciplinary oncology committee, and it was decided to perform a complete pelvic exenteration with inguinal lymph node dissection and total penectomy.

The surgery consisted of two phases:

(i) Phase I: A complete pelvic exenteration with iliac-obturator lymph node dissection was done

(ii) Phase II: Incision was made with a cold scalpel over the limits of the mass in the cutaneous plane. The bulbar urethra and the corpora cavernosa were removed from their roots. Penile degloving was performed, and the penis was extracted through the perineal incision, thus achieving an en bloc removal of all tumor tissue. Osteotomy and resection of both ischiopubic branches were performed for on block removal of surgical piece (Figure 1). Bilateral inguinal lymphadenectomy was performed

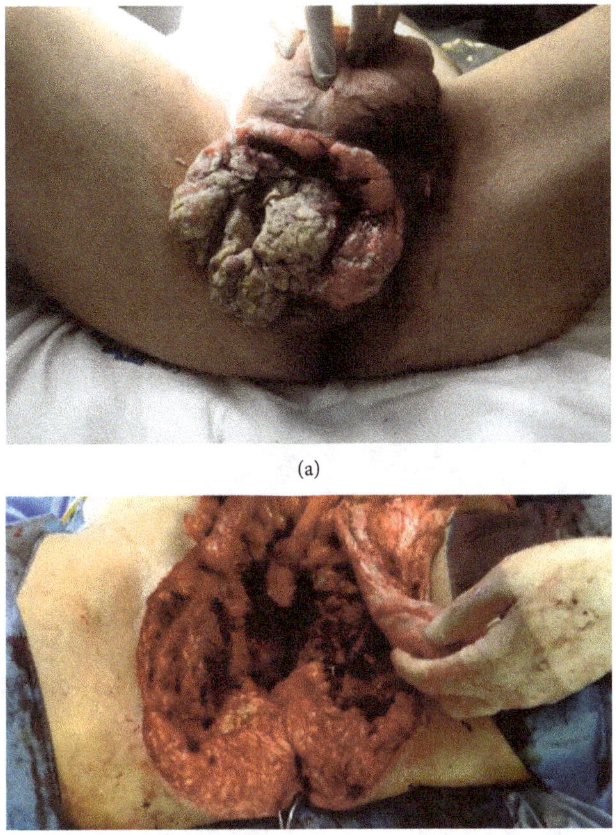

(a)

(b)

FIGURE 1: Locally advanced perineal carcinoma. (a) A voluminous and heterogeneous perineal mass. (b) Total penectomy and pelvis exenteration with resection of both ischiopubic branches.

A vacuum-assisted closure system (VAC) was placed to perform a delayed closure.

Perineal closure was performed with the help of the plastic surgery department with a latissimus dorsi flap and a PTFE-polypropylene mesh. The patient remained hospitalized for 3 months. The functional recovery was excellent, allowing the patient the autonomy necessary to continue home rehabilitation.

The pathological result of specimen resulted in a well-differentiated squamous cell carcinoma of the perineal region of 11 cm in diameter that massively infiltrates the soft tissues of the perineum, spreading and infiltrating the penile root, prostatic capsule, and perianal and peri-bladder adipose tissue, affecting the bone fragments of the pubis and ischium without infiltrating the cortex. Two lymph node metastases were observed in the left inguinal lymph node dissection piece containing 7 lymph nodes in total. The patient subsequently received adjuvant treatment with four cycles of carboplatin and gemcitabine. After 3 year of follow-up, he continues with periodic reviews with PET-CT

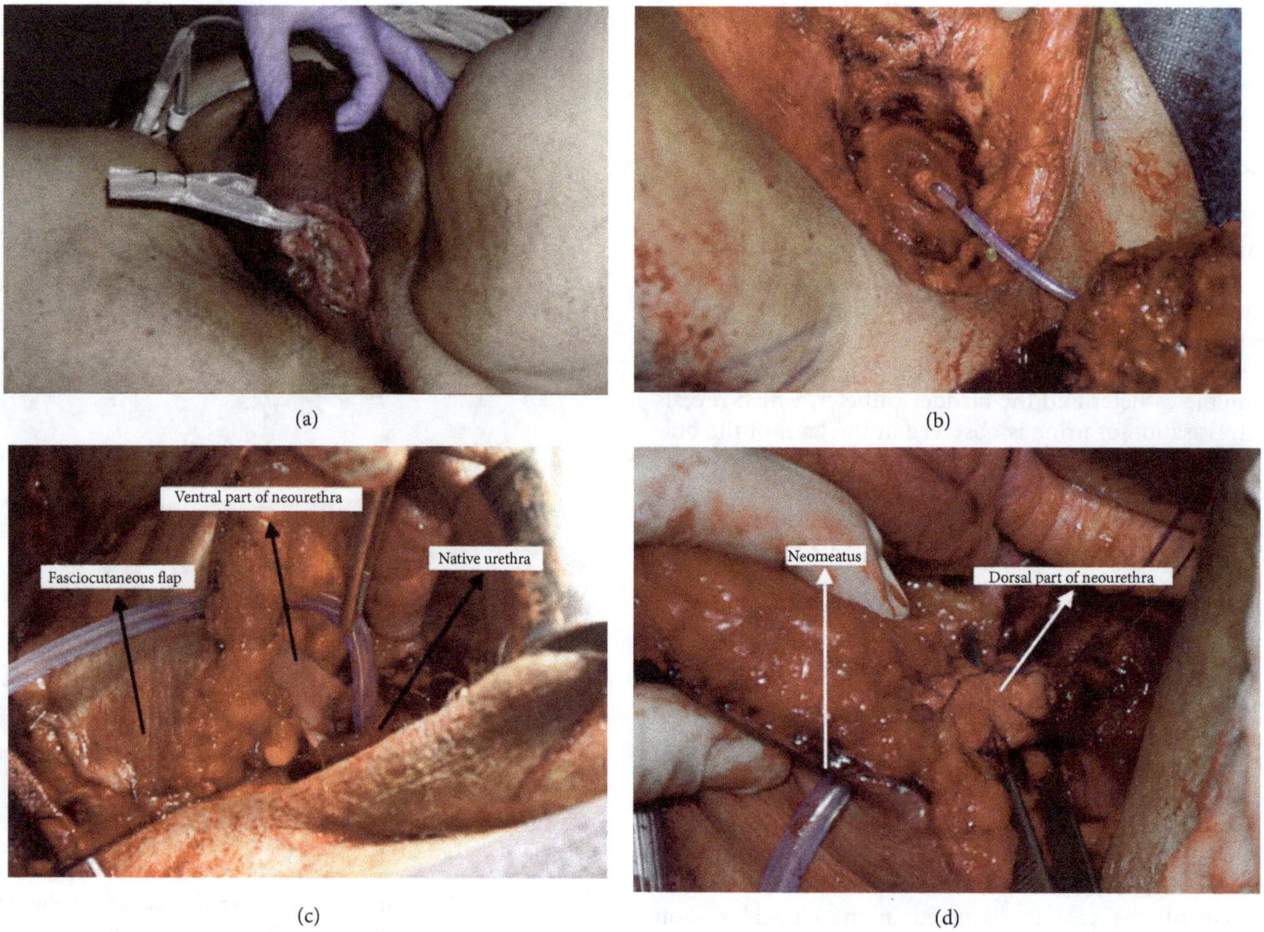

FIGURE 2: En-bloc excision of carcinoma and reconstruction of perineal defect. (a) Perineal wound indurated on palpation with drainage of purulent material. (b) En-bloc excision of tumor tissue. The prostatic apex can be seen. (c) Ventral side of neourethra. (d) Double buccal mucosa tubular graft. The neourethra is passed through the fasciocutaneous flap.

without recurrence of his disease with excellent functional recovery.

2.2. Case 2. A 67-year old male patient with a medical history of diabetes mellitus, chronic kidney disease, and dyslipidemia who consults for urinary discomfort, dysuria, and frequency for three months was associated with a perineal abscess. The cystography shows a contrast extravasation at the level of the bulbar urethra compatible with urethral fistula, and the endoscopic examination shows a devitalized bulbar urethra with a stenotic area that prevents the endoscope from passing. During the exploration, abundant saline solution was observed through the perineum. Surgical drainage of the collection was performed as well as placement of a bladder and suprapubic catheter. Microbiological examination did not show growth of bacteria or fungi, despite which he was treated with piperacillin/tazobactan. In the first month of follow-up, the patient returned to the emergency room due to pain at the scrotal level and at the root of the penis associated with the recurrence of the collection, so it was decided to perform a new drainage of the abscess and a Friedrich of the perineal wound.

The anatomopathological outcomes of the latter revealed the existence of a well-differentiated squamous cell carcinoma in areas of abundant keratinization that widely infiltrate the skin and soft tissue. On physical examination, the patient presents a perineal wound with drainage of purulent material, indurated on palpation, and adhered to deep planes.

CT scan and MRI reveal a mass with irregular borders with a maximum diameter of 84 mm that invades both corpora cavernosa and the corpus spongiosum, reaching the urethral bulb. The existence of metastases was excluded. After discussing the case in the multidisciplinary tumor committee, the surgical treatment was decided.

The surgical procedure consisted of different phases. Phase I: Total penectomy was performed, and en bloc removal of tumor tissue was done (Figures 2(a) and 2(b)). Phase II: Neourethra was performed with a double buccal mucosa graft, and internal pudendal fasciocutaneous flap was performed to cover the dead space and provide vascular support to the neourethra (Figures 2(c) and 2(d)).

The procedure lasted 9 hours and the estimated blood loss was 500 cc. During the postoperative period, the patient remained with the urinary catheter through the neourethra,

Table 1: Literature review.

Literature	Age	Presentation	Metastasis in other organs at diagnosis	Treatment	Follow up (months)
Chiec et al. 2014	52	Buttock pain	Liver, lung	Chemoradiation (cisplatin; 6000 centigray in 30 fractions)	12
Creta et al. 2017	78	Urethral stricture and perineal abscess	—	Palliative colostomy	3
Present	62	Urethral stricture and perineal abscess	Inguinal lymph nodes	Surgery + chemotherapy (carboplatin/gemcitabine)	36
Present	67	Urethral stricture and perineal abscess	—	Surgery + immunotherapy (cemiplimab 350 mg IV)	9
Present	78	Urethral stricture and perineal abscess	—	Surgery	30
Present	78	Penile pain, perineal abscess	Inguinal lymph nodes	Surgery + chemotherapy (cisplatin + 5-Fluoracil)	17

a suprapubic catheter, and a rectal catheter to keep the receiving area of the flap as dry as possible. The patient was discharged on the twelfth day after surgery. During admission, he presented with a superficial dehiscence of the skin of the flap that was successfully treated with local paraffin dressings.

The patient presented a satisfactory postoperative period, being able to remove the urinary catheter and suprapubic catheter at 3 weeks prior urethrography, achieving spontaneous urination without involuntary leakage of urine.

The histological study reveals a moderately differentiated squamous cell carcinoma with keratinization and pleomorphic areas. The tumor shows neurotropism and frequent mitotic figures. The surgical edges were not compromised.

The patient received three cycles of adjuvant treatment with immunotherapy (cemiplimab 350 mg every 21 days), because was not subsidiary to treatment with platinum for renal failure. At 7 months postoperatively, he was diagnosed with pulmonary metastases associating massive pleural effusion that required thoracentesis in addition to pelvic and local lymph node disease. He passed out 9 months after surgery.

2.3. Case 3. A 78-year-old male patient with history of high blood pressure, dyslipidemia, and bulbar urethral stricture was treated by urethroplasty with dura graft in 1989. Subsequently, he underwent periodical dilations due to a recurrence of the stricture. The patient has perineal abscesses on multiple occasions that required surgical drainage. In the last drainage, a mamelon lesion suspected of carcinoma was observed adjacent to the perineal collection. The pathological result of the lesion reveals the existence of a well-differentiated squamous cell carcinoma. The extension study confirms the existence of a perineal collection that extends through both corpora cavernosa measuring 79 × 15 mm with solid and necrotic areas. In the first instance, the patient underwent a resection of the perineal tumor and a radical cystoprostatectomy. Subsequently, the perineal defect was covered with a fasciocutaneous flap. The pathological examination revealed the existence of a squamous cell carcinoma that affected both corpora cavernosa and corpus spongiosum, the perineal soft tissues, and the prostatic apex, leaving the surgical margins free of tumor. After one year of follow-up, the patient presented on imaging tests a recurrence in the pelvic bed that seemed to infiltrate the right ischiopubic branch and the right lateral wall of the rectum. The case is discussed in the multidisciplinary tumor committee, and the surgical treatment is decided. The patient underwent an abdominoperineal amputation, resection of the previous fasciocutaneous flap, and partial resection of the right ischiopubic branch. The perineal defect is covered with an anterolateral flap of the thigh.

The patient was discharged at 3 weeks without complications in the immediate postoperative period. After 2 years and 6 months of follow-up, the patient remains free of disease and with a complete functional recovery.

2.4. Case 4. A 78-year-old male patient with history of high blood pressure, a renal tumor that underwent partial nephrectomy, and a carcinoma in situ in the glans was treated by resurfacing. During the follow-up, the patient reported perineal and penile pain of months of evolution. The imaging tests performed revealed an abscess with a solid pole in the infrapubic region that affects the left corpus cavernosum. A core needle biopsy of the solid area was performed, diagnosing squamous cell carcinoma.

In the extension study, multiple indeterminate pulmonary nodules were identified. In the preoperative study, a significant growth of the perineal mass was observed, reaching 75 mm in its maximum diameter and affecting the left ischiopubic branch, adductor muscles, and ipsilateral gracilis. Pathological left inguinal lymph nodes were also observed.

Penile exploration and negative glans biopsy ruled out possible recurrence of penile carcinoma. The case was discussed in the multidisciplinary tumor committee, and the surgical treatment was decided.

The patient underwent total penectomy, resection of left isquiopubic branch, and partial resection of adductor muscles of the thigh and left inguinal lymph node dissection.

The perineal defect was covered with a contralateral gracilis flap.

The patient required postoperative wound debridement due to partial necrosis of the wound. The patient was discharged 3 weeks after the intervention with good functional recovery. The histological study revealed the existence of a moderately differentiated squamous cell carcinoma with a maximum diameter of 7.5 that affects the root of the penis and both corpora cavernosa. Inguinal lymph node dissection showed one metastatic node of the six resected. The patient received adjuvant chemotherapy treatment with cisplatin and 5-FU. At 6 months of follow-up, the patient presented a single left inguinal lymph node, subjected to excision with pathological results of metastasis of squamous cell carcinoma. After 17 months of follow-up, the patient presented pulmonary progression of the disease under treatment with the fourth line of chemotherapy treatment.

3. Discussion

We present a series of cases of 4 patients diagnosed with perineal squamous cell carcinoma undergoing surgical treatment. The uniqueness of this series of cases is supported by the lack of published case reports describing men patients with this malignancy treated surgically (Table 1). The two cases previously described were treated, one of them with chemoradiotherapy and the other with palliative treatment given the advanced state of the disease [1, 4]. From the published literature regarding squamous cell CUP in the pelvic region, the patients described were all women [1].

Carcinomas of unknown primary origin represent 3-5% of all malignancies and are defined as a heterogeneous group of tumors for which the primary origin cannot be established at the time of diagnosis. Within them, squamous carcinoma of unknown primary origin represents between 5 and 10% and is more frequent in the head and neck region, although they are also described at the uterine level and in iliac lymph nodes [1]. The presence of this type of tumors in the pelvic cavity is very rare, and the majority of cases described have occurred in women; there are only two cases reported in the literature of perineal carcinoma of unknown origin in men [1, 4].

Regarding the pathophysiology of these tumors, several articles have been written relating the inflammatory status with an increase in IL-1β that stimulates the NF-κB pathway, highly involved in angiogenic and protumorigenic processes [5].

Patients with chronic infections of the perineal region, suppurative hydrosadenitis [6], urethral fistula, or any inflammatory/infectious process with a torpid evolution at this level should make us rule out the existence of an epidermoid carcinoma.

Transperineal biopsy proved to be a valid option for histological diagnosis. In experienced hands, the transperineal route allows to access to the small pelvis in complex situations [4]. Based on the limited literature data, it appears that squamous CUP outside of the head and neck region have a more favorable prognosis compared to other CUP and that these malignancies may respond well to a combination of surgical resection, when feasible, local radiotherapy, and platinum-based systemic chemotherapy [1].

Treatment regimens remain controversial, with limited cases to allow for consensus. Surgical intervention remains the leading form of therapy; however, approaches are case specific, depending on the location of the tumor and the degree of invasiveness [3].

In general, CUP has a poor prognosis, with a median survival time of less than six months and only about 15% of patients surviving after 1 year [1]. In our series, although with a very small number of cases, we have an overall survival of 75% with a median follow-up of 23 months which is much longer than those published to date.

4. Conclusion

Squamous cell CUP located in the male pelvis represent a rare entity, so the ideal diagnostic work-up, the optimal treatment strategies, and prognosis are not well determined. Radical surgical treatment, followed by adjuvant chemotherapy in patients with a localized tumor and with good baseline status, appears to be the best treatment regimen, achieving higher survival rates than those published to date.

References

[1] L. Chiec, S. Verma, A. Kendler, and K. N. Abdel, "Male pelvic squamous cell carcinoma of unknown primary origin," *Case Reports in Oncological Medicine*, vol. 2014, Article ID 953698, 5 pages, 2014.

[2] M. Neagu, C. Constantin, C. Caruntu, C. Dimitru, M. Surcel, and S. Zurac, "Inflammation: a key process in skin tumorigenesis," *Oncology Letters*, vol. 17, no. 5, pp. 4068–4084, 2019.

[3] S. J. Moore, O. Rashidipour, and R. B. Moore, "Primary metastatic squamous cell carcinoma of the male urethra presenting with scrotal abscess and subsequent development of Fournier`s gangrene," *Clinical Medicine Insights: Case Reports*, vol. 9, pp. 83–86, 2016.

[4] M. Creta, V. Mirone, S. MeoDi, R. Buonopane, N. Longo, F. Fusco, N. R. Forte, and V. Imperatore, Eds., "A rare case of male pelvic squamous cell carcinoma of unknown primary origin presenting as perineal abscess and urethral stenosis," *Archivio Italiano di Urologia, Andrologia*, vol. 89, no. 2, p. 154, 2017.

[5] V. Paulitschke, C. Gerner, E. Hofstätter et al., "Proteome profiling of keratinocytes transforming to malignancy," *Electrophoresis*, vol. 36, no. 4, pp. 564–576, 2015.

[6] J. J. Kohorst, K. K. Shah, C. L. Hallemeier, C. L. Baum, and M. D. Davis, "Squamous cell carcinoma in perineal, perianal, and gluteal hidradenitis suppurativa: experience in 12 patients," *Dermatologic Surgery*, vol. 45, no. 4, pp. 519–526, 2019.

25

Functional Bladder Paraganglioma Treated by Partial Cystectomy

Amine Hermi ,[1] Hamza Ichaoui ,[1] Aziz Kacem,[1] Houcem Hedhli,[1] Faten Gargouri,[2] Ramzi Khiari,[1] and Samir Ghozzi[1]

[1]*Faculty of Medicine of Tunis, University Tunis El Manar, Department of Urology, Military Hospital of First Instruction of Tunis, Tunisia*
[2]*Faculty of Medicine of Tunis, University Tunis El Manar, Department of Pathology, Military Hospital of First Instruction of Tunis, Tunisia*

Correspondence should be addressed to Amine Hermi; hermiamine@gmail.com

Academic Editor: David Duchene

Paraganglioma is a rare neuroendocrine tumor that arises from the autonomic nervous system. The urinary bladder paraganglioma accounts for less than 0.1% of bladder tumors. It remains a challenging entity to diagnose and treat due to its rareness and the lack of specific symptoms. Treatment modalities include transurethral resection and cystectomy (partial or total). The authors report a new case of an isolated paraganglioma of the urinary bladder in a 52-year-old female patient that underwent partial cystectomy. This case aims to remind the clinical, histological and therapeutic features of this rare tumor.

1. Introduction

Pheochromocytoma is a tumor developed from the chromaffin tissues of the sympathetic nervous system. It is commonly localized in the adrenal medulla. However, in about 10% of cases, pheochromocytomas may occur in ectopic or extra adrenal sites, extending from head to pelvis. Ectopic pheochromocytoma is called paraganglioma.

The urinary bladder is a rare localization of paragangliomas, accounting for less than 1% of all pheochromocytomas. It occurs in all age groups, more commonly in females [1].

It can be nonfunctional or functional by catecholamine secreting. It may be difficult for urologists to pinpoint the exact diagnosis.

Histological examination is often the only key leading to diagnosis. This neoplasm is usually benign but can occasionally show malignant behavior.

In presenting this case, we aim to provide a complete overview of etiology, symptom, diagnosis and possible treatments of paraganglioma of the urinary bladder, in order to write up a useful article for urologists that could have to manage similar cases.

2. Case Presentation

A 62 year-old-woman, complaining from micturition lipothymia for six months, was admitted in our hospital. She had no significant past medical history, and there was no history of headaches, palpitations, profuse sweating, hypertension or gross hematuria. Her family history was unremarkable.

Physical examination was normal, and blood pressure was within normal range at 120/80 mmHg. Cytobacteriological examination of the urine was negative. The patient was not anemic and the white cell count was within normal range. There was no renal failure.

An abdominal ultrasonographic examination was performed initially, which depicted an approximately 40 mm heterogeneous mass along the anterior wall of the bladder with abundant internal flow at Doppler interrogation (Figure 1).

An abdominal computed tomography (CT) scan, with intravenous administration of contrast medium, revealed a 32 mm heterogenous lobulated anterior bladder wall mass. The mass showed intense uniform enhancement with contrast study. There was no sign of any lymphadenopathy or metastatic invasion (Figure 2).

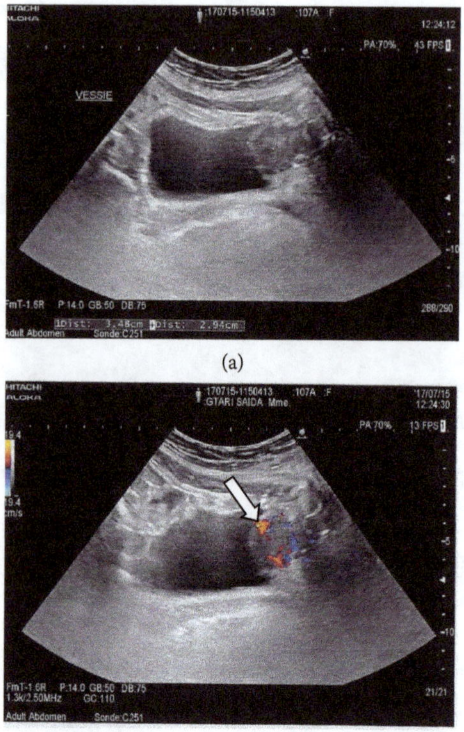

(a)

(b)

Figure 1: (a) Sagittal gray-scale ultrasound image of the urinary bladder shows a heterogeneous 40 mm mass along the anterior wall of the bladder. (b) Sagittal color Doppler ultrasound image demonstrates marked flow within the bladder mass (arrow).

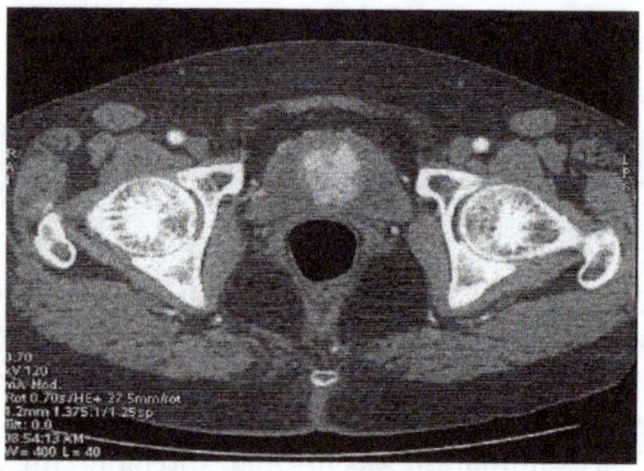

Figure 2: Transverse computer tomography image showing an avidly enhancing mass in the anterior urinary bladder wall.

Further imaging with Iodine-123-meta-iodobenzylguanidine (I-123 MIBG) scintiscan confirmed the presence of bladder pheochromocytoma without metastatic disease (Figure 3).

The 24-hour urine metanephrine and normetanephrine measurement was within normal levels.

The patient underwent a complete and deep transurethral resection of the bladder tumor. A solid submucosal mass was seen on the left lateral wall near the neck of the urinary bladder, with normal mucosal covering. The resection was complete and tissue was submitted to histopathological examination. During the procedure, the patient became severely hypertensive. Her blood pressure raised up to 236/118 mmHg and pulse rate dropped to 46/min. This episode was controlled with intraoperative intravenous antihypertensive and atropine. Postoperative recovery was uneventful.

The histological examination of the tumor confirmed the diagnosis of vesical paraganglioma showing tumorous small cells with a positive immunostaining for synaptophysin and anti-CD 56 (Figure 4).

The patient underwent partial cystectomy (Figure 5). The surgical margin of the removed specimen was negative. Postoperative recovery was uneventful.

On a recent follow-up at 12 months, her cystoscopy examination did not reveal any evidence of recurrence. Her radiological assessment (thoracic-abdomino-pelvic CT) was negative for metastatic disease.

3. Discussion

Paraganglioma or extra-adrenal pheochromocytoma of the urinary bladder arises from chromaffin tissue of the sympathetic nervous system within the layers of the bladder wall. It is a very rare localization of extra renal pheochromocytoma. However, in the genitourinary tract, the urinary bladder is the most common site (79.2%), followed by the urethra (12.7%), pelvis (4.9%), and ureter (3.2%) [2]. Paraganglioma of the urinary bladder was first reported in 1953 by Zimmerman [3], and since that time there have been fewer than 200 cases described.

Bladder pheochromocytoma occurs more frequently in women than in men, and mainly during the third decade of life [4].

It is most commonly situated at the dome or the trigone of the bladder and may be nonfunctional or functional. They remain usually benign, but about 20% of paragangliomas may show malignant behavior [4].

Functional paragangliomas secrete catecholamines, which may lead to symptoms similar to a hyperfunctioning adrenal pheochromocytoma, such as headaches, palpitations, dizziness, and sweating. These symptoms occur by in spells or paroxysm. They are mainly precipitated by micturition, overdistention of the bladder, defecation, sexual activity, ejaculation, or bladder instrumentation. Painless hematuria is the presenting complaint in about 60% of reported cases [4]. However, it has been estimated that 17% of bladder pheochromocytomas patient are hormonally nonfunctional, so less symptomatic.

On most imaging modalities a bladder paraganglioma is indistinguishable from other tumor types specially in ultrasound and CT examination. If the bladder tumor is submucosal, and shows marked enhancement after contrast administration and markedly increased, homogeneous signal intensity on T2-weighted magnetic resonance images. Paraganglioma should be considered in the differential diagnosis, although these tumors usually show less hyperintensity than the typical adrenal pheochromocytoma [5].

Metaiodobenzylguanidine scintigraphy demonstrates high specificity for pheochromocytoma but this nuclear medicine scan is less sensitive compared to magnetic resonance imaging [5].

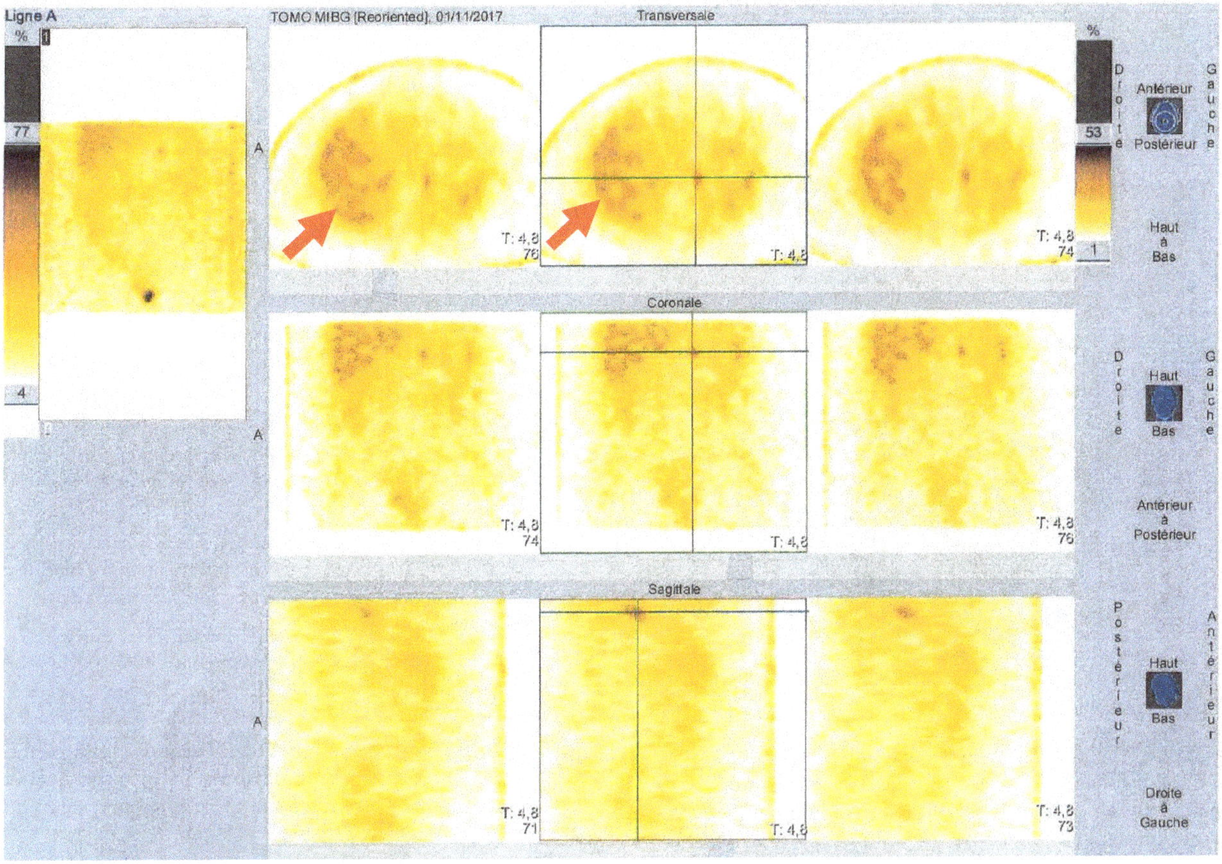

FIGURE 3: Iodine-123-meta-iodobenzylguanidine (I-123 MIBG) scintiscan showing intense tracer uptake in the anterior side of the bladder consistent with bladder paraganglioma (arrow).

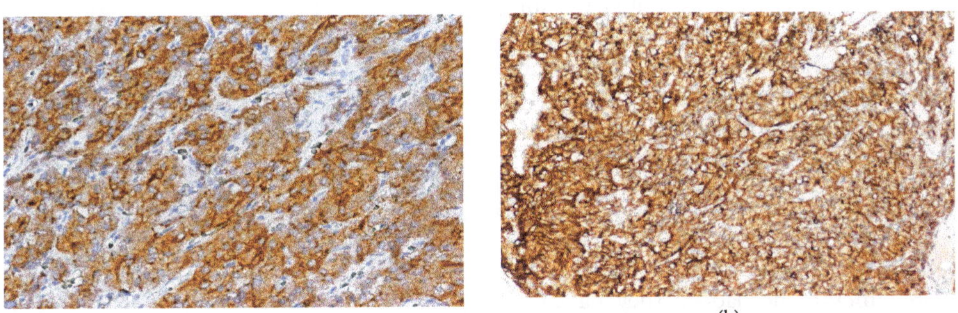

(a) (b)

FIGURE 4: (a) Tumor cells are strongly stained with synaptophysin (×200). (b) Tumorous small cells with a positive immunostaining for anti CD56 (×100).

Surgical resection is the treatment of choice. To avoid hypertensive crisis during the mass manipulation, preoperative treatment with alpha and beta-blocking agents is required, starting 1–3 weeks before surgery [6]. The cystoscopic appearance of a submucosal tumor with an intact surface, yellow at the cut, should raise the suspicion of bladder paraganglioma.

Histological examination of the tumor tissue will confirm diagnosis with diffuse, strong positivity for neuron-specific enolase (NSE), synaptophysin, and/or chromogranin. Histologically, it is often misdiagnosed as urothelial carcinoma, malignant melanoma and granular cell tumor [7].

Between 5% and 15% of the paragangliomas of the urinary bladder are said to be malignant. However, no histological criteria have been established to distinguish between benign and malignant tumors. Only the appearance of local invasion or distant metastases confirms that the tumor is cancerous [8].

Forty gray external beam radiation therapy in patients with paragangliomas has shown clinically significant symptomatic relief for at least one year or until death. For patients in which surgery or local radiation therapy is not viable, palliative system options include 131-iodine-labeled meta-iodobenzylguanidine (131I-MIBG) therapy and cytotoxic chemotherapy [9].

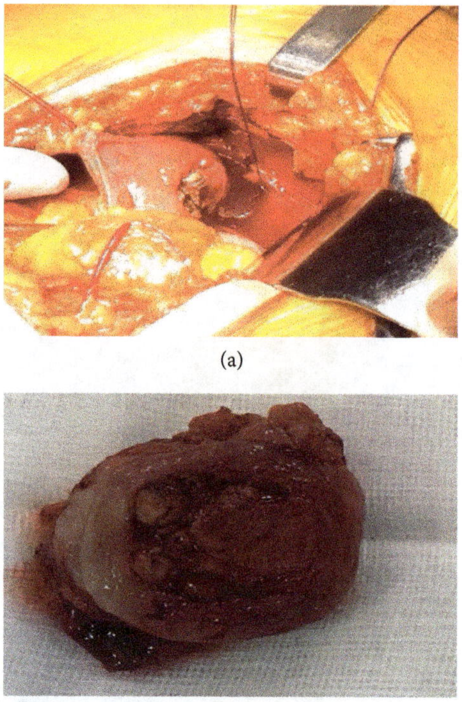

(a)

(b)

FIGURE 5: (a) The surgically resected lesion is well defined and polypoid, and it appears to be vasc. (b) Macroscopic view of bladder paraganglioma. The tumour is red-brown in colour, lobulated and well-circumscribed.

Most of bladder paragangliomas grow slowly and have a good prognosis. Regular follow-up is necessary to evaluate the bladder function after partial cystectomy as well as the surveillance for late recurrences. It must be lifelong and include cystoscopy and imaging study. No consensus has been established for the frequency of these measures: nevertheless, we suggested at least an annual follow-up for those patients who are asymptomatic or whenever clinically indicated [10].

4. Conclusions

Paragangliomas are rare tumors of the bladder. They may present clinical, radiology and pathological features similar to bladder cancer. There are typical symptoms due to catecholamine secretion especially associated with micturation periods. They are rarely malignant and most of the tumors are treated successfully with partial cystectomy. Other treatment modalities such transurethral resection can be considered as effective first-line treatments. Moving forward, it would be helpful to standardize the reporting guidelines of pheochromocytomas cases to better understand the natural process and outcomes.

References

[1] Loveys, F. W., C. Pushpanathan, and S. Jackman, "Urinary bladder paraganglioma: AIRP best cases in radiologic-pathologic correlation," *RadioGraphics*, vol. 35, no. 5, pp. 1433–1438, 2015.

[2] A. M. Hanji, V. S. Rohan, J. J. Patel, and R. A. Tankshali, "Pheochromocytoma of the urinary bladder: a rare cause of severe hypertension," *Saudi Journal of Kidney Diseases and Transplantation*, vol. 23, no. 4, p. 813, 2012.

[3] I. J. Zimmerman, R. E. Biron, and H. E. Macmahon, "Pheochromocytoma of the urinary bladder," *New England Journal of Medicine*, vol. 249, no. 1, pp. 25–26, 1953.

[4] C.-C. Tsai, W.-J. Wu, K.-S. Chueh et al., "Paraganglioma of the urinary bladder first presented by bladder bloody tamponade: two case reports and review of the literatures," *The Kaohsiung Journal of Medical Sciences*, vol. 27, no. 3, pp. 108–113, 2011.

[5] S. M. Bhalani, D. D. Casalino, and A. M. Manvar, "Paraganglioma of the bladder," *Journal of Urology*, vol. 186, no. 1, pp. 279–280, 2011.

[6] V. De Pasquale and A. Magistrelli, "Diomedi Camassei F. Caione P. Unusual bladder mass in a 14-year-old boy: bladder paraganglioma," *Urologia Internationalis*, vol. 86, no. 1, pp. 117–120, 2011.

[7] A. Sangwaiya, V. Kaira, S. Samal, R. Sen, V. Gupta, and J. Sharma, "Nonfunctioning paraganglioma of the urinary bladder: a rare entity," *Clinical Cancer Investigation Journal*, vol. 4, no. 2, p. 268, 2015.

[8] P. L. M. Dahia, "Evolving concepts in pheochromocytoma and paraganglioma," *Current Opinion in Oncology*, vol. 18, no. 1, pp. 1–8, 2006.

[9] W. Li, B. Yang, J.-P. Che et al., "Diagnosis and treatment of extra-adrenal pheochromocytoma of urinary bladder: case report and literature review. International Journal of," *Clinical and Experimental Medicine*, vol. 6, no. 9, pp. 832–839, 2013.

[10] R. A. Maddocks and W. T. Fagan, "Paraganglioma of bladder with recurrence ten years later," *Urology*, vol. 7, no. 4, pp. 430–432, 1976.

Isolated Fungal Balls in Urinary Bladder Presenting as Acute Retention of Urine

Tariq Hameed, Sudhir Kumar Jain, Faiz Manzar Ansari, and Amrita Dua

Department of Surgery, Maulana Azad Medical College, Delhi, India

Correspondence should be addressed to Tariq Hameed; drtariqhameed@gmail.com

Academic Editor: Fumitaka Koga

A 52-year-old male presented to surgery emergency with acute retention of urine. Patient was relieved in the emergency setting by catheterization and bladder irrigation. Urine was sterile; however, microscopy revealed field full of RBCs (>50/high-power field) and pus cells (>20/hpf). Cystoscopy revealed fungal balls in the urinary bladder which upon histopathological examination showed *Aspergillus* species. Patient was managed with systemic voriconazole and bladder wash with diluted povidone iodine. Predisposing factors diabetes mellitus and benign prostatic hyperplasia were medically managed, and patient recovered well. This case stresses the importance of considering isolated fungal urinary infections in predisposed individuals.

1. Introduction

Fungal ball in urinary bladder is an uncommon entity, the first case being reported way back in 1961 and around 20 cases have since then been reported in literature [1]. Tissue invasion of *Aspergillus* is rare and occurs most commonly in the setting of immunosuppression [2]. Isolated bladder infection with *Aspergillus* presenting as fungal balls is extremely rare [3]. Here, we present a case with urinary bladder fungal balls without disseminated disease or renal involvement who presented as progressive dysuria along with hematuria.

2. Case Presentation

A 52-year-old male presented to surgery emergency with acute retention of urine for 12 hours. He also complained of progressive dysuria and gross hematuria along with low-grade fever for the last 15 days. Patient had a history of lower urinary tract symptoms (LUTS) for the last 6 months. Patient was a shopkeeper by occupation with no known comorbidities or significant family history. On physical examination, patient was febrile with enlarged prostate on digital rectal examination and palpable bladder per abdomen. A Foley catheter was inserted, and bladder irrigation with diluted povidone iodine was started after obtaining urine samples.

Urine routine examination showed field full of RBCs (>50/high power field) and pus cells (>20/hpf). Urine culture was sterile. His WBC counts were 12,000/microlitre with absolute eosinophil count of 850. Blood sugar charting was deranged with fasting blood sugar 174 mg/dL and postprandial blood sugar 228 mg/dL. HbA1c was 11.2 g%. He was previously unaware of his diabetic status. USG abdomen showed hyperechogenic contents in the urinary bladder and thickened bladder wall ~7 mm (Figure 1); bilateral kidneys were normal without any abnormal echogenic focus or hydronephrosis.

To evaluate the cause of acute retention of urine, hematuria, and LUTS, patient was taken up for cystoscopy which showed membranous urethritis, median lobe prostatic enlargement, and white fluffy cotton-like balls in the bladder (Figure 2). Bladder wash fluid was sent for both bacterial and fungal culture, and fluffy balls were sent for histopathological examination (HPE). HPE showed fungal hyphae which were septate with acute angle branching and PAS stain positivity suggestive of *Aspergillus* (Figure 3). No growth was identified on Sabouraud's dextrose agar inoculation of bladder wash fluid. To screen the patient for immunodeficiency, an enzyme immune assay test for HIV 1 and 2 was done and found out to be negative. Additional tests for confirmation of *Aspergillus*-like galactomannan antigen and β-D-glucan

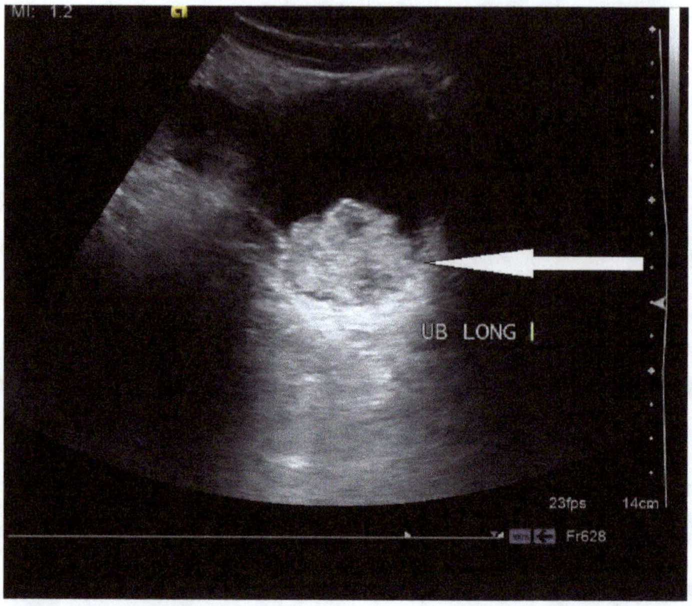

FIGURE 1: Ultrasonography showing hyperechogenic contents in the urinary bladder and thickened bladder wall.

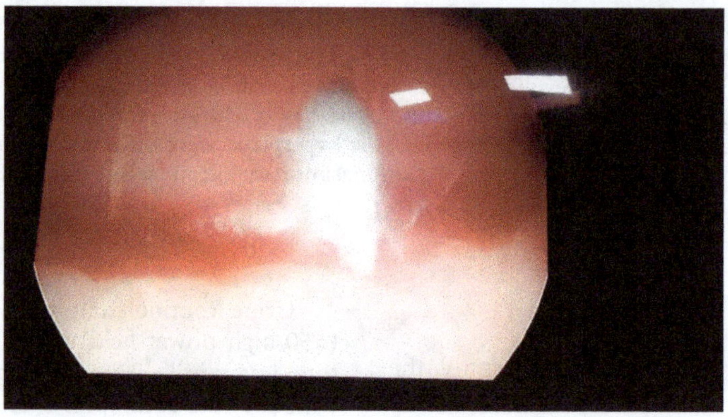

FIGURE 2: Cystoscopy showing fungal balls in the urinary bladder.

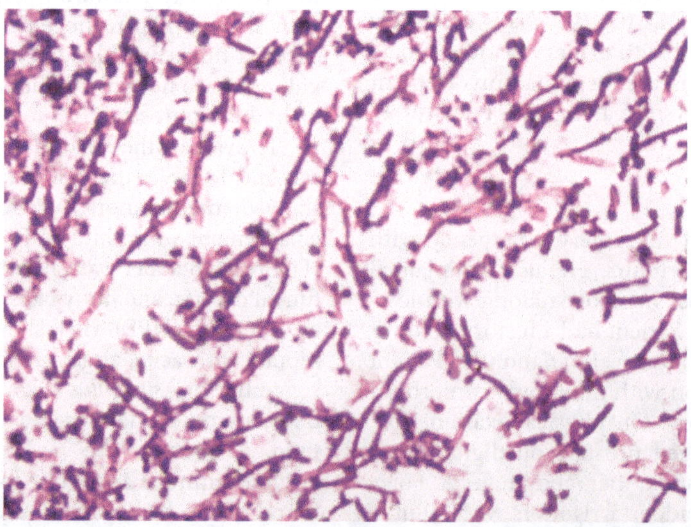

FIGURE 3: HPE showing septate fungal hyphae with acute angle branching.

were not performed in view of financial constraints for the patient. Patient was treated with systemic voriconazole and bladder irrigation with diluted povidone iodine. He was asymptomatic after 14 days of treatment. Check cystoscopy was performed after 4 weeks, and urinary bladder and urethra were normal without any evidence of fungal balls.

3. Discussion

Aspergillus are ubiquitous fungal molds found in organic matter. More than 100 species of *Aspergillus* have been identified while around 40 species are pathogenic to humans. Amongst them, *Aspergillus fumigatus* is the most commonly identified species. *Aspergillus* commonly affects the lungs, followed by the liver, spleen, heart, bones, central nervous system, ear, and paranasal sinuses [4, 5]. Fungal balls or bezoars are not common in the urinary bladder, and in majority of cases, *Candida albicans* has been found to be the causative agent [2, 6]. It is usually seen in immunocompromised states like hematological malignancies, in neutropenic patients following bone marrow or organ transplantation, or those receiving high dose of corticosteroids or cytotoxic drugs. Diabetes is also a risk factor for aspergillosis [7]. For urinary tract aspergillosis, additional risk factors are prolonged indwelling catheter, obstructive uropathy, or any surgical procedure. In the urinary tract, kidneys are most commonly involved, and isolated bladder involvement is very rare [3, 8, 9]. Diagnosis can be established through urine cytology and repeated fungal culture in case of resistant urinary tract infection (UTI) in predisposed individuals. In vitro fungal culture is positive in only around 50% of cases as fungus gets altered and is not viable, viability of fungal tissues in fungal balls is usually poor [10]. For invasive *Aspergillus* infection, galactomannan antigen and β-D-glucans are employed; they are quite sensitive and specific [11]. Managing urinary fungal infections is a tedious job. No definitive guidelines exist. Intravenous fluconazole/voriconazole, local irrigation with povidone iodine and amphotericin B, and cystoscopic removal of fungal balls and even operative methods are employed [12]. Under lying conditions like neurogenic bladder, diabetes mellitus, and prostatic hyperplasia must be taken care of.

4. Conclusion

Fungal infections of urinary tract even though rare should always be kept as differential diagnosis in patients of persistent UTI. In case of sterile pyuria with lower urinary tract symptoms, fungal cystitis should be considered as a possible diagnosis. Early diagnosis and complete treatment is required to control the dissemination of disease and to have a favourable prognosis. Fungal balls very rarely can also cause acute retention of urine in setting of severe lower urinary tract symptoms.

References

[1] E. R. Chisholm and J. A. Hutch, "Fungus ball (*Candida albicans*) formation in the bladder," *The Journal of Urology*, vol. 86, no. 5, pp. 559–562, 1961.

[2] P. B. Irby, M. L. Stoller, and J. W. McAninch, "Fungal bezoars of the upper urinary tract," *The Journal of Urology*, vol. 143, no. 3, pp. 447–451, 1990.

[3] S. Sakamoto, J. Ogata, Y. Sakazaki, and K. Ikegami, "Fungus ball formation of aspergillus in the bladder. An unusual case report," *European Urology*, vol. 4, no. 5, pp. 388-389, 1978.

[4] N. S. Raja and N. N. Singh, "Disseminated invasive aspergillosis in an apparently immunocompetent host," *Journal of Microbiology, Immunology, and Infection*, vol. 39, no. 1, pp. 73–77, 2006.

[5] A. O. Soubani and P. H. Chandrasekar, "The clinical spectrum of pulmonary aspergillosis," *Chest*, vol. 121, no. 6, pp. 1988–1999, 2002.

[6] C. A. Kauffman, "Candiduria," *Clinical Infectious Diseases*, vol. 41, Supplement 6, pp. S371–S376, 2005.

[7] A. S. Merseburger, M. Oelke, J. Hartmann, A. Stenzl, and M. A. Kuczyk, "Intracranial aspergillosis in a non-immunocompromised patient treated for muscle-invasive bladder cancer," *International Journal of Urology*, vol. 11, no. 8, pp. 666–668, 2004.

[8] E. Dervisoglu, E. Dikmen, D. Filinte, and A. Yilmaz, "Isolated bladder aspergillosis as the primary presentation of non-oliguric acute renal failure," *Scandinavian Journal of Urology and Nephrology*, vol. 42, no. 2, pp. 189–191, 2008.

[9] S. Siddappa, K. Mythri, R. Kowsalya, and M. Shivalingaiah, "An unusual case of non-disseminated bladder aspergillosis in a setting of transitional cell carcinoma," *Indian Journal of Medical Microbiology*, vol. 30, no. 1, pp. 106–108, 2012.

[10] B. Willinger, A. Obradovic, B. Selitsch et al., "Detection and identification of fungi from fungus balls of the maxillary sinus by molecular techniques," *Journal of Clinical Microbiology*, vol. 41, no. 2, pp. 581–585, 2003.

[11] G. Desoubeaux, E. Bailly, and J. Chandenier, "Diagnostic de l'aspergillose pulmonaire invasive : actualites et recommandations," *Médecine et Maladies Infectieuses*, vol. 44, no. 3, pp. 89–101, 2014.

[12] S. Lechmiannandan, E. H. Goh, B. W. Teoh, and K. A. Git, "A rare case of fungus balls of the urinary bladder due to Candida Tropicalis," *UroToday International Journal*, vol. 5, no. 4, article art 30, 2012.

27

Delayed Presentation of Iliac Vein Injury: A Severe Complication at Retropubic Midurethral Sling Arm Removal

Pansy Uberoi and Forrest Jellison

San Antonio Uniformed Services Health Education Consortium, USA

Correspondence should be addressed to Forrest Jellison; fjellison@gmail.com

Academic Editor: Tun-Chieh Chen

Midurethral slings are the most common treatment for female stress urinary incontinence. Perioperative vascular injuries during placement of a retropubic midurethral sling (RMUS) are uncommon but have been described. The objective of this case report is to describe a complication of delayed presentation from a vascular injury at the time of retropubic sling arm removal not previously documented in the literature. This life-threating complication should be considered and precautions should be taken at retropubic sling arm removal. Prevention is accomplished by proper visualization of pelvic vasculature and/or eliminating tension on sling before excision.

1. Introduction

Retropubic midurethral mesh slings (RMUS) are a standard treatment option for the management of stress urinary incontinence. The recent American Urologic Association guideline for surgical management of female stress urinary incontinence (SUI) described MUS as the most widely studied with follow-up data over more than 15 years [1]. Despite its well documented safety and efficacy, the RMUS is associated with complications. Common complications can be divided into intraoperative and postoperative issues, and the management and report outcomes are well described [2, 3]. Intraoperative hemorrhage has been described with significant vessel injury found less than 0.7% and hematoma has been described in approximately 2% of patients [4]. Delayed and asymptomatic vascular injuries have not been reported.

In this case report, we describe the asymptomatic delayed presentation of a RMUS located in the wall of the external iliac vein that leads to catastrophic bleeding requiring emergent repair at the time of sling arm removal.

2. Case Presentation

A 69-year-old female underwent placement of RMUS in May 2014 for SUI by a surgeon from another institution. She developed de novo left groin/inner thigh pain, vaginal pain, and abdominal pain at the site of left sling arm and de novo overactive bladder and dysfunctional voiding. After follow-up and discussion with her original surgeon, they decided to proceed with a sling incision six months from her sling placement. After the sling revision, her pain and urinary symptoms did not improve, and she was self-referred to our institution for evaluation.

After a thorough evaluation that included examination, cystoscopy, labs, CT scan, and Urodynamics (UDS) that revealed pertinent findings of trigger point tenderness at the left suprapubic trocar incision site and vaginally in the left levator muscles, the left trocar incision site was unusually more superior and lateral than is typically found on examination, and UDS findings demonstrated urodynamic stress incontinence and bladder outflow obstruction. After extensive counseling, patient underwent transvaginal and suprapubic removal of the remaining left retropubic arm and remaining suburethral portion of the sling.

3. Interventions/Surgical Course

Approximately one year after her RMUS, she was taken to the operating room with the plan for excision of the remaining suburethral portion of the mesh sling and partial removal of the left retropubic arm. We made an inverted U-incision and then identified the suburethral portion of the mesh sling. During her suburethral revision, the right side of her sling was partially excised without entering the retropubic space, and we noted that the remaining left portion of the mesh sling was nearly penetrating the urethral mucosa. This portion of the sling was nearly penetrating the mucosal layer, located submucosally with extensive fibrosis that required a small urethrotomy to excise it completely. The urethrotomy was closed primarily with absorbable suture and left a martius flap was interposed to provide tissue coverage.

Attention was then taken to the removal of the left retropubic arm of the sling. The incision scar from the trocar of the remaining left portion of the sling was identified to be 5 cm superior and 6 cm lateral to the pubic symphysis, and, during vaginal exploration, the sling was noted to enter the obturator internus and iliococcygeus muscles. Given the location of the trocar site, preoperatively we discussed partial removal of the left arm of the mesh to the level of the abdominal fascia without removal of RMUS retropubic arms as they are potentially located adjacent to the iliac vessels. We removed the suburethral sling from a vaginal approach to where it entered the retropubic space, and the sling was embedded into the periosteum and then we began the removal of the sling abdominally to the level of the rectus fascia. A 3 cm mini-Gibson incision was used in the left lower abdomen over the scar from initial sling placement to allow for adequate exposure and reduce morbidity of a larger incision. The sling was dissected free to the level of the abdominal fascia. Careful attention was paid not to injure sounding structures, and the sling was pulled on traction superiorly and excised under direct visualization.

Immediately after excision of the abdominal arm of the sling, approximately 200 ml of blood loss was experienced. Bleeding was controlled with direct pressure to the area. Expeditiously, the abdominal incision was extended from a mini-Gibson to a full Gibson to allow visualization of bleeding. After obtaining exposure, the source of bleeding was identified with the sling embedded in the wall of the vein creating a traction injury in the medial wall of the left external iliac vein. The remaining visible sling was excised from the external iliac vein, and the venotomy was repaired with primary closure. Intraoperatively Vascular Surgery team was consulted and examined the repaired vein and determined that lumen diameter was adequate and assessed for any thrombus. She was taken to the ICU postoperatively where, after extubation, she complained of worsened left lower extremity pain which, at that time, also appeared to have some purple discoloration in her left foot. Her symptoms were consistent with acute venous congestion from a left external vein thrombus that was diagnosed on CT arteriogram and venogram. The patient returned to the operative room with the Vascular Surgery team. A small remaining intraluminal portion of mesh was identified and removed from the sling in the external iliac vein and was associated with the thrombus. Venotomy, thrombectomy, and excision of mesh were performed, and the vein was subsequently repaired with a contralateral saphenous vein patch.

4. Aftercare

After recovery from her surgery and completion of her course of anticoagulation she underwent placement of an autologous rectus fascia pubovaginal sling for her persistent SUI. She noted significant improvement in her SUI and since the prior surgery reported complete resolution of vaginal and leg pain, with 70% improvement in abdominal pain, symptoms at 18-month follow-up.

5. Discussion

Despite its reported safety and efficacy for treatment of female stress urinary incontinence, placement of retropubic midurethral mesh sling has known complications. Management and outcomes of these complications are well described in the literature [2, 3]. Vascular injury with MUS placement is rare, and most are identified intraoperatively as active extravasation of blood or hemodynamic instability. However, this case represents delayed recognition of vascular injury at the time of sling removal. It was unexpected to find that the sling is transverse through the wall of the external iliac vein, due to there being no reported vascular complications at sling placement or any vascular complications postoperatively.

In our literature search, one case of delayed diagnosis of external iliac vein injury was noted. However, the patient described in that report sustained several complications at index surgery and presented with back and abdominal bloating and gross hematuria with sling perforation and bladder stones. At the time of reoperation, the surgeon had decided to perform a laparotomy and remove the entire retropubic sling as per her request, and intraoperatively it was noted that the sling penetrated into bladder lumen, created scar tissue surrounding the obturator nerve, and was intraluminal in the contralateral external iliac vein [5].

Although the overall frequency of vascular injury during MUS placement is rare, a comprehensive knowledge of pelvic anatomy is necessary to prevent injury [6]. Sufficient surgical experience and training are paramount to the prevention of morbidity and increased safety. The AUA/SUFU position statement is that surgeons are to be trained rigorously in the pelvic anatomy and in recognition of complications [7]. In this case, the patient reported that the outside surgeon had stated that he had minimal experience performing retropubic midurethral slings.

In our case, the patient experienced a life-threatening complication during the removal of the retropubic arms of the sling. A venotomy resulted from traction of the sling on the external iliac vein tension prior to excision. We suspect that the RMUS was into but not through the intimal layer of the vessel during placement (Figure 1). Given the possible proximity of sling arms to pelvic vessels, open/laparoscopic laparotomy should be considered by the operating surgeon when removing suprapubic sling arms to prevent vascular injury and to identify such injuries if they occur. Although still investigational, there is possibly a role for pelvic/translabial ultrasound in perioperative planning [8, 9]. Alternately, if we had placed minimal tension when pulling on the sling before excising it, this would have resulted

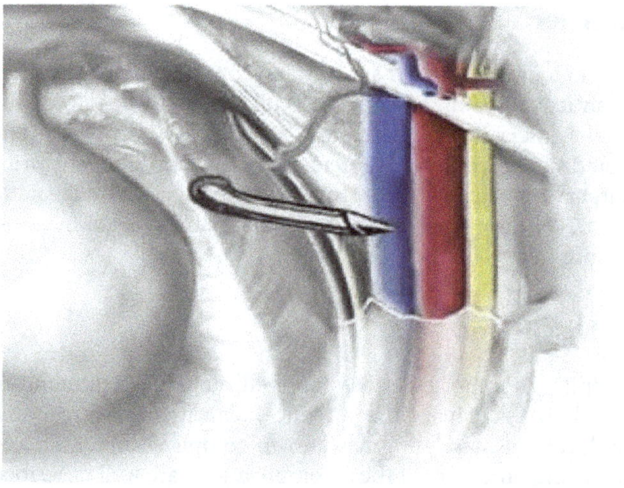

FIGURE 1: Trocar position relative to external iliac vein at placement.

in no vascular injury. Additionally, this would have resulted in using the planned 3 cm incision and would have decreased the morbidity due to the incision size.

In conclusion, prevention of vascular injury is vital when removing the retropubic sling arms even when the patient has no prior vascular complications at sling placement. This is accomplished by proper visualization of pelvic vasculature and/or minimizing tension on sling during excision.

Disclosure

This research was presented at 96th Annual Meeting of the South Central Section of the AUA, October 2017. The views expressed are those of the author(s) and do not reflect the official views or policy of the Department of Defense or its components.

References

[1] K. C. Kobashi, M. E. Albo, R. R. Dmochowski et al., "Surgical treatment of female stress urinary incontinence: AUA/SUFU guideline," *The Journal of Urology*, vol. 198, no. 4, pp. 875–883, 2017.

[2] V. Kershaw, R. Nicholson, P. Ballard, A. Khunda, S. Puthuraya, and E. Gouk, "Outcome of surgical management for midurethral sling complications: a multicentre retrospective cohort study," *International Urogynecology Journal*, 2019.

[3] D. Lee, C. Bacsu, B. Dillon, and P. E. Zimmern, "Complications following the insertion of two synthetic mid-urethral slings and subsequent removal," *LUTS: Lower Urinary Tract Symptoms*, vol. 10, no. 3, pp. 259–265, 2018.

[4] B. Çetinel and T. Tarcan, "Management of complications after tension-free midurethral slings," *Korean Journal of Urology*, vol. 54, no. 10, pp. 651–659, 2013.

[5] M. F. Aslam and M. A. Denman, "Case report: delayed diagnosis of vascular injury with a retropubic midurethral sling," *Obstetrics & Gynecology*, vol. 122, pp. 444–446, 2013.

[6] T. W. Muir, P. K. Tulikangas, M. F. Paraiso, and M. D. Walters, "The relationship of tension-free vaginal tape insertion and the vascular anatomy," *Obstetrics and Gynecology: TVT and Vascular Anatomy*, vol. 101, no. 5, 2003.

[7] "AUA position statement on the use of vaginal mesh for the surgical treatment of stress urinary incontinence (SUI)," https://www.auanet.org/guidelines/use-of-vaginal-mesh-for-the-surgical-treatment-of-stress-urinary-incontinence.

[8] K. Y. Kim, J. W. Cheng, J. K. Shen, H. Wagner, and A. Staack, "Translabial ultrasound evaluation of pelvic floor structures and mesh in the urology office and intraoperative setting," *Urology*, vol. 120, article 267, 2018.

[9] K. A. Viragh, S. A. Cohen, L. Shen, N. Kurzbard-Roach, S. Raz, and S. S. Raman, "Translabial US: preoperative detection of midurethral sling erosion in stress urinary incontinence," *Radiology*, vol. 289, no. 3, pp. 721–727, 2018.

28

A Rare Case Report of Giant Urinary Bladder Stone Causing Recurrent Dysuria in a Woman

Rojan Adhikari, Hari Prasad Baral, Utsav Bhattarai, Ravi Kiran Gautam, Kiran Jung Kunwar, Dipesh Shrestha, and Bijay Mansingh Katwal

Department of Urology and Kidney Transplant, Shahid Dharmabhakta National Transplant Centre, Bhaktapur, Nepal

Correspondence should be addressed to Rojan Adhikari; rojanadhikari@gmail.com

Academic Editor: Tun-Chieh Chen

Background. Large urinary bladder stones are not common and even less common in females. We report a case of large bladder stone presented with acute retention of urine in a female patient. *Case Report.* A 62-year-old female presented in emergency department with retention of urine for 12 hours with history of recurrent UTIs for last 1 year. She was also complaining of mild dull lower abdominal pain for last 6 months. She had no history of incontinence of urine and fever. On physical examination, hard mass was palpable on suprapubic region on palpation of abdomen. Urine culture shows Escherichia coli for which antibiotics was given. An X-ray kidney ureter bladder showed a radio-opacity in the pelvic region measuring 9 × 8 cm in size. Ultrasonography revealed bilateral mild hydronephrosis with a large bladder stone. Open cystolithotomy was performed, and the stone was taken out. Stone biochemical analysis showed predominantly urate crystals. Patient had uneventful postoperative course, and she was discharged on 4th postoperative day and was followed up for 1 months after operation. *Conclusions.* Large urinary bladder stones are not common and even less common in females. Clinician should have think regarding large bladder stone as a cause of recurrent lower urinary tract symptoms like dysuria and should assess renal function for proper treatment. Open cystolithotomy is choice of operation in large bladder stone.

1. Introduction

Bladder stones (BS) comprised of 5% of all urinary tract stones. The aetiology of bladder stones is multifactorial. Bladder stones can be classified as primary, secondary, or migratory. Primary calculus are stones which passes from kidney or ureter and lodges in the urinary bladder while secondary calculus are formed inside the bladder [1]. Primary stones occur in the absence of other urinary tract pathology, whereas secondary bladder stones occur in the presence of other urinary tract abnormalities, such as bladder outlet obstruction (BOO), neurogenic bladder, chronic urinary tract infection, foreign bodies, and bladder diverticula. In male, the bladder stones are usually related with urinary obstruction, urinary retention, urinary tract infections, foreign body retention, and enlargement of prostate. While in female, it can occur secondary to bladder outlet obstruction, neurogenic voiding dysfunction, urinary tract infections (UTIs), or foreign bodies. The prevalence of bladder stone is very high in male in comparison to female population. Nearly, about 5% of all bladder stone occur in women. Giant urinary bladder calculi are defined as stones with weight more than 100 g and dimensions larger than 4 cm in diameter [2] . Giant or massive bladder stone is an uncommon condition which usually take long time to form. The presenting symptoms and signs varies with dysuria, lower urinary tract symptoms (LUTS), hematuria, pyuria, and recurrent urinary tract infections. Large bladder stones are common in developing countries because the initial symptoms of lower urinary tract symptoms are usually overlooked [3].

Our patient who is from rural part of Nepal experienced recurrent dysuria without any additional workup and

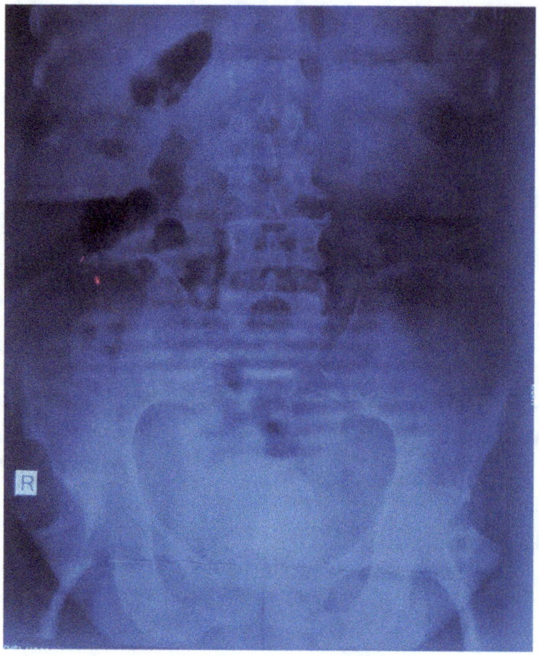

Figure 1: X-ray pelvis with bladder stone.

received empirical treatment despite of recurrent symptoms. Here, we report an unusual case of giant urinary bladder stone causing recurrent dysuria in a female patient.

2. Case Report

A 62-year-old female presented as an emergency patient with retention of urine for 12 hours. She had history of hesitancy at urination, increase frequency, interruption of urinary stream, urgency, and feeling of incomplete voiding for last 1 year. She was complaining of mild dull lower abdominal pain for last 6 months, intermittent in nature, no radiation, and aggravated while micturition. She had burning micturition on and off. She had no history of incontinence of urine and fever. She smoked cigarette 20 pack per year and left 10 years back. She denied any history of significant weight loss and hematuria. She is hypertensive under medication for 5 years and has chronic pulmonary obstructive disease for 2 years. On physical examination, her vital signs were stable. Hard mass was palpable on suprapubic region on palpation of abdomen. However, there was no renal angle tenderness present, and digital rectal examination was not done. Her blood investigation showed normal white blood cell count, blood urea nitrogen, and serum creatinine. Urine analysis indicated a very high white blood cell count and few red blood cells. Urine culture shows Escherichia coli for which antibiotics ciprofloxacin was given.

An X-ray kidney ureter bladder showed a radio-opacity in the pelvic region measuring 9 × 8 cm in size (Figure 1). Ultrasonography revealed bilateral mild hydronephrosis with a large bladder stone. After aseptic urine, cystoscopy was performed which shows no any lower urinary tract obstruction and large bladder stone almost occupying the bladder. No additional stones were noticed in the urinary

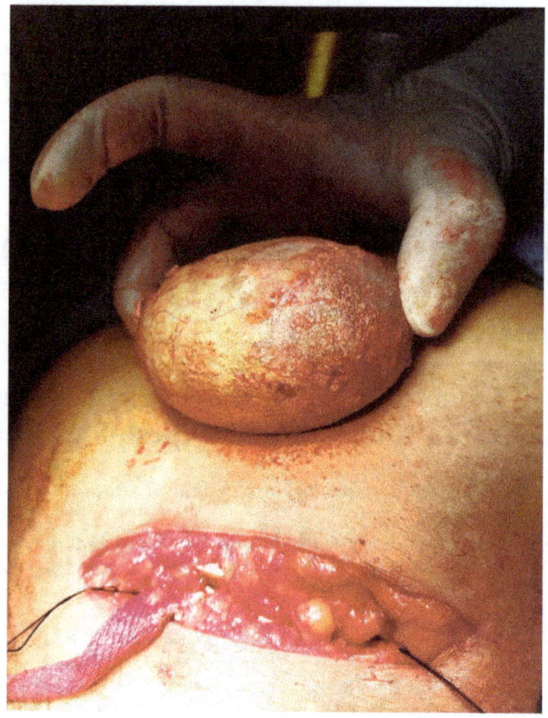

Figure 2: Stone after removal from bladder.

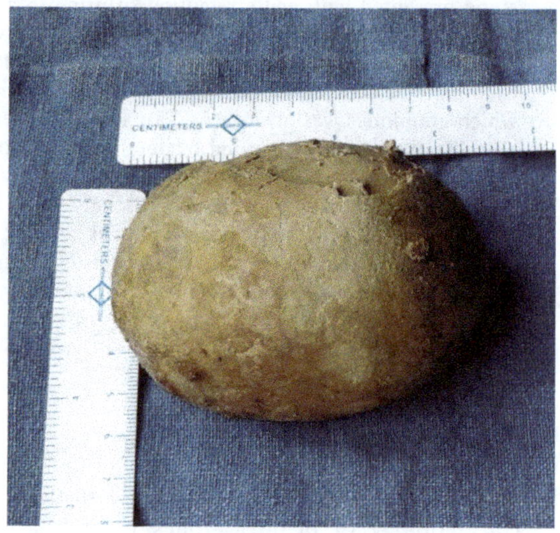

Figure 3: Size of bladder stone.

tract. After optimization, open cystolithotomy was performed under spinal using a suprapubic, midline incision. A transverse incision was given in the bladder, and the stone was taken out (Figure 2). The bladder mucosa was erythematous and edematous, with no evidence of masses. The ureteral orifices were visible with normal pouring of urine. Bladder mucosa biopsy was not taken. The bladder was closed in two layers, and a suprapubic catheter of 12Fr and urethral Foley catheter of 16Fr were kept. A retrieved stone was of size 9 × 6 × 7 cm (Figure 3) and a weight of 300 gm. Stone biochemical analysis showed predominantly urate crystals.

After optimization, open cystolithotomy was performed under spinal anesthesia. Patient had uneventful postoperative course, and she was discharged on 4th postoperative day with suprapubic catheter and urethral catheter in situ. Suprapubic catheter was removed on 10th postoperative day, and urethral catheter was removed on 14th POD in outpatient department. She was followed up for 1 month after operation and no any residual stone seen and patient had normal urination.

3. Discussion

Bladder stones are commonly contained with mixed composition. Struvite (ammonium magnesium phosphate) stone is the most common stone in presence of history of recurrent urinary tract infections with urea-splitting organisms such as Proteus, Klebsiella, Serratia, and Enterobacter species that produce alkaline urine [4]. While calcium oxalate is most common without history of UTIs. Nearly, 50% of bladder stones are composed of ammonium urate [5]. They are normally related with a positive urinalysis for nitrite, leukocyte esterase, and blood.

X-ray, ultrasound, computed tomography (CT) scan, or cystoscopy are common methods to make diagnosis of bladder stone [3].

Nowadays, it is fact that open approach is being replaced by newer techniques aimed to be less invasive [6]. There is a broad spectrum of modalities for treatment of bladder stones like open cystolithotomy, transurethral cystolithotripsy, shock wave lithotripsy, and percutaneous cystolithotripsy [7]. For our patient, we choose open cystolithotomy as the size of stone is extremely large and choosing other option may lead to retain of stone fragment as described in the literature [8]. Fortunately, the bladder stone was not adherent to the bladder wall, and we can easily take out. We present this case as there is no any bladder outlet obstruction, bilateral ureteric orifice compromised with bladder stone causing mild hydroureteronephrosis, and the bladder stone in female is rare.

4. Conclusions

Large urinary bladder stones are not common and even less common in females. Clinician should have think regarding large bladder stone as a cause of recurrent lower urinary tract symptoms like dysuria and should assess renal function for proper treatment. Open cystolithotomy is choice of operation in large bladder stone.

References

[1] I. Sorokin, C. Mamoulakis, K. Miyazawa, A. Rodgers, J. Talati, and Y. Lotan, "Epidemiology of stone disease across the world," *World Journal of Urology*, vol. 35, no. 9, pp. 1301–1320, 2017.

[2] R. Ishtiaq, A. Randhawa, L. Zulfiqar, and N. Shabbir, "An uncommon cause of dysuria in a female patient: huge urinary bladder stones," *Cureus*, vol. 9, no. 10, article e1788, 2017.

[3] O. Hasan, A. Ellis, R. Powers, and P. Vidal, "Vesical megalithiasis," *Urology Case Reports*, vol. 23, pp. 41–43, 2019.

[4] K. Stav and P. L. Dwyer, "Urinary bladder stones in women," *Obstetrical & Gynecological Survey*, vol. 67, no. 11, pp. 715–725, 2012.

[5] C. Y. Wai, V. Margulis, B. R. Baugh, and J. I. Schaffer, "Multiple vesical calculi and complete vaginal vault prolapse," *American Journal of Obstetrics and Gynecology*, vol. 189, no. 3, pp. 884-885, 2003.

[6] A. Cicione, S. Manno, R. Damiano et al., "Bladder stone management: an update," *Minerva Urologica e Nefrologica= The Italian Journal of Urology and Nephrology*, vol. 70, no. 1, pp. 53–65, 2018.

[7] F. C. M. Torricelli, E. Mazzucchi, A. Danilovic, R. F. Coelho, and M. Srougi, "Surgical management of bladder stones: literature review," *Revista do Colégio Brasileiro de Cirurgiões*, vol. 40, no. 3, pp. 227–233, 2013.

[8] İ. N. Tahtalı and T. Karataş, "Giant bladder stone: a case report and review of the literature," *Turkish Journal of Urology*, vol. 40, no. 3, pp. 189–191, 2014.

29

Ureteral Diaphragmatic Hernia Treated with Ureteral Stenting: A Case Report and Review of the Literature

Tateki Yoshino,[1] **Ayako Itakura**,[1] **Shinnosuke Fujikawa**,[1] **Tomoyuki Sugitani**,[1] **Kazuo Kawakami**,[1] **Emi Ishibashi**,[2] **Koji Kodama**,[2] **and Shota Oshima**[1]

[1]*Department of Urology, Shimane Prefectural Central Hospital, Shimane, Japan*
[2]*Department of Radiology, Shimane Prefectural Central Hospital, Shimane, Japan*

Correspondence should be addressed to Tateki Yoshino; uroltateki@yahoo.co.jp

Academic Editor: David Duchene

Ureteral diaphragmatic hernia through diaphragmatic defects is an exceptionally rare subset of ureteral hernia with only fourteen such cases reported in English manuscripts. An 85-year-old woman was introduced to our department with right flank pain, fever elevation, and nausea. Urinalysis showed bacteriuria, and *Escherichia coli* was detected in the urine culture. Blood analysis revealed abnormal findings, including elevated WBC count (10,510/μl) and C-reactive protein (0.28 mg/dl). Computed tomography (CT) of the abdomen demonstrated a defect of the right diaphragmatic crus containing a dilated right ureter with associated hydronephrosis. Retrograde pyelography showed hydronephrosis and dilated ureter loops through the defect of diaphragmatic crus, known as a "curlicue sign," and the diagnosis was right ureteral diaphragmatic hernia. A ureteral stent was placed on her right side, and the ureter was reducted into the retroperitoneal space. After six months, the ureteral stent was removed, with no subsequent recurrence of the ureteral diaphragmatic hernia at seven months. We reviewed all cases in the literature published in English of ureteral diaphragmatic hernia. While the etiology of ureteral diaphragmatic hernia is unknown, our present case and previous reports suggest that a ureteral diaphragmatic hernia may occur due to hepatic atrophy and/or an elevated position of the right kidney.

1. Introduction

Ureteral hernias are a rare occurrence normally identified incidentally on imaging or during surgical hernia correction and can be a cause of ureteral obstruction [1]. These hernias can occur in several locations including the inguinal, femoral, obturator, sciatic, and thoracic regions [2]. The rarest location of a ureteral hernia is through a defect in the diaphragmatic muscle [3] with fourteen such cases reported since 1958 in the English language literature [4, 5]. Ureteral diaphragmatic hernias have been found in the the retrocrural area [2, 6] and through congenital Bochdalek foramen [3, 5, 7–14]. Clinical presentation is varied, from incidental radiographic finding to obstructive pyelonephritis and urosepsis. Management has ranged from conservative to ureteral stenting or surgical repair.

In this report, we present a case of right ureteral diaphragmatic hernia containing an incarcerated right proximal ureter with subsequent obstructive pyelonephritis. We review all cases of ureteral diaphragmatic hernia published in the literature in English and discuss optimal treatment methods and the etiology.

2. Case Report

An 85-year-old woman, with a medical history of hypertension, dyslipidemia, reflux esophagitis, osteoporosis, and kyphosis, was introduced to our department with right flank pain, fever elevation, and nausea. Her mental condition appeared stable. The patient's temperature was 37.7°C, pulse rate 72/min, and respiration 22/min. She was 148 cm in height, weighed 37.8 kg, with a BMI of 17.2 kg/m^2, and suffered from kyphosis. The pharynx and bilateral tonsils were not swollen, and there was no evidence of rales of the lungs. However, right costovertebral angle tenderness was notable.

Urinalysis showed bacteriuria. *Escherichia coli* and *Streptococcus* were detected in the urine culture. Abnormal findings of a complete blood count and laboratory examination included an elevated WBC count (10,510/μl) and C-reactive protein (0.28 mg/dl) and serum creatinine of 0.98 mg/dl. Ultrasound examination revealed right hydronephrosis, and subsequent CT of the abdomen revealed a right diaphragmatic hernia of a part of the urinary tract, causing moderate to severe hydronephrosis (Figures 1(a) and 1(b)); there were no signs of intraperitoneal lesions. Retrograde pyelography in combination with an inserted guidewire demonstrated ureteral loops known as a "curlicue sign" through the defect of the diaphragmatic crus, (Figure 2(a)), and our diagnosis was a right ureteral diaphragmatic hernia with associated hydronephrosis and obstructive pyelonephritis. For drainage of bacteriuria and improved renal function, a ureteral stent was placed on the patient's right side using cystoscopic guidance. At the time of ureteral manipulation by stent, the incarcerated ureter was reducted to the retroperitoneal cavity (Figure 2(b)).

A CT done one year previously on our patient showed neither a right ureteral diaphragmatic hernia nor hydronephrosis; however, it did reveal the higher position of the right kidney due to hepatic atrophy (Figure 3(a)), and a defect of the right diaphragmatic crus, which eventually developed into the hernia orifice (Figure 3(b)).

Based on the diagnosis of pyelonephritis and the results of the urine culture, we administered antibiotics and placed an indwelling Foley catheter. Treatment resulted in reduced inflammation and hydronephrosis, and improvement of the ureteral diaphragmatic hernia was confirmed by CT. The stent was removed at six months after placement, and at seven months after removal, there had been no recurrence of pyelonephritis or right ureteral diaphragmatic hernia.

3. Discussion

It is a rarity to encounter a ureteral hernia. Pollack et al. reported that 120 reports of ureteral hernias had been confirmed at the time of their case-series publication in 1975 [15]. While the exact number of ureteral hernias is unknown, recent publications have documented less than 200 cases [10]. Common locations of ureteral hernias are the inguinal, femoral, sciatic, obturator, and thoracic regions. Ureteral inguinal hernias occur most commonly (42-64%) in these regions [15], while the rarest ureteral hernia, the ureteral thoracic hernia, occurs through a muscular diaphragmatic defect.

We conducted a retrospective review of reported cases, and published papers were retrieved from Medline, PubMed and Google Scholar. Literature review and a case report revealed 14 documented cases of ureteral diaphragmatic hernia [4, 5], making, to our knowledge, the current case the 15th such patient diagnosed and reported. Clinical data of these 15 cases were reviewed and are summarized in Table 1, and aggregate results are set out in Table 2.

A majority of the reviewed 15 cases occurred in the elderly, with the diagnosis mean age being 75.6 years; 10 (66.6%) of the 15 were female. The right side was the diseased side in all cases; some ureteral hernias presented with symptoms attributable to the ureteral hernia/urinary tract obstruction while others were detected incidentally. Symptomatic cases presented with flank pain, renal dysfunction, gross hematuria, nausea, pyelonephritis, and urosepsis. Of the 15, 8 cases (53.3%) presented with right flank pain [3, 5, 7, 8, 11, 12, 14], while 7 (46.6%) were incidental findings in a workup for azotemia [10], contralateral flank pain [9], renal [2] and ureteral stones [16], vomiting and loose stools [4], a PET-CT scan for the workup of a lung nodule [6], and one presented as septic obstructive pyelonephritis [13]. With relation to the hernia orifice, 10 cases were herniated through the right Bochdalek foramen [3, 5, 7–14] and the other 5 were located in the retrocrural region [2, 6], diaphragm [4, 16], or diaphragmatic crus.

Ten of the cases were diagnosed by CT combined with pyelography (retrograde, antegrade, and intravenous) [2, 8–14, 16], four were by CT only [3–6] and one was solely by retrograde pyelography [7]. A curlicue sign, referring to the loop or spiral configuration of the herniated ureteral segment, was identified in all cases.

Of these 15 cases, 3 (20.0%) were managed conservatively [4, 5, 10], 4 (26.6%) underwent surgical repair [2, 3, 7, 8], and 7 (46.6%) were treated by ureteral stent [3, 11–14, 16]. Two cases did not report management [6, 9]. In the last 10 years, there has been only one reported case of surgical repair [3] and the 7 cases here of ureteral stenting were also reported in that period [3, 11–14, 16]. Within the 7 ureteral stent cases, one was followed by surgical repair due to failure of ureteral reduction by stenting [3]; a second required a transient nephrostomy due to difficulties with retrograde stenting [13]; and a third case underwent intrarenal surgery with stenting [16]. Two cases required ureteral stent removal: one had no relapse of ureteral hernia [14], while the second experienced a relapse of the ureteral hernia but no urinary tract obstruction was observed [12].

In cases of obstruction and resultant pain or pyelonephritis, drainage becomes imperative. Attempt at retrograde ureteral stenting is reasonable and minimally invasive [12] and was done with notable success in the reduction of an incarcerated ureter in 6 of the 7 stented cases. As the mean age of the stented-case patients undergoing ureteral stenting was higher (84.0 years) than the overall average (75.6), minimally invasive management by ureteral stenting may be the treatment of choice by doctors caring for extremely elderly patients.

Open surgery was done in 4 of the 15 cases, two of which underwent surgical repair via the retroperitoneal approach [3, 7]. Lin et al. [3] reported that the incarcerated ureteral segment was mobilized out of the diaphragmatic defect and returned to the retroperitoneal cavity, and the diaphragmatic defect was closed using interrupted 0 silk sutures; resection and anastomosis of the redundant proximal ureteral segment and nephropexy were also done. Due to the difficulty of locating

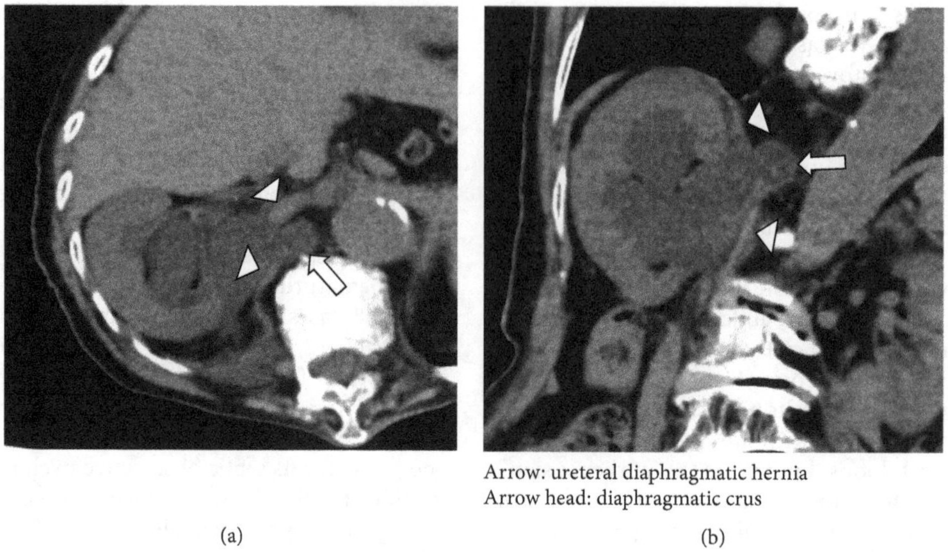

Figure 1: CT of the abdomen shows a diaphragmatic hernia of a part of urinary tract resulting in moderate-severe hydronephrosis ((a) axial and (b) coronal).

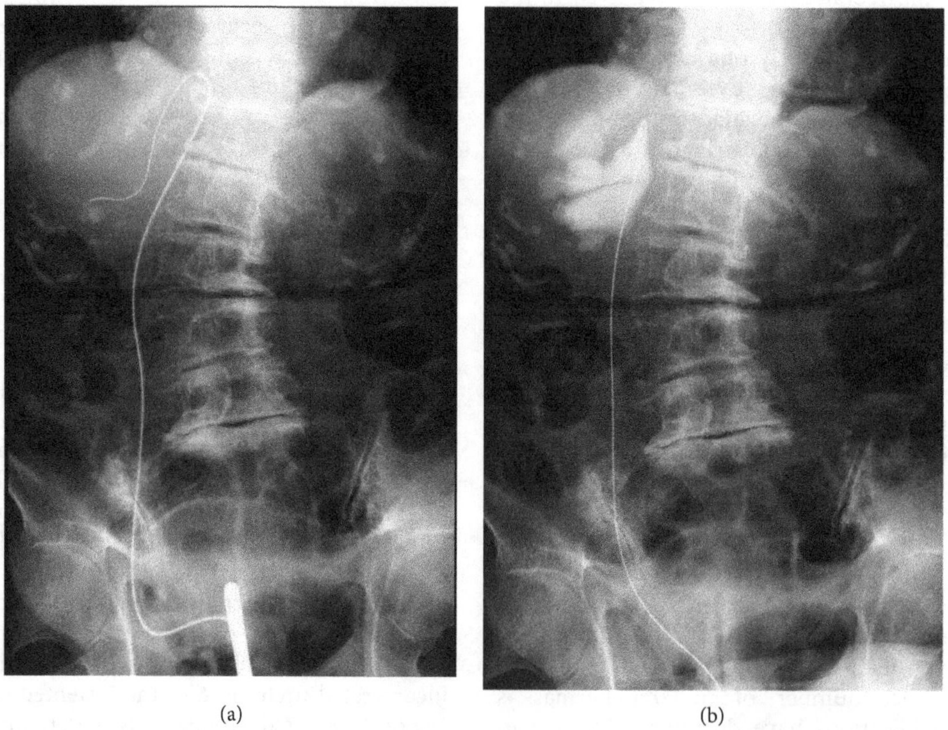

Figure 2: Insertion of guidewire at retrograde pyelography demonstrated ureteral loops through the diaphragm, known as a "curlicue sign" (a). At the time of ureteral manipulation by stent, the incarcerated ureter was reducted to the retroperitoneal cavity (b).

a small hernia orifice, it may be important for surgical repair to be done before an incarcerated ureter is reducted to the retroperitoneal cavity. Laparoscopic surgical repair may be more optimal than open surgery as the operative field is similar to that for retroperitoneoscopic nephrectomy.

In all 15 cases of ureteral diaphragmatic hernia, the herniation lateralized to the right-side; however, the etiology of this disorder characteristic is unknown [3].

Bochdalek hernias in adults are thought to be more prevalent on the left side than the right. It has been postulated that the liver normally obstructs any right-sided defect [17]. If there is hepatic atrophy or deformity, the liver no longer shields the diaphragm completely. Thus, the exposed diaphragm may be susceptible to right diaphragmatic herniation [17, 18]. In our present case, as hepatic atrophy was seen on CT examination, the patient likely had an exposed

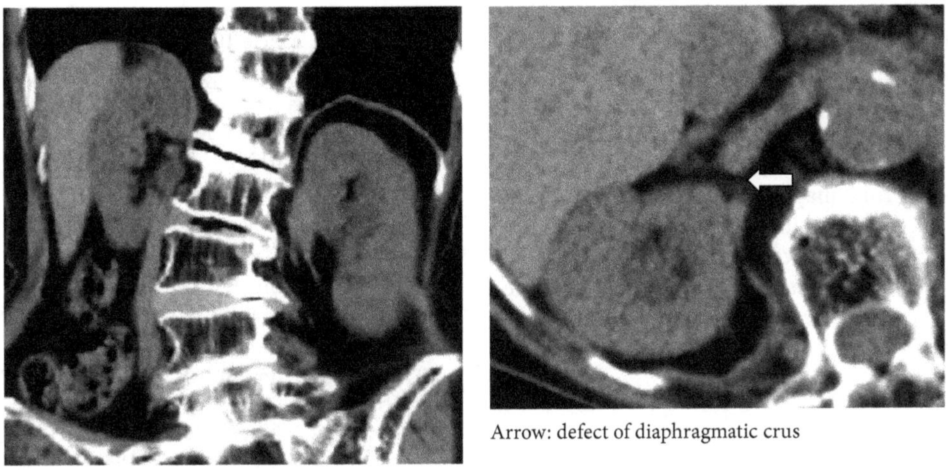

(a) (b)

FIGURE 3: Previous CT of the abdomen revealed the right kidney in a higher position than the left one ((a) coronal) and a defect of the right diaphragmatic crus which eventually became the hernia orifice ((b) axial).

TABLE 1: Review of ureteral diaphragmatic hernia reported in the literature in English.

No.	Author	Year	Age/gender	Laterality	Presentation	Hernia orifice	Treatment
1	Swithinbank	1958	60/F	R	Right flank pain	BF	Surgical repair
2	Paterson	1989	75/M	R	Right flank pain	BF	Surgical repair
3	Chawla	1994	56/M	R	Workup for left flank pain	BF	NA
4	Catalano	1998	63/F	R	Workup for renal stones	Retrocrural	Surgical repair
5	Sukumar	2010	75/F	R	Workup for azotemia	BF	Conservative
6	Balakrishnan	2011	83/F	R	Right flank pain	BF	Ureteral stenting
7	Song	2011	75/M	R	Right flank pain	BF	Ureteral stenting
8	Osman	2012	65/M	R	Right flank pain	BF	Conservative
9	Hatzidakis	2014	86/F	R	Septic obstructive pyelonephritis	BF	PNS→ureteral stenting
10	Almeida	2015	82/F	R	Workup for lung nodule	Retrocrural	NA
11	Dru	2016	94/F	R	Right flank pain	BF	Ureteral stenting
12	Lin	2017	81/F	R	Right flank pain	BF	Ureteral stenting→surgical repair
13	Beland	2019	84/F	R	Workup for ureteral stone	DP	Ureteral stenting
14	Heidar	2019	71/M	R	Workup for vomiting	DP	Conservative
15	Current case	2021	85/F	R	Right flank pain, fever	DC	Ureteral stenting

BF: Bochdalek foramen; DP: diaphragm; DC: diaphragmatic crus; NA: not available.

TABLE 2: Aggregate results of ureteral diaphragmatic hernia including present case.

Age, years old	Median: 75.0, mean: 75.6 (range: 56-94)
Gender, case	Female: 10 (66.6%), male: 5 (33.3%)
Diseased side, case	Right: 15 (100%)
Presentation, case	Rt. flank pain: 8 (53.3%), incidental: 7 (46.6%)
Diagnosis, case	CT+pyelography (RP, IVP, AP): 10 (66.6%) CT only: 4, RP only: 1 "Curlicue sign" was identified in all cases
Hernia orifice, case	Bochdalek foramen: 10 (66.6%), others: 5 (33.3%)
Treatment, case	Conservative: 3 (20.0%) Ureteral stenting: 7 (46.6%) Surgical repair: 4 (26.6%)

diaphragmatic area. In support of this, the high position of the right kidney due to hepatic atrophy and a defect of the right diaphragmatic crus which later became a hernia orifice had been identified on CT one year previously. In at least 6 (including ours) of the 15 cases (40.0%), the right kidney was in a higher position [3, 9, 10, 14, 16]. Consequently, the ureteral diaphragmatic hernia may be caused as a result of hepatic atrophy and/or high position of the right kidney.

Based on the above results, we can speculate that since the right upper urinary tract was close to the defect of the right diaphragmatic crus, increased intra-abdominal pressure may have caused the right ureter to eventually herniate through the defect.

4. Conclusions

Ureteral hernias are generally an exceptional occurrence, with ureteral diaphragmatic hernia being even more exceedingly rare in the literature. Imaging studies such as CT and/or pyelography are imperative for the diagnosis of ureteral diaphragmatic hernia. Management strategies depend on the clinical context. In cases of obstructive pyelonephritis or renal dysfunction, drainage is essential. A trial with retrograde ureteral stenting is reasonable and minimally invasive and has a notable success rate. While the etiology of ureteral diaphragmatic hernia remains unknown, our present case and previous reports suggest that the ureteral diaphragmatic hernia may be the result of hepatic atrophy and/or a high position of the right kidney.

Consent

Written informed consent was obtained from the patient for publication of this case report and any accompanying images.

Authors' Contributions

T. Y., T. S., and S. O. conducted the literature review. E. I. and K. K. diagnosed the patient and were responsible for retrieval of radiologic images. A. I., S. F., and K. K. helped write the manuscript. T. Y. edited the final version of the manuscript. All authors read and approved the final manuscript before submission.

References

[1] E. S. Allam, D. Y. Johnson, S. G. Grewal, and F. E. Johnson, "Inguinoscrotal herniation of the ureter: description of five cases," *International Journal of Surgery Case Reports*, vol. 14, pp. 160–163, 2015.

[2] O. Catalano, A. Nunziata, B. Cusati, and A. Siani, "Retrocrural loop of the ureter: CT findings," *American Journal of Roentgenology*, vol. 170, no. 5, pp. 1293-1294, 1998.

[3] F. C. Lin, J. S. Lin, S. Kim, and J. R. Walker, "A rare diaphragmatic ureteral herniation case report: endoscopic and open reconstructive management," *BMC Urology*, vol. 17, no. 1, p. 26, 2017.

[4] N. A. Heidar, H. Elsemesmani, A. Elamine, and M. Natout, "A rare case of isolated ureteral diaphragmatic herniation: case report and review of literature," *Case Report in Urology*, vol. 2019, article 1092018, 4 pages, 2019.

[5] N. Osman, S. Venugopal, G. Doyle, and C. S. Powell, "Bochdalek's hernia causing functional upper ureteric obstruction," *British Journal of Medical&Surgical Urology*, vol. 5, no. 2, pp. 90–92, 2012.

[6] L. Almeida, F. Carvalhaes, A. Bitencourt, and F. Moreira, "Ureteral hernia mimicking retrocrural lymphadenopathy in 18F-FDG PET/CT," *Clinical Nuclear Medicine*, vol. 40, no. 8, pp. e415–e416, 2015.

[7] A. H. Swithinbank, "Intrathoracic deviation of a ureteric loop," *British Journal of Surgery*, vol. 45, no. 192, pp. 379–381, 2005.

[8] I. S. Paterson and E. W. Lupton, "Periureteric junction obstruction secondary to renal pelvic incarceration in a congenital diaphragmatic hernia," *British Journal of Urology*, vol. 64, no. 5, pp. 548-549, 1989.

[9] K. Chawla and D. J. Mond, "Progressive bochdalek hernia with unusual ureteral herniation," *Computerized Medical Imaging and Graphics*, vol. 18, no. 1, pp. 53–58, 1994.

[10] S. Sukumar, P. G. Kumar, and A. Thomas, "Thoracic curlicue: a case of ureteral herniation," *Indian Journal of Urology*, vol. 26, no. 1, pp. 131-132, 2010.

[11] V. Balakrishnan and G. Neerhut, "Right sided Bochdalek hernia causing ureteric obstruction," *BJU International*, 2011, http://www.bjui.co.uk/ContentFullItem.aspx?id=769&SectionType=1&title=Right-sided-Bochdalek-hernia-causing-ureteric-obstruction.

[12] Y. S. Song, C. Hassani, and P. M. Nardi, "Bochdalek hernia with obstructive uropathy," *Urology*, vol. 77, no. 6, p. 1338, 2011.

[13] A. Hatzidakis, A. Kozana, D. Glaritis, and C. Mamoulakis, "Right-sided Bochdalek hernia causing septic ureteric obstruction. Percutaneous treatment with placement of a nephroureteral double pigtail," *BMJ Case Reports*, vol. 2014, 2014.

[14] C. J. Dru and D. Y. Josephson, "Bochdalek-type diaphragmatic hernia leading to high-grade kidney obstruction," *Urology*, vol. 97, pp. e17–e18, 2016.

[15] H. M. Pollack, G. L. Popky, and M. L. Blumberg, "Hernias of the ureter—an anatomic-roentgenographic study," *Radiology*, vol. 117, no. 2, pp. 275–281, 1975.

[16] L. E. Beland, M. A. Henry, T. Solomon, and K. Ogan, "Obstructing nephrolithiasis in an 84-year-old patient with a diaphragmatic herniated ureter," *Urology*, vol. 124, pp. e1–e3, 2019.

[17] P. P. S. Chui and C. T. T. Tan, "Sudden death due to incarcerated Bochdalek hernia in an adult," *Annales of the Academy of Medicine, Singapore*, vol. 22, no. 1, pp. 57–60, 1993.

[18] K. Kyoku, Y. Okuda, S. Hashimoto, A. Hara, K. Akiyama, and T. Goya, "A case of adult right sided Bochdalek hernia needed emergency operation with bowel obstruction," *KMJ Kitakanto Medical Journal*, vol. 71, no. 1, pp. 53–58, 2021.

30

Initial Diagnosis and Detection of Very Late Local Recurrence of a Ductal Prostate Cancer due to a Ureteral Stone

Manolis Pratsinis,[1] Charlotte Düwel,[2] Olivia Köhle,[1] Annette Enzler-Tschudy,[3] Hans-Peter Schmid,[1] and Patrick Betschart[1]

[1]*Department of Urology, Cantonal Hospital St. Gallen, St. Gallen, Switzerland*
[2]*Department of Urology, Klinikum Rechts der Isar, Technical University of Munich, Munich, Germany*
[3]*Department of Pathology, Cantonal Hospital St. Gallen, St. Gallen, Switzerland*

Correspondence should be addressed to Manolis Pratsinis; manolis.pratsinis@gmail.com

Academic Editor: Shiou-Sheng Chen

We report the case of a 74-year-old patient in whom a ductal prostate cancer was incidentally endoscopically diagnosed in the course of ureteral stenting due to a left distal ureteral stone. The initial PSA was 0.8 μg/l and the digital rectal examination was not suspicious. A radical prostatectomy was performed, and the ensuing follow-up was unremarkable with no signs of recurrence. Fourteen years later, the patient presented with an obstructive pyelonephritis due to a left-sided ureteral stone requiring ureteral stenting. An exophytic tumor was seen in the lining of vesicourethral anastomosis and surgically excised after the pyelonephritis subsided. The histopathological and immunohistochemical analysis revealed a ductal cancer of the prostate consistent with a late local recurrence. Serum PSA was below the limit of detection. Re-staging performed by an MRI of the pelvis, thoracoabdominal CT scan, and gallium-68 PSMA-PET did not reveal any other signs of disease. The ensuing follow-up is planned with regular flexible cystoscopy and computed thoracoabdominopelvic CT scans.

1. Introduction

The majority of prostate cancers are adenocarcinomas, with histological variants seen in 5–10% of carcinomas [1]. Ductal adenocarcinoma is the most common histological variant with pure ductal adenocarcinoma accounting for 0.4–0.8% of prostate cancer cases and mixed ductal adenocarcinoma seen in up to 5% of cases. The initial clinical manifestation is often hematuria and/or obstructive urinary symptoms as ductal adenocarcinomas classically arise in the central prostatic ducts [2]. Compared with acinar adenocarcinomas of the prostate, the serum prostate-specific antigen (PSA) level of ductal adenocarcinomas was seen to be 30% lower in a multivariate linear regression analysis of the SEER database performed by Morgan et al. in 2010 [3]. In the same study, ductal adenocarcinomas were also more likely high grade and had distant disease at initial presentation. Furthermore, even those patients with localized disease at diagnosis had a 2.4-fold increase of disease-specific mortality, highlighting the aggressive natural history of ductal adenocarcinomas compared with acinar adenocarcinomas [3].

In localized disease, radical prostatectomy or external beam radiation therapy is recommended. Optimal management poses a challenge for clinicians, as ductal adenocarcinomas may not express PSA, potentially delaying the diagnosis of disease and complicating follow-up.

2. Case Presentation

The at-the-time 60-year-old patient was referred to our clinic 14 years ago due to persistent left-sided flank pain for over six months. The patient described intermittent radiating pain to the left groin and denied micturition disorders such as urinary discomfort or gross hematuria. Left-sided hydronephrosis was seen on renal ultrasound, and a kidney, ureter, bladder (KUB) plain film radiography was performed demonstrating an 8 mm large opaque structure in projection of the distal ureter, suspicious for a ureteral stone as well as a 10 mm large bladder stone. Stone therapy with transurethral lithotripsy and ureteral stenting on the left was planned. During cystoscopy, an exulcerating lesion with whitish, fibrinous necrotic slough was seen left of verumontanum, with no other lesions apparent. The bladder stone was disintegrated and removed using a grasping forceps, and a biopsy of the tumor was performed. The ureteral stone was pushed back into the left renal pelvis and a double-pigtail stent was inserted. Further stone treatment was performed by extracorporeal shock wave lithotripsy with removal of the ureteral stent after radiological disintegration of the stone was seen.

The histopathological analysis revealed a ductal adenocarcinoma of the prostate. Digital rectal examination of the prostate was not suspicious, and total serum PSA was 0.8 μg/l. The tumor markers carcinoembryonic antigen (CEA), carbohydrate antigen 19-9 (CA 19-9), and cancer antigen 125 (CA 125) were normal. Staging was conducted with a pelvic MRI, thoracoabdominal CT scan, and bone scintigraphy without evidence of metastasis. A radical prostatectomy with extended pelvic lymphadenectomy was performed, with ductal adenocarcinoma seen in both prostate lobes without extraprostatic extension, nodal metastasis, or positive surgical margins, corresponding to a pT2c, pN0, cM0, Gleason score 7b (4 + 3), R0 stage. The postoperative course was uneventful, and the patient was subjected to regular clinical follow-up with digital-rectal examination and serum PSA control. Serum PSA was not detectable in the first postoperative control and remained below the limit of detection throughout the whole duration of follow-up. The patient had persistent postoperative stress urinary incontinence, which required the use of 1-2 pads per day with an otherwise unremarkable follow-up.

Fourteen years after the initial diagnosis, the now 74-year-old patient was admitted to the emergency department with fever and left-sided flank pain. A computed tomography of the abdomen revealed an 8 mm stone in the distal left ureter with consecutive dilation of the left ureter and perirenal stranding of the left kidney indicating obstructive pyelonephritis. Intravenous antibiotic therapy was initiated, and the immediate ureteral stenting of the left ureter was performed with a double-pigtail stent. During cystoscopy, a solitary 15 mm large tumorous lesion was seen on the left side of vesicourethral anastomosis, which was not resected due to the urosepsis. The patient quickly recovered from the infection and was subjected to a transurethral resection of the tumor and semirigid ureteroscopy for stone removal. The tumorous lesion of the bladder was resected in toto and the ureterolithiasis successfully removed.

The histological analysis revealed a ductal adenocarcinoma consistent with a local recurrence of the known ductal adenocarcinoma of the prostate (Figure 1). Immunohistochemical analysis revealed a low focal PSA positivity and androgen receptor (AR) positivity in approximately 60% of tumor cells (Figure 2). The Ki67 proliferation index was 3%.

Imaging with a pelvic MRI, thoracoabdominal CT scan, and a gallium-68 PSMA-PET scan revealed no signs of metastasis. The case was discussed at our multidisciplinary tumor board, and external beam radiation therapy of the prostate bed was recommended to reduce the risk of recurrence. The patient wished to abstain from further therapy so as not to worsen the preexisting stress urinary incontinence. A flexible cystoscopy was performed 3 months postoperatively demonstrating an unremarkable vesicourethral anastomosis. Further follow-up is scheduled with annual cystoscopies and thoracoabdominopelvic CT scans.

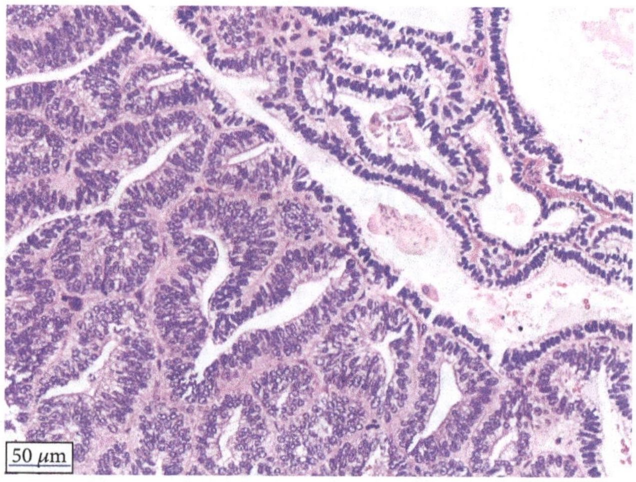

Figure 1: Hematoxylin and eosin staining. Ductal adenocarcinoma of the prostate with pseudoendometrioid growth pattern, focally even reminiscent of secreting endometrium.

3. Discussion

In the reported case, a very late local recurrence was incidentally detected fourteen years after initial diagnosis. Prior to that, regular follow-up had been performed with digital rectal examinations and serum PSA detection, with no signs of local recurrence and a serum PSA which was below detection level. Furthermore, the Ki67 proliferation index of the resected local recurrence was very low at 3%, indicating a very slowly growing disease, which may partially explain the long latency period between primary diagnosis and recurrence.

As with the initial diagnosis, the recurrence was only detected due to left-sided ureterolithiasis. Chung et al. performed a retrospective population-based case-control study to assess the association of prostate cancer and urinary calculi. While they were able to show that the incidence of prior urinary calculi was higher in patients with newly diagnosed prostate cancer compared with the control group (21% vs. 14.1%), no significant relationship was seen in regard to ureter calculi [4].

The treatment of localized disease of ductal adenocarcinomas of the prostate consists of radical prostatectomy or external beam radiation therapy. When compared with acinar adenocarcinomas of the prostate, ductal cancers were more likely to present with advanced disease and a lower PSA indicating the challenging diagnosis [3]. Patients who were subjected to surgical treatment by radical prostatectomy appeared to have a higher risk of extraprostatic extension,

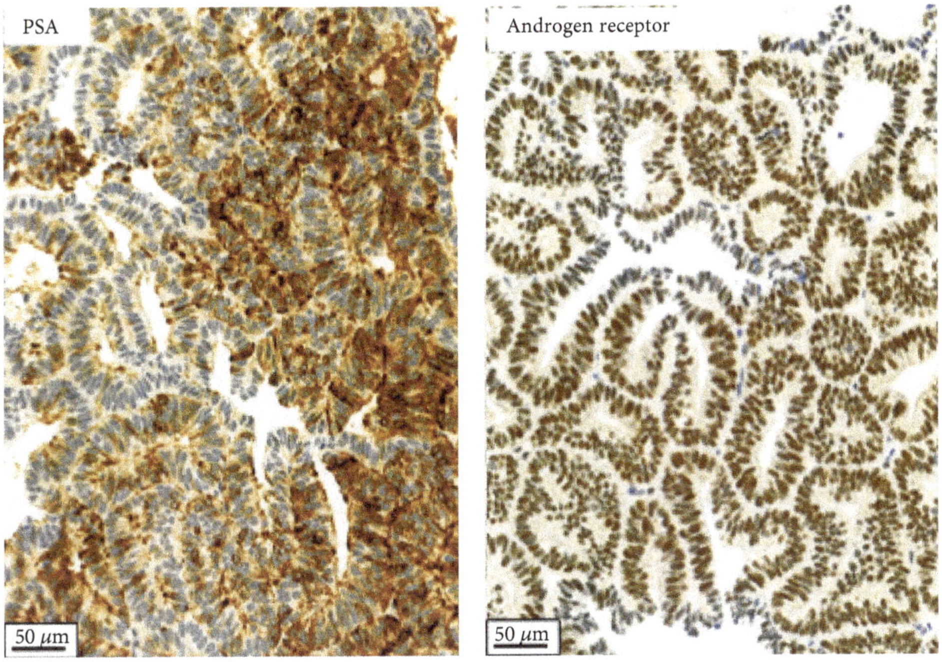

(a) (b)

FIGURE 2: Immunohistochemical staining. Ductal adenocarcinoma of the prostate with focal expression of PSA (a). Nuclear expression of androgen receptor in approximately 60% of tumor cells (b).

positive surgical margins [5, 6], and a higher local recurrence rate [7] when compared with acinar adenocarcinomas of the prostate. Nonetheless, there is currently no recommended specific alterations of follow-up compared with acinar adenocarcinomas of the prostate in the latest prostate cancer guidelines of the European Association of Urology [8]. A recent retrospective analysis of twenty-seven patients treated with radiotherapy and androgen deprivation therapy by Bergamin et al. recommended including regular CT scans in follow-up as local recurrences and metastasis occurred at undetectable PSA levels [9], but prospective data regarding the optimal follow-up is lacking.

4. Conclusion

Ductal adenocarcinomas of the prostate are rare histological variants and should be treated as a separate tumor entity with an individualized management. When localized disease is present, a radical prostatectomy or external beam radiation therapy can be performed. The further follow-up has to be tailored to the individual patient, as PSA is not a reliable tool for assessing the existence of disease. Furthermore, regular thoracoabdominopelvic imaging, for instance, with regular CT or MRI scans as well as flexible cystoscopies should be considered.

Consent

The author retains written patient consent and copies of the consent can be provided on request.

References

[1] J. I. Epstein, A. L. Cubilla, and P. A. Humphrey, "Tumors of the prostate gland, seminal vesicles, penis, and scrotum," in *AFIP Atlas of Tumor Pathology Series*, p. 4, American Registry of Pathology, Silver Spring, MD, USA, 2011.

[2] J. D. Hertel and P. A. Humphrey, "Ductal adenocarcinoma of the prostate," *The Journal of Urology*, vol. 186, no. 1, pp. 277-278, 2011.

[3] T. M. Morgan, C. J. Welty, F. Vakar-Lopez, D. W. Lin, and J. L. Wright, "Ductal adenocarcinoma of the prostate: increased mortality risk and decreased serum prostate specific antigen," *The Journal of Urology*, vol. 184, no. 6, pp. 2303–2307, 2010.

[4] S. D. Chung, S. P. Liu, and H. C. Lin, "Association between prostate cancer and urinary calculi: a population-based study," *PLoS One*, vol. 8, no. 2, article e57743, 2013.

[5] H. Samaratunga, D. Duffy, J. Yaxley, and B. Delahunt, "Any proportion of ductal adenocarcinoma in radical prostatectomy specimens predicts extraprostatic extension," *Human Pathology*, vol. 41, no. 2, pp. 281–285, 2010.

[6] D. A. Brinker, S. R. Potter, and J. I. Epstein, "Ductal adenocarcinoma of the prostate diagnosed on needle biopsy: correlation with clinical and radical prostatectomy findings and progression," *The American Journal of Surgical Pathology*, vol. 23, no. 12, pp. 1471–1479, 1999.

[7] S. M. Tu, A. Lopez, D. Leibovici et al., "Ductal adenocarcinoma of the prostate: clinical features and implications after local therapy," *Cancer*, vol. 115, no. 13, pp. 2872–2880, 2009.

[8] N. Mottet, R. C. N. van den Bergh, E. Briers et al., "EAU – ESTRO – ESUR – SIOG guidelines on prostate cancer," 2019,

https://uroweb.org/wp-content/uploads/EAU-ESUR-ESTRO-SIOG-Guidelines-on-Prostate-Cancer-large-text-V2.pdf.

[9] S. Bergamin, T. Eade, A. Kneebone et al., "Ductal carcinoma of the prostate: an uncommon entity with atypical behaviour," *Clinical Oncology*, vol. 31, no. 2, pp. 108–114, 2019.

Total Penectomy for Recurrent Chordoma of the Corpus Cavernosum

Lennert Eismann,[1] Sabine Kess,[2] Christian G. Stief,[1] and Frank Strittmatter[1]

[1]*Department of Urology, Ludwig-Maximilians-University, Munich, Germany*
[2]*Department of Gynecology and Obstetrics, University Hospital of Heidelberg, Heidelberg, Germany*

Correspondence should be addressed to Lennert Eismann; lennert.eismann@med.uni-muenchen.de

Academic Editor: Francesco M. Solivetti

Chordomas are rare low malignant neoplasm arising from remnants of the notochord with predilection site of the clivus or the os sacrum. Standard therapy is radical excision and adjuvant radiation. Due to invasive growth and adjacent to vital structures resection is often incomplete, and therefore, local recurrence is frequent. First, to the best knowledge of our authors, we present a 70-year-old man with a recurrent chordoma infiltrating the corpus cavernosum. Asymptomatic recurrence was diagnosed by magnet resonance imaging according to the standard follow-up. Our interdisciplinary tumor board recommended surgical resection. We performed a total penectomy and perineal urethrostomy to achieve negative resection margins and preserve best quality of life for the patient.

1. Introduction

Chordoma is a rare malignancy with an incidence reported up to 0.08/100,000 person per year with a predominance in male patients according to the Surveillance, Epidemiology, and End Results (SEER) [1]. They arise from the notochord along the axial skeleton and occur most frequently in the os sacrum and the skull base region [1]. According to the histopathology, chordomas are considered low-grade malignant neoplasms; therefore, slow but locally aggressive growth patterns explain late clinical appearance [2]. Independent of primary tumor location, standard therapy remains radical en bloc resection [3]. Total resection is often not feasible due to infiltration of surrounding vital structures [1]. Local recurrence is frequently seen after incomplete resection or after violation of tumor capsule [1, 4]. The 5-year local relapse rate for completely resected sacral chordoma remains 30% [5]. Local recurrence determines patient's survival [1]. In 5% of patients suffering from chordomas, distant metastasis in the lungs, bone, skin, and the central nervous system are reported at initial diagnosis [1].

Here, we report about a rare case of local recurrence of a sacral chordoma after multiple resections. The patient was referred to our urological department for surgical treatment of a clinically inapparent recurrence located on the basis of the corpora cavernosa. We performed a complete resection of the recurrent chordoma by total penectomy and perineal urethrostomy.

2. Case Presentation

A 70-year-old patient was referred to our Department of Urology, Faculty of Medicine, Munich Germany, for a surgical treatment of a recurrent chordoma located at the radix penis. The primary chordoma of the os sacrum was diagnosed in 1996 and primarily resected. In the following eight years, the patient underwent three resections (R2) of local recurrences before starting medical therapy with imatinib 400 mg per day in 2009. In 2014, a dorsal complete compartment resection was performed for a fifth local recurrence (R0). Imatinib was paused until in the same year, a single pulmonary metastasis was diagnosed and treated by surgery (R0). Consequently, the medical therapy with imatinib was restarted. In the following year, a local recurrence of the proximal femur was diagnosed. Furthermore, the complete resection (R0) of the gluteal metastases was performed in

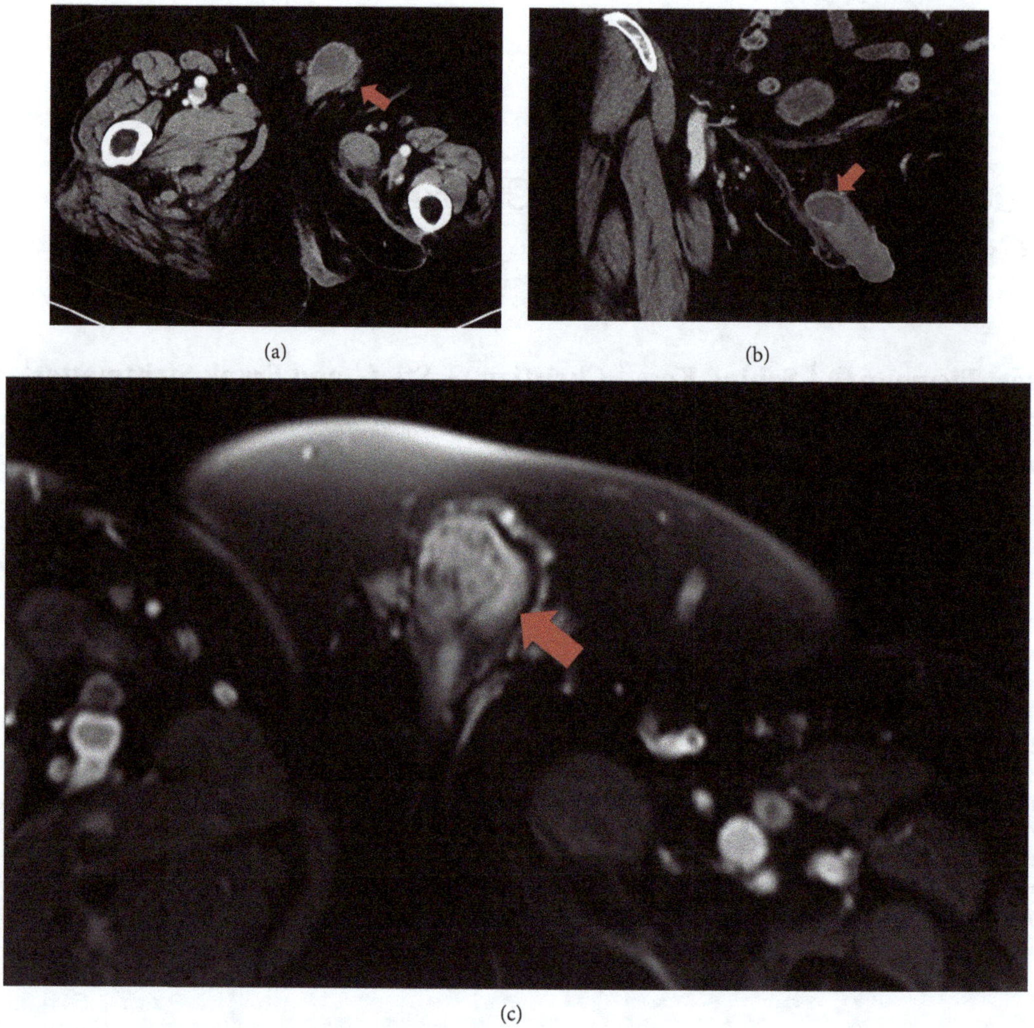

FIGURE 1: Preoperative MR imaging: (a) axial, (b) coronal, and (c) axial in T1 perfusion. Red arrows mark chordoma metastasis at the right corpus cavernosum of the penis as solid mass of about 2.3 × 3.0 cm.

2017. In February 2019, another pulmonary metastasis was treated by atypical pulmonary resection (R0).

The follow-up computer tomography (CT) and magnet resonance imaging (MRI) indicated a suspicious lesion of the radix penis (Figure 1). Therefore, a biopsy was taken to prove the seventh local recurrence. The histopathology showed a chondroid chordoma. Clinically, the recurrence was unapparent. The interdisciplinary tumor board advised a surgical treatment.

2.1. Surgical Treatment. For preoperative preparation, a standard blood sample was taken, an abdominal CT scan in order to plan surgical procedure was performed and, antibiotic perioperative prophylaxis was given. We performed a total penectomy and perineal urethrostomy (Figures 2(a) and 2(b)). The intraoperative surgical margin was negative. Postoperatively, a transurethral catheter was used for 5 days to decrease risk of infection and to improve wound healing. A total inpatient stay of 7 days was noted. We reevaluated wound healing and functional outcome 14 days postoperatively.

2.2. Histopathology Findings. The macroscopic preparation showed an asymmetric indurated lesion with a maximal expansion of 4.1 × 2.5 × 2.6 cm. The resection margin to the corpus cavernosum was measured 0.3 cm and to the corpus spongiosum 1.9 cm. The tumor showed a suppressive, but not infiltrative growth of the corpus cavernosum.

The microscopic evaluation revealed a microcystic and partly solid tumor embedded in a myxoid and chondroid matrix (Figures 2(c) and 2(d)). In the center of the tumor, hemorrhagic and necrotic parts were identified. The tumor cells were voluminous and rich of vacuoles with rough chromatin.

3. Discussion

Local recurrence of chordoma is common even after aggressive surgical excision of primary tumor depending on surgical margins [4, 6]. Incomplete resection in initial therapy is a prognostic predictor for poor overall survival [7]. The literature describes 49% of disease-free survival after 15 years for negative surgical margins in comparison to 7% after R1 status

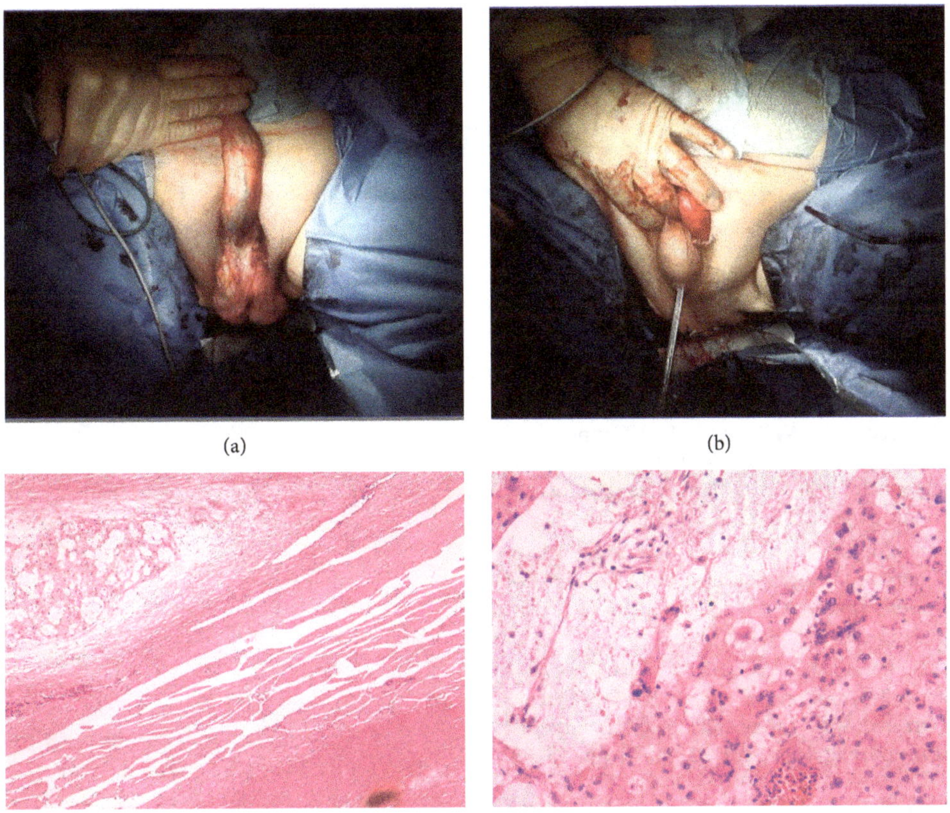

FIGURE 2: (a) First, the penis was denudated and the corpora cavernosa was separated before complete penectomy was performed. (b) In the last step, the urethra was diverted through the perineum. In the histology findings, the hematoxylin and eosin section shows corpora cavernosa infiltrated by typical physaliferous vacuolated large chordoma cells embedded in a myxoid stroma in images (c) and (d) (magnification 20x).

in sacral chordomas [5]. Postoperative follow-up to detect recurrence is important before reaching a size to become clinically apparent [8]. The treatment of recurrence remains the surgical resection and/or radiotherapy [4]. The literature describes that local recurrence of the os sacrum and mobile spine is highly related to tumor-related death [9]. Treatment options have to be chosen carefully by an interdisciplinary team to preserve best quality of life [4].

Most penile tumors are squamous cell carcinoma [10]. Metastases of the penis are uncommon, most frequently are primary malignancies from the urogenital tract [11]. Depending on tumor stage and location of the tumor, there are various treatment options [10]. The gold standard in advanced tumor stage is total penectomy and perineal urethrostomy [12]. Also, perineal urethrostomy is the last treatment option for benign urethral disease such as urethral strictures [13]. Despite invasiveness of total penectomy particularly affecting sexuality [14], Barbagli et al. reports a satisfaction after perineal urethrostomy in cases of urethral stricture of 78% [15].

There is one case that reported of a primary vaginal chordoma treated successfully by surgery; other than that, no chordomas of the genital region have been described so far [16].

We describe the first case of a recurrent chordoma located at the corpus cavernosum treated with total penectomy and perineal urethrostomy. For best oncological outcome, wide resection margins were achieved and perineal urethrostomy was performed to preserve continence.

4. Conclusions

The treatment of chordoma and its recurrence disease demands an aggressive surgical excision for best long-term survival in consideration of conserving vital structures and preserving best quality of life.

References

[1] B. P. Walcott, B. V. Nahed, A. Mohyeldin, J.-V. Coumans, K. T. Kahle, and M. J. Ferreira, "Chordoma: current concepts, management, and future directions," *The Lancet Oncology*, vol. 13, no. 2, pp. e69–e76, 2012.

[2] V. Colia and S. Stacchiotti, "Medical treatment of advanced chordomas," *European Journal of Cancer*, vol. 83, pp. 220–228, 2017.

[3] S. Stacchiotti and J. Sommer, "Building a global consensus approach to chordoma: a position paper from the medical and patient community," *The Lancet Oncology*, vol. 16, no. 2, pp. e71–e83, 2015.

[4] S. Stacchiotti, A. Gronchi, P. Fossati et al., "Best practices for the management of local-regional recurrent chordoma: a

position paper by the Chordoma Global Consensus Group," *Annals of Oncology*, vol. 28, no. 6, pp. 1230–1242, 2017.

[5] S. Radaelli, S. Stacchiotti, P. Ruggieri et al., "Sacral chordoma: long-term outcome of a large series of patients surgically treated at two reference centers," *Spine*, vol. 41, no. 12, pp. 1049–1057, 2016.

[6] P. Ruggieri, A. Angelini, G. Ussia, M. Montalti, and M. Mercuri, "Surgical margins and local control in resection of sacral chordomas," *Clinical Orthopaedics and Related Research®*, vol. 468, no. 11, pp. 2939–2947, 2010.

[7] M. X. Zou, J. Li, X. B. Wang, and G. H. Lv, "Prognostic significance of resection degree in skull base chordoma: a systematic review and meta-analysis," *World Neurosurgery*, vol. 100, pp. 692–694, 2017.

[8] S. A. Hanna, W. J. S. Aston, T. W. R. Briggs, S. R. Cannon, and A. Saifuddin, "Sacral chordoma: can local recurrence after sacrectomy be predicted?," *Clinical Orthopaedics and Related Research*, vol. 466, no. 9, pp. 2217–2223, 2008.

[9] P. Bergh, L.-G. Kindblom, B. Gunterberg, F. Remotti, W. Ryd, and J. M. Meis-Kindblom, "Prognostic factors in chordoma of the sacrum and mobile spine: a study of 39 patients," *Cancer*, vol. 88, no. 9, pp. 2122–2134, 2000.

[10] E. Marchionne, C. Perez, A. Hui, and A. Khachemoune, "Penile squamous cell carcinoma: a review of the literature and case report treated with Mohs micrographic surgery," *Anais Brasileiros de Dermatologia*, vol. 92, no. 1, pp. 95–99, 2017.

[11] K. Zhang, J. Da, H.-j. Yao et al., "Metastatic tumors of the penis: a report of 8 cases and review of the literature," *Medicine*, vol. 94, no. 1, p. e132, 2015.

[12] A. Simonato, A. Lissiani, S. Galli, A. Bozzola, A. Gregori, and F. Gaboardi, "Total penectomy with perineal urethrostomy for carcinoma of the penis," *European Urology Supplements*, vol. 1, no. 1, p. 193, 2002.

[13] N. Lumen, M. Beysens, C. Van Praet et al., "Perineal urethrostomy: surgical and functional evaluation of two techniques," *BioMed Research International*, vol. 2015, Article ID 365715, 6 pages, 2015.

[14] R. Sosnowski, M. Kulpa, M. Kosowicz et al., "Quality of life in penile carcinoma patients - post-total penectomy," *Central European Journal of Urology*, vol. 69, no. 2, pp. 204–211, 2016.

[15] G. Barbagli, M. De Angelis, G. Romano, and M. Lazzeri, "Clinical outcome and quality of life assessment in patients treated with perineal urethrostomy for anterior urethral stricture disease," *The Journal of Urology*, vol. 182, no. 2, pp. 548–557, 2009.

[16] S. L. Wei He, X. Gan, and L. Hu, "Chordoma of vagina a case report and review of the literature," *International Journal of Clinical and Experimental Medicine*, vol. 11, no. 5, pp. 5164–5170, 2018.

32

Vulvar Pyogenic Granuloma in Adult Female Population: A Case Report and Review of the Literature

Nastaran Mahmoudnejad,[1] **Alireza Zadmehr**,[2] **and Mohammad Hamidi Madani**[3]

[1]*Assistant Professor of Urology, Fellowship of Female Urology, Labbafinejad Hospital, Urology and Nephrology Research Center, Shahid Beheshti University of Medical Sciences (SBMU), Tehran, Iran*
[2]*Resident of Urology, Labbafinejad Hospital, Urology and Nephrology Research Center, Shahid Beheshti University of Medical Science (SBMU), Tehran, Iran*
[3]*Department of Urology, Labbafinejad Hospital, Shahid Beheshti University of Medical Science (SBMU), Tehran, Iran*

Correspondence should be addressed to Mohammad Hamidi Madani; m.hamidimadani70@gmail.com

Academic Editor: Tun-Chieh Chen

Pyogenic granuloma (PG) is an uncommon lesion of unknown etiology. It may be formed following a minor injury. They result from a reactive or inflammatory process consisting of proliferating vascular channels, immature fibroblastic connective tissue, and scattered inflammatory cells rather than neoplastic process. Bleeding is the most common symptom of the lesion. They may be seen in all age groups, and there is no clear predominance of a gender. Vulvar PGs can be confused with other polypoid or sessile lesions of the genital site. There are only a few cases of female genital PGs reported in the literature. Herein, we describe the first case of vulvar (clitoral) PG in an Iranian patient and a brief review of the literature in this regard.

1. Introduction

Lobular capillary hemangioma or pyogenic granuloma (PG) is a common acquired benign vascular lesion of the skin and mucous membranes. [1–3] PG is one of the most common vascular tumors in all ages and may be formed following a minor injury. [3] This hypervascularized lesion grows rapidly in a couple of weeks or months and usually presents as an erythematous, pedunculated, exophytic, or sessile lesion, with a smooth or lobulated surface [1–4]. PGs may be seen at different areas including the head, neck, and extremities or in the oral mucosa cavity during pregnancy [3–6]. Vulvar PG is a rare finding, and to our best knowledge, only twelve cases in adult female population have been described in the literature [3, 4, 6–12]. Herein, we introduce the first vulvar PG in an Iranian female patient and a brief review of the literature in this regard.

2. Case Presentation

A 54-year-old married woman complained of an easy bleeding, nontender, relatively fast growing clitoral lesion since 6 months ago. She did not mention any genital injury or trauma lately. In past medical history, we did not find anything contributory. Physical examination revealed a 2.5×0.5 cm, pedunculated, erythematous, granulation tissue-like appearance lesion beneath the clitoral hood (Figure 1). Vaginal examination was unremarkable, and routine lab tests were all within normal limits. She underwent surgical excision of the lesion under local anesthesia. We did not use any electrocautery in the region, and base of the mass was repaired with separate absorbable 3-0 sutures. She was discharged from the hospital at the same day. Postoperative course was uneventful. Histopathological evaluation revealed a 19.98 mm polypoid lesion with surface ulceration, composed

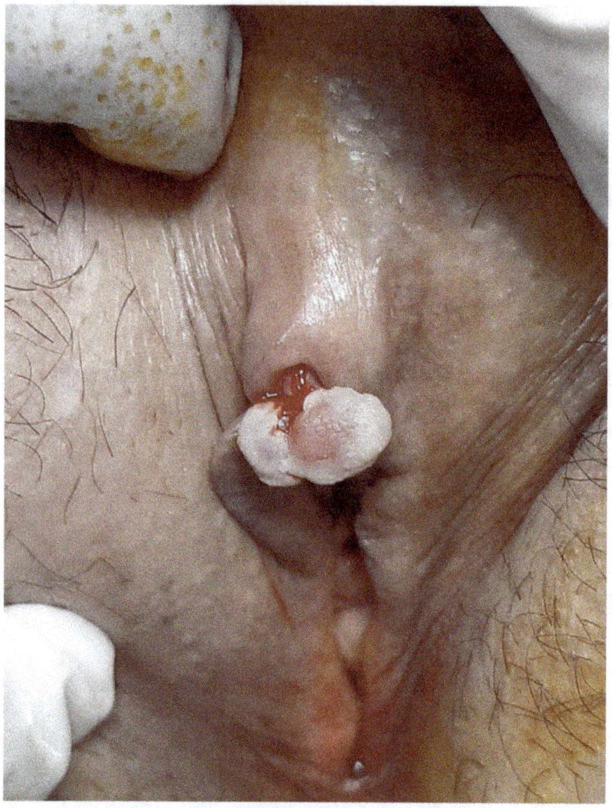

Figure 1: A 2.5×0.5 cm pedunculated and easy bleeding lesion beneath the clitoral hood.

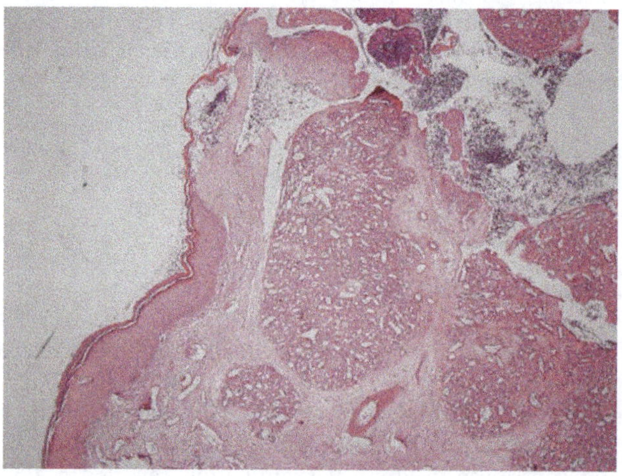

Figure 2: Ulcerated skin with a lobular growth pattern of capillary sized vessels (H&E, ×40).

of lobular configuration of capillaries within inflamed stroma compatible with PG (Figure 2). In the six-month postoperative visit, there was no recurrence or scar tissue at the surgical site. Tactile and sexual sensation of the clitoris was preserved.

3. Discussion

PG results from a reactive or inflammatory process, and it consists of proliferating vascular channels, immature fibroblastic connective tissue, and scattered inflammatory cells rather than neoplastic process. The exact etiology and pathogenesis of these lesions are not fully understood. However, it is assumed that minor trauma (in 50% of patients), chronic local irritation, hormonal influences, viral oncogenes, underlying microscopic arteriovenous malformation, and production of angiogenic factors may play a role in formation of them [5]. PG has variable variants including disseminated, subcutaneous, intravenous, and systemic medication-induced subtypes [9]. Bleeding is usually the leading symptom for a visit to the doctor's office. It can be profuse and refractory to conservative treatment [13].

These lesions may be seen in all age groups, and according to our literature review, there is no clear predominance of a gender [13]. Based on Arikan et al.'s study, there was a higher frequency of PG in the second decade of life and a female predilection of 2 : 1 [3]. A 10-year retrospective analysis of 82 cases by Akamatsu et al. [1] revealed a slight male gender preponderance in overall patients, and the head and neck areas, including the oral cavity and nasal mucosa, were the most affected sites in both sexes.

PGs are considered to be benign. However, vulvar PGs can cause confusion with some benign and malignant genital lesions including warts, giant condylomas, Kaposi's sarcoma, basal cell carcinoma, malignant melanoma, lymphomas, bowenoid papulosis, verrucous carcinoma, acquired tufted angioma, epithelioid hemangioendothelioma and bacillary angiomatosis [4, 13]. Approximately 63% of the patients may have an associated underlying systemic disorder like rheumatoid arthritis, hematological malignancies, and inflammatory bowel disease. In "localized genital" PGs, underlying systemic diseases are extremely rare [6]. Various cutaneous pathologies including port wine stains, psoriasis, eczema, burns, erythroderma, insect bites, and even cutaneous changes following retinoid therapy may be accompanied by PGs [9].

Invasive and minimally invasive treatments of PGs include surgical excision, curettage followed by electrocauterization, cryotherapy with liquid nitrogen, sclerotherapy, radiosurgery, silver nitrate cautery, microembolization, and lasers. Photodynamic therapy with 5-aminolevulinic acid has been used for single PG either [8, 13]. Several oral or topical treatments of PGs have been described in the literature. They include 5% imiquimod cream, timolol, propranolol, prednisolone, and clobetasol [5, 8, 11].

The current patient did not have an underlying cutaneous or systemic disease. She did not mention any trauma or minor surgeries at the vulvar region. Since the lesion was located just beneath the clitoral hood, we preferred not to use electrocautery in order to avoid probable thermal injury of clitoral neurovascular bundle. In the 6-month follow-up of the patient, tactile and sexual sensation of the clitoris was preserved and there was no recurrence at the surgical site. To our best knowledge, this is the first published report of vulvar PG in Iran. Due to the special role of the clitoris in female sexual function, we believe that in the management of the clitoral lesions, special care should be given to preserving dorsal clitoral

Table 1: Reports of vulvar pyogenic granuloma in the literature.

Cases/first author	Year	Age	Description of lesions	Symptom/underlying disease	Treatment
(1) Somesh Gupta et al. [4]	2000	57	Multiple large pedunculated, papillomatous lesions, on the left labia major	Bleeding	Surgical excision
(2) Kian-Mei Chong et al. [11]	2005	52	Reddish, 3 × 2 mm, ulcerated papule on the right labia major	Bleeding	Surgical excision
(3) Deniz Cemgil Arikan et al. [3]	2011	57	Multiple large 2-4 cm, papillomatous, pedunculated, and lobulated lesions on the labia major and clitoris	Bleeding	Surgical excision
(4) Vani Malhotra et al. [9]	2012	52	A single 3 × 3 cm lesion with smooth surface on the left labia major	Pain	Surgical excision
(5) Masataka Satoh et al. [6]	2013	74	Granulomatous vulvar ulcer	Pain	Oral prednisolone
(6) F. Abreu-Dos-Santos et al. [12]	2016	51	Lobulated reddish 2 cm ulcerated lesion on the upper part of the right labia major	Bleeding	Surgical excision
(7) Mónica Vences Carranza et al. [7]	2017	55	Single exophytic hemispherical, erythematous 5 mm, pedunculated, smooth surface lesion on the left side of labia major	Bleeding	Surgical excision
(8) Mónica Vences Carranza et al. [7]	2017	54	Multiform erythematous 2.5 mm diameter, hard pedunculated lesion on the right side of labia major	—	Surgical excision
(9) Mónica Vences Carranza et al. [7]	2017	—	Multiple exophytic erythematous 0.5 cm in diameter, pedunculated lesions of the vulva and clitoral hood	Previous history of lichen sclerosis	Surgical excision
(10) Shivani Ranjan and BD Thakur [8]	2018	23	Solitary cherry red pedunculated lesion on the lower aspect of the left labia major	Pain and bleeding	Surgical excision
(11) Shivani Ranjan and BD Thakur [8]	2018	48	A single, erythematous, pedunculated lesion with lobulated surface on the left labia major	Bleeding	Surgical excision
(12) Carlos Cuenca-Barrales et al. [10]	2018	18	Multiple ulcerated exophytic dome-shaped lesions in the intergluteal fold and pubic region	Previous history of acne	Reduction of isotretinoin dosage and topical application of clobetasol
(13) Present case	2020	54	Solitary pedunculated, granulation tissue-like lesion, beneath the clitoral hood	Spotting	Surgical excision

nerve and associated vascular content. Meticulous dissection and minimizing electrocautery usage should be considered.

Complete surgical excision and primary closure are the most advised and acceptable treatment of vulvar PGs (Table 1). Since the definitive diagnosis of PG is made by histopathologic examination, a skin biopsy prior to any conservative or ablational therapy is recommended.

4. Conclusion

Although the vulva is a rare location of PG formation, it should be considered as a differential diagnosis of any polypoid or sessile lesion at this site. Since it sometimes may occur with underlying diseases or malignant conditions, taking medical history and performing physical examination are recommended. Complete surgical excision and primary closure of the lesion are the medical treatment of choice with very low recurrence rate. In clitoral PGs, in order to avoid compromising the neurovascular bundle of the clitoris, meticulous dissection and preventing usage of electrocauterization are highly suggested.

Consent

The patient provided written informed consent for publication of the photographs in medical journals.

References

[1] T. Akamatsu, U. Hanai, M. Kobayashi, and M. Miyasaka, "Pyogenic granuloma: a retrospective 10-year analysis of 82 cases," *The Tokai Journal of Experimental and Clinical Medicine*, vol. 40, no. 3, pp. 110–114, 2015.

[2] F. Akbulut, T. Akbulut, F. Kucukdurmaz, E. Sonmezay, A. Simsek, and G. Gurbuz, "Huge pyogenic granuloma of the penis," *Case reports in Urology*, vol. 2015, Article ID 263168, 2 pages, 2015.

[3] D. C. Arikan, G. Kiran, H. Sayar, B. Kostu, A. Coskun, and H. Kiran, "Vulvar pyogenic granuloma in a postmenopausal woman: case report and review of the literature," *Case Reports in Medicine*, vol. 2011, Article ID 201901, 3 pages, 2011.

[4] S. Gupta, B. D. Radotra, and B. Kumar, "Multiple, genital lobular capillary haemangioma (pyogenic granuloma) in a young woman: a diagnostic puzzle," *Sexually transmitted infections*, vol. 76, no. 1, pp. 51-52, 2000.

[5] E. S. Sills, D. J. Zegarelli, M. M. Hoschander, and W. E. Strider, "Clinical diagnosis and management of hormonally responsive oral pregnancy tumor (pyogenic granuloma)," *The Journal of reproductive medicine*, vol. 41, no. 7, pp. 467–470, 1996.

[6] M. Satoh and T. Yamamoto, "Genital pyoderma gangrenosum: report of two cases and published work review of Japanese cases," *The Journal of Dermatology*, vol. 40, no. 10, pp. 840–843, 2013.

[7] M. Vences-Carranza, M. González-González, and E. Figueroa-Benítez, "Granuloma piógeno en la vulva," *Dermatología Revista Mexicana*, vol. 62, no. 5, pp. 423–429, 2018.

[8] S. Ranjan and B. D. Thakur, "Vulvar pyogenic granuloma: a rare location," *Indian Journal of Clinical and Experimental Dermatology*, vol. 4, no. 4, pp. 346-347, 2018.

[9] V. Malhotra, S. Nanda, M. Chauhan, N. Malhotra, P. Malhotra, and M. Juneja, "Pyogenic granuloma of the vulva: a rare presentation," *Journal of Gynecologic Surgery*, vol. 28, no. 3, pp. 238–240, 2012.

[10] C. Cuenca-Barrales, T. Ródenas-Herranz, L. Linares-Gonzalez, and R. Ruiz-Villaverde, "Pyogenic granuloma in an atypical location following isotretinoin treatment," *Sultan Qaboos University Medical Journal*, vol. 18, no. 3, article e409, pp. 409–e410, 2018.

[11] K. M. Chong, T. C. Yeh, and J. L. Hwang, "Vulvar lobular capillary hemangioma (pyogenic granuloma)," *Taiwanese Journal of Obstetrics and Gynecology*, vol. 44, no. 1, pp. 94-95, 2005.

[12] F. Abreu-Dos-Santos, S. Câmara, F. Reis, T. Freitas, H. Gaspar, and M. Cordeiro, "Vulvar lobular capillary hemangioma: a rare location for a frequent entity," *Case reports in obstetrics and gynecology*, vol. 2016, Article ID 3435270, 3 pages, 2016.

[13] U. Wollina, D. Langner, K. França, S. Gianfaldoni, T. Lotti, and G. Tchernev, "Pyogenic granuloma – a common benign vascular tumor with variable clinical presentation: new findings and treatment options," *Open access Macedonian journal of medical sciences*, vol. 5, no. 4, pp. 423–426, 2017.

33

Leptomeningeal Carcinomatosis in Urothelial Carcinoma of the Urinary Bladder: A Report of a Patient with a Fulminant Course Who Died of Cancer after Definitive Therapies

Masayuki Tomioka,[1] Makoto Kawase,[1] Daiki Kato,[1] Manabu Takai,[1] Koji Iinuma,[1] Kengo Horie,[1] Keita Nakane,[1] Natsuko Suzui,[2] Tatsuhiko Miyazaki,[2] and Takuya Koie[1]

[1]*Department of Urology, Gifu University Graduate School of Medicine, Gifu, Japan*
[2]*Department of Pathology, Gifu University Graduate School of Medicine, Gifu, Japan*

Correspondence should be addressed to Takuya Koie; goodwin@gifu-u.ac.jp

Academic Editor: Fumitaka Koga

A 45-year-old Japanese man visited a community hospital with the chief complaint of asymptomatic macrohematuria. He was diagnosed with muscle-invasive bladder cancer (MIBC), and he received intra-arterial chemotherapy followed by radiation therapy at another institution. Twenty-eight months after chemoradiotherapy, magnetic resonance imaging (MRI) revealed MIBC recurrence. After neoadjuvant chemotherapy, robot-assisted radical cystectomy was performed. Pathological examination indicated high-grade urothelial carcinoma with lymphovascular invasion, a positive surgical margin, and skip lesions of cancer cells in the perivesical adipose tissue. Three months after surgery, he was brought to our hospital in an ambulance with the chief complaint of rotatory vertigo and was speaking inarticulately. Head and whole spine MRI revealed meningeal metastasis along both the vestibulocochlear nerves and cauda equina. Analysis of the cerebrospinal fluid revealed malignant cells. The patient was diagnosed with leptomeningeal carcinomatosis originating from the MIBC. He received whole-brain radiotherapy followed by the administration of pembrolizumab. Unfortunately, the patient's condition quickly deteriorated, and he died of cancer 4 months after surgery.

1. Introduction

Leptomeningeal carcinomatosis (LMC) is defined as malignant cell infiltration in the pia mater and arachnoid membrane [1]. Although LMC occurs in 3%–5% of cancer patients [1], only 0.03% of patients with genitourinary (GU) cancer are diagnosed with LMC [2]. In addition, only four cases of an initial diagnosis of LMC originating from bladder cancer (BC) without other metastatic sites have been reported to date [3]. Herein, we present a patient with LMC that developed at the time of the initial diagnosis of muscle-invasive BC (MIBC). The patient underwent a fulminant course and died of BC after definitive therapies.

2. Case Presentation

A 45-year-old Japanese man visited a community hospital with a chief complaint of asymptomatic macrohematuria. Cystoscopy revealed multiple papillary nonpedunculated tumors ranging from the left lateral wall to the anterior wall of the urinary bladder. Histopathological diagnosis revealed high-grade urothelial carcinoma (UC) of the bladder with carcinoma in situ (CIS). At this point, the patient did not exhibit lymph node involvement or distant metastases. Bladder cancer (BC) was classified as clinical T2bN0M0 according to the staging system defined in the American Joint Committee on Cancer Staging Manual [4]. Although radical cystectomy (RC) was recommended, the patient hoped to

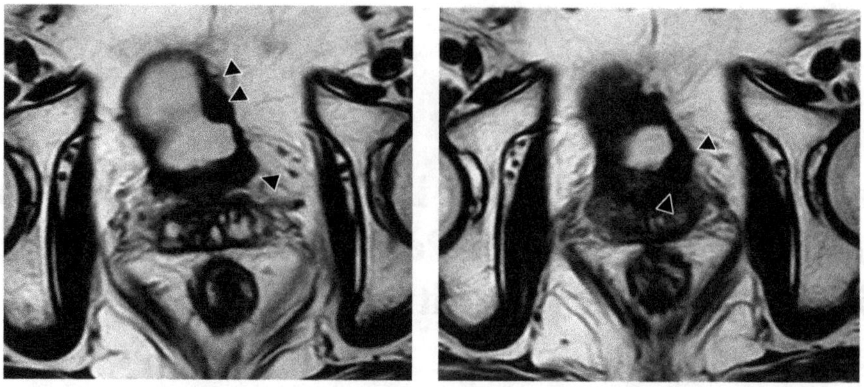

(a) (b)

FIGURE 1: T2-weighted magnetic resonance image showing multiple recurrent tumors with muscle layer infiltration at the left laterally wall (a) and the neck (b) of the urinary bladder (arrows).

preserve the urinary bladder. The patient received one cycle of intra-arterial chemotherapy using a combination of gemcitabine and cisplatin (GC) followed by radiation therapy (36 Gy in 2 Gy fractions) for the urinary bladder at another institution [5]. Subsequently, there was no evidence of the disease.

Twenty-eight months after chemoradiotherapy, magnetic resonance imaging (MRI) revealed multiple recurrent tumors with muscle layer infiltration of the left lateral wall and the neck of the urinary bladder (T2-weighted image; Figures 1(a) and 1(b)). Transurethral resection of the bladder tumor was performed, and the histopathological diagnosis was a high-grade UC with muscle layer invasion. RC was recommended again; therefore, the patient visited our hospital to undergo RC. Before surgery, he received two courses of GC (1000 mg/m^2 gemcitabine on days 1, 8, and 15 and cisplatin 70 mg/m^2 on day 2) as neoadjuvant chemotherapy (NAC) every 21 days [6]. Preoperative computed tomography (CT) after NAC showed that the BC was stable, and lymph node involvement and distant metastasis were not identified. Robot-assisted RC followed by intracorporeal ileal neobladder reconstruction was performed [6]. Pathological examination of the surgical specimen indicated high-grade UC, pathological stage T4a, with lymphovascular invasion, positive surgical margin, and skip lesions of the UC in the perivesical adipose tissue (Figure 2). Therefore, we decided to perform more careful observation of this patient without adjuvant chemotherapy.

However, he was brought to our hospital in an ambulance with the chief complaint of rotatory vertigo and speaking inarticulately 3 months after surgery. Dynamic contrast-enhanced MRI showed LMC of the cerebrum, mesencephalon, and cerebellum (Figure 3(a)). Infiltrating tumor cells were identified along the cerebral cortex on T2 fluid-attenuated inversion-recovery images (Figure 3(b)). In addition, T2-weighted MRI revealed meningeal metastasis along both the vestibulocochlear nerves and cauda equina (Figures 4(a) and 4(b)). Whole-body CT could not identify pelvic lymphadenopathy or metastasis to other organs. A lumbar puncture was performed, and analysis of the cerebrospinal fluid revealed malignant cells (Figure 5). The patient

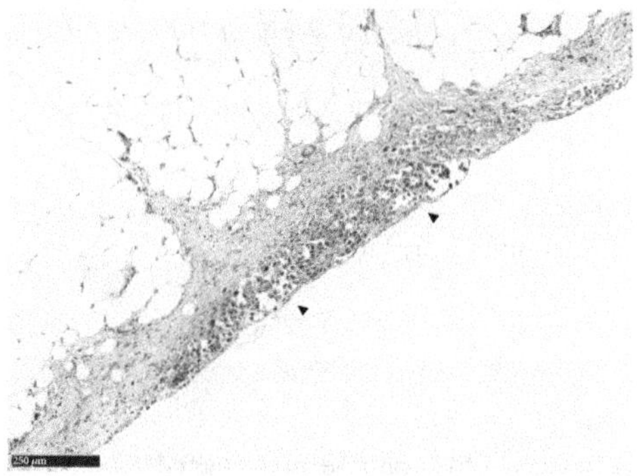

FIGURE 2: Pathological examination of the surgical specimen with skip lesions of cancer cells in the perivesical adipose tissue (arrows).

was diagnosed with LMC originating from the MIBC. Thereafter, his level of consciousness decreased without warning. Immediately, the patient was started on dexamethasone (6.6 mg) intravenously, and his level of consciousness recovered temporarily. Hence, he received whole-brain radiotherapy (30 Gy) followed by the administration of pembrolizumab (200 mg). Unfortunately, the patient's condition quickly deteriorated, and he died of BC one month after the diagnosis of LMC.

3. Discussion

LMC is diagnosed in 1%–5% of patients with solid tumors, 5%–15% of patients with leukemia and lymphoma, and 1%–2% of patients with primary brain tumors [7]. Autopsy studies have demonstrated that 19% of patients with cancer and neurological signs and symptoms have evidence of meningeal involvement [8]. Regarding the primary site, carcinomas of unknown origin constitute 1%–7% of all cases of LMC, even though small cell lung cancer and melanoma have the highest rates of LMC (11% and 20%, respectively) [9]. Regarding LMC originating from genitourinary cancer, in the MD Anderson Cancer Center database, only 31 (0.03%) patients were diagnosed with LMC among 93,960 patients diagnosed with GU cancer [2]. Umezawa et al. reported 33 cases of LMC originating from BC [3]. Four patients

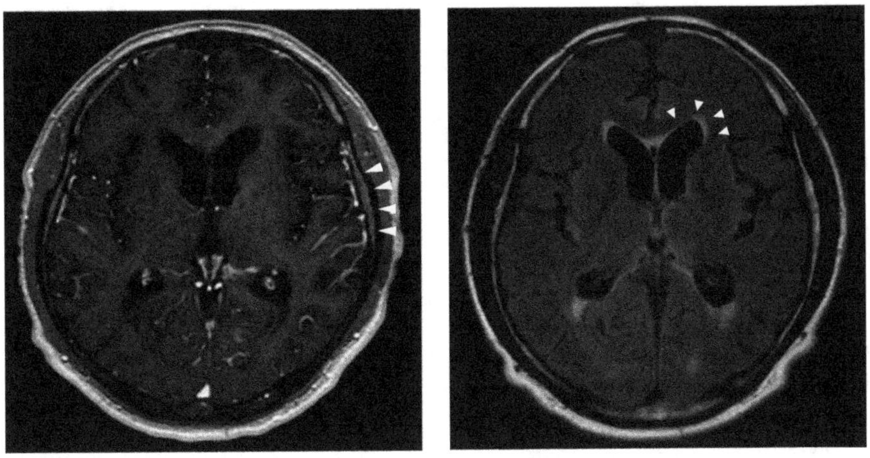

(a) (b)

FIGURE 3: Dynamic contrast-enhanced MRI showing LMC of the cerebrum, mesencephalon, and cerebellum (a). Infiltrating tumor cells can be identified along the cerebral cortex on T2 fluid-attenuated inversion-recovery imaging (b) (arrows).

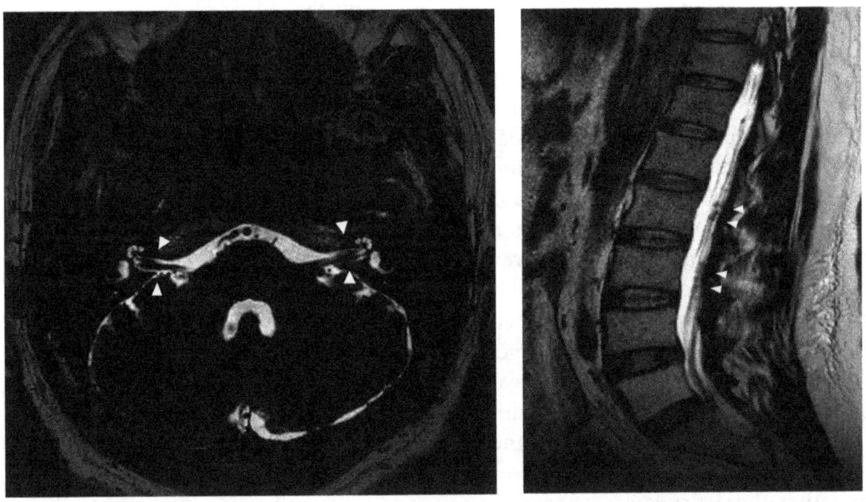

(a) (b)

FIGURE 4: T2-weighted MRI showing vestibulocochlear nerves metastasis (a) and cauda equina metastasis (b) (arrows).

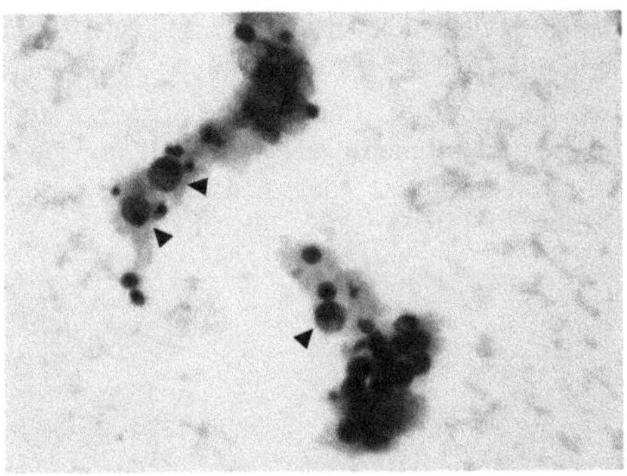

FIGURE 5: Analysis of the cerebrospinal fluid showing malignant cells (arrows).

(16.7%) had already developed LMC at the initial diagnosis [3]. Conversely, 20 patients (60.6%) were diagnosed with LMC during treatment for BC, and 16 (48.5%) developed LMC without progression of the primary or metastatic sites [3]. For patients with BC who have severe systemic disease, the possible diagnosis of LMC may not have been pursued because of the overall poor prognosis of these patients [2]. Therefore, the true frequency of LMC may be difficult to estimate for patients with systemic BC or those who are frequently treated with several drugs.

LMC is usually a late manifestation of systemic disease, and most often occurs in patients after extensive therapy with surgery, radiation, and chemotherapy [10]. Tumor metastasis to the meninges typically occurs by one of four mechanisms: meningeal seeding from preexisting hemispheric central nervous system (CNS) metastases, direct extension from subdural or epidural tumors, direct extension from sites outside but adjacent to the CNS, and hematogenous spread [11]. Once cancer cells enter the subarachnoid space, they are transported by cerebrospinal fluid (CSF) flow, resulting in disseminated and multifocal neuraxis seeding of the leptomeninges [12]. In addition, tumor infiltration is most prominent at the base of the brain and on the dorsal surface of the spinal cord, especially the cauda equina [7, 13]. In our case, the nature of the metastasis to the leptomeninges remains unclear. The cause of unprecedented LMC without metastasis to regional lymph nodes or other organs suggests that the lymphatic or venous flow of the urinary bladder may have changed after receiving intra-arterial chemotherapy followed by radiation therapy for the urinary bladder before surgery.

To date, the optimal treatment for LMC remains poorly defined. For this reason, the prognosis of LMC from BC is worse, and the median survival from diagnosis to death is 35 days (interquartile range, 16–134 days) [3]. Therefore, the treatment of LMC is typically palliative and rarely curative based on four prospective randomized trials in LMC [12]. In addition, the therapeutic management strategies employed for LMC are similar to those employed for brain metastasis. Radiation therapy is used in the treatment of LMC for palliation of symptoms, decreasing bulky disease, and correcting CSF flow abnormalities [12]. However, whole neuraxis radiation is rarely indicated because it is associated with significant systemic toxicity, including severe myelosuppression and mucositis, and is not curative [12]. Conversely, systemic or intrathecal chemotherapy is a treatment modality that can medicate the entire neuraxis, multiple lymph nodes, and other organs [12]. Methotrexate (MTX) is a key drug for the treatment of LMC and is administered as a systemic and/or intrathecal chemotherapeutic agent [14]. However, most chemotherapeutic agents administered systemically have poor CSF penetration and do not reach therapeutic levels [12]. Recently, the effectiveness of molecular targeted therapy or immune checkpoint inhibitors, including bevacizumab for breast cancer, intrathecal trastuzumab for human epidermal growth factor receptor 2-positive breast cancer, and nivolumab for lung adenocarcinoma, has been reported [15–17]. It is unclear whether these drugs are effective for treating LMC originating from BC. Although pembrolizumab was used for the treatment of LMC in our case, the treatment effect was not completely achieved. It may have been better to have chosen a chemotherapy regimen, including methotrexate if possible, although the patient's condition was very poor. A promising strategy for LMC should be devised in the near future.

References

[1] B. Gleissner and M. Chamberlain, "Neoplastic meningitis," *Lancet Neurology*, vol. 5, no. 5, pp. 443–452, 2006.

[2] S. Yust-Katz, S. Mathis, and M. D. Groves, "Leptomeningeal metastases from genitourinary cancer: the University of Texas MD Anderson Cancer Center experience," *Medical Oncology*, vol. 30, no. 1, p. 429, 2013.

[3] Y. Umezawa, S. Shirotake, G. Kaneko et al., "Meningeal carcinomatosis from bladder cancer: a case report and review of the literature," *Mol Clin Oncol*, vol. 10, no. 5, pp. 506–510, 2019.

[4] American Joint Committee on Cancer, "Urinary bladder," in *AJCC Cancer Staging Manual*, S. B. Edge, D. R. Byrd, and C. C. Compton, Eds., pp. 497–505, Springer, New York, 7th edition, 2010.

[5] H. Azuma, T. Inamoto, K. Takahara et al., "Novel bladder preservation therapy with Osaka Medical College regimen," *The Journal of Urology*, vol. 193, no. 2, pp. 443–450, 2015.

[6] T. Koie, C. Ohyama, K. Makiyama et al., "Utility of robot-assisted radical cystectomy with intracorporeal urinary diversion for muscle-invasive bladder cancer," *International Journal of Urology*, vol. 26, no. 3, pp. 334–340, 2019.

[7] M. C. Chamberlain, "Carcinomatous meningitis," *Archives of Neurology*, vol. 54, no. 1, pp. 16-17, 1997.

[8] J. P. Glass, M. Melamed, N. L. Chernik, and J. B. Posner, "Malignant cells in cerebrospinal fluid (CSF): the meaning of a positive CSF cytology," *Neurology*, vol. 29, no. 10, pp. 1369–1375, 1979.

[9] W. R. Wasserstrom, J. P. Glass, and J. B. Posner, "Diagnosis and treatment of leptomeningeal metastases from solid tumors: experience with 90 patients," *Cancer*, vol. 49, no. 4, pp. 759–772, 1982.

[10] M. J. Glantz and B. C. Walters, "Diagnosis and outcome measures in trials for neoplastic meningitis: a review of the literature and clinical experience," *Neurosurgical Focus*, vol. 4, no. 6, p. e4, 1998.

[11] M. C. Chamberlain, "Neoplastic meningitis," *Current Neurology and Neuroscience Reports*, vol. 8, no. 3, pp. 249–258, 2008.

[12] M. C. Chamberlain, "Neoplastic meningitis," *The Oncologist*, vol. 13, no. 9, pp. 967–977, 2008.

[13] R. Boyle, M. Thomas, and J. H. Adams, "Diffuse involvement of the leptomeninges by tumour–a clinical and pathological study of 63 cases," *Postgraduate Medical Journal*, vol. 56, no. 653, pp. 149–158, 1980.

[14] E. Le Rhun, M. Weller, D. Brandsma et al., "EANO-ESMO Clinical Practice Guidelines for diagnosis, treatment and follow-up of patients with leptomeningeal metastasis from solid tumours," *Annals of Oncology*, vol. 28, no. 4, pp. iv84–iv99, 2017.

[15] P. F. Wu, C. H. Lin, C. H. Kuo et al., "A pilot study of bevacizumab combined with etoposide and cisplatin in breast cancer patients with leptomeningeal carcinomatosis," *BMC Cancer*, vol. 15, no. 1, p. 299, 2015.

[16] F. Zagouri, T. N. Sergentanis, R. Bartsch et al., "Intrathecal administration of trastuzumab for the treatment of meningeal carcinomatosis in HER2-positive metastatic breast cancer: a systematic review and pooled analysis," *Breast Cancer Research and Treatment*, vol. 139, no. 1, pp. 13–22, 2013.

[17] M. Gion, J. Remon, C. Caramella, J. C. Soria, and B. Besse, "Symptomatic leptomeningeal metastasis improvement with nivolumab in advanced non-small cell lung cancer patient," *Lung Cancer*, vol. 108, pp. 72–74, 2017.

Effectiveness of Steroid Pulse Therapy for Systemic Side Effects after Bacillus Calmette-Guérin Intravesical Instillation Therapy: A Series of Five Cases

Tatsuya Umemoto,[1] Jun Naruse,[2] Yukio Usui,[3] Hidenori Zakoji,[1] Hideshi Miyakita,[2] and Akira Miyajima[4]

[1]*Department of Urology, Tokai University Hachioji Hospital, 1838 Ishikawa-machi, Hachioji, Tokyo 192-0032, Japan*
[2]*Department of Urology, Tokai University Oiso Hospital, 21-1, Gakkyo, Oiso-machi, Naka-gun, Kanagawa 259-0198, Japan*
[3]*Department of Urology, Shizuoka City Shimizu Hospital, Miyakami 1231, Shimizu Ward Shizuoka City, Shizuoka 424-8636, Japan*
[4]*Department of Urology, Tokai University School of Medicine, 143 Shimokasuya, Isehara, Kanagawa 259-1193, Japan*

Correspondence should be addressed to Hidenori Zakoji; hzakohji@tokai.ac.jp

Academic Editor: Fumitaka Koga

Introduction. Bacillus Calmette-Guérin (BCG) instillation is an established therapy for the treatment of carcinoma in situ (CIS) of the bladder and prevention of recurrence after transurethral resection of bladder tumor noninvasive bladder cancer. However, serious systemic side effects may occur in less than 5% of patients with BCG intravesical instillation. Systemic side effects can sometimes be fatal and require early and accurate treatment. We describe five cases wherein steroid pulse therapy was effective for treating the systemic side effects after BCG intravesical instillation. *Case Presentations.* BCG intravesical instillation was used to prevent the recurrence of nonmuscle invasive bladder cancer and treat CIS of the bladder; the dose used was 40–80 mg each time, and the Tokyo strain was used. The patients developed fever, impaired consciousness, arthralgia, conjunctival hyperemia, and symptoms of cystitis. The median time from installation to side effect manifestation was 6 days (0–8). One to two courses of steroid pulse therapy were administered (1 course in 3 days), and the dose of methylprednisolone was 500–1000 mg/day. BCG sepsis was observed in one case; however, in the other four cases, one course of steroid pulse therapy showed a rapid improvement in symptoms. In the case of BCG sepsis, hemodialysis and mechanical ventilation were required because of septic shock and acute renal failure. Antituberculosis drugs (isoniazid, rifampicin, and ethambutol) were started promptly; however, no improvement was noticed. Two courses of steroid pulse therapy improved the patient's general condition, and hemodialysis and mechanical ventilation were no longer required. All patients survived without relapse of symptoms. *Conclusion.* Our cases suggest that early steroid pulse therapy may be effective for rapid symptom improvement of the systemic side effects of BCG instillation therapy.

1. Introduction

Bacillus Calmette-Guérin (BCG) instillation is an established therapy for the treatment of carcinoma in situ (CIS) of the bladder and prevention of recurrence after transurethral resection of bladder tumor (TURBT) for noninvasive bladder cancer [1–7]. BCG is an attenuated strain of *Mycobacterium bovis* that induces a cell-mediated immune response and induces attacks on malignant cells [8]. BCG infusion causes various side effects, such as symptoms of cystitis, nausea, fever, and hematuria; however, they are mostly mild. Additionally, it does have known severe side effects, including pneumonitis/hepatitis (0.7%), BCG sepsis (0.4%), and even death [9]. BCG infection is one of the side effects of BCG infusion therapy [10], which is classified into local infection, disseminated infection, and ectopic infection. The characteristics and treatment methods of each are shown in Table 1 [9]. Similarly, infection of aortic aneurysms has been reported as an ectopic

Table 1: Types of Bacillus Calmette-Guérin infections and treatments.

	Type of BCG infection	Treatment
Local	Infection of the bladder, kidney, renal pelvis, ureter, prostate, and epididymis.	Discontinue BCG. Administer isoniazid, rifampicin, and ethambutol for 3–6 months.
Systemic	Hematogenous dissemination of BCG to the systemic organs (BCG sepsis, hepatitis, and cerebromeningitis, among others).	Discontinue BCG. Administer isoniazid, rifampicin, and ethambutol for six months.
Ectopic	Ectopic infection of aneurysms and artificial organs (artificial joints, etc.), among others.	Administer isoniazid and rifampicin for one year. Consider excision of the infected area.

BCG = Bacillus Calmette-Guérin.

infection [11]. In clinical practice, mild local side effects are most likely to improve rapidly with the discontinuation of BCG administration; however, systemic side effects are often difficult to treat. Table 2 shows the management of side effects (local and systemic) after BCG perfusion therapy based on a partial excerpt from the European Association of Urology guidelines [11]. The guidelines show that systemic side effects include persistent high-grade fever (>38.5°C for >48 hours), arthralgia and/or arthritis, BCG sepsis, and allergic reactions. Nonsteroidal anti-inflammatory drugs (NSAIDs) are the first treatment choice for joint symptoms; however, if they are ineffective, the use of antituberculosis drugs and high-dose quinolones is recommended. Although antituberculosis drugs and quinolones are highly recommended for other systemic side effects, steroids are recommended for only BCG sepsis. We describe our experience of five cases wherein steroid pulse therapy was effective for the treatment of BCG instillation-induced systemic side effects.

2. Case Presentations

In all cases, BCG intravesical instillation therapy was started at six weeks or more after the operation. Table 3 shows the characteristics of all patients. The median of the number of BCG therapy sessions performed before the manifestation of severe side effects was 4 (range, 3-8 sessions). According to Gonzales et al., stratification is proposed within three months from the first dose, and this likely applied to cases 1–4 due to the early presentation [10]. Case 5 was excluded because the patient received 14 courses of BCG maintenance therapy, and the side effect was caused by iatrogenic trauma.

2.1. Case 1. A 60-year-old woman underwent 80 mg BCG (Tokyo strain) intravesical instillation therapy for high-grade pTa bladder cancer. She presented with fever (>48 hours), knee joint pain, and conjunctival hyperemia after receiving four infusions. She was administered 10 mg/day of prednisolone (as per 0.2 mg/kg body weight), an NSAID (loxoprofen sodium hydrate, 180 mg/day), and antituberculosis drugs (isoniazid (INH), 300 mg/day; rifampicin (REP), 450 mg/day; and ethambutol (EB), 750 mg/day) because she was diagnosed with BCG-induced Reiter syndrome. She was administered steroid pulse therapy (methylprednisolone, 1000 mg/day) for three days because high white blood cell (WBC) and C-reactive protein (CRP) levels and fever persisted. After the third day of administration, fever, joint pain, and inflammation improved quickly. Subsequently, the dose of prednisolone was gradually reduced to a maintenance dose of 30 mg (as per 0.6 mg/kg body weight), and the symptoms did not recur.

2.2. Case 2. A 66-year-old woman underwent 80 mg BCG intravesical instillation therapy for bladder urothelial CIS. She presented with knee joint pain, conjunctival hyperemia, and urethritis after receiving eight infusions. She was administered prednisolone (30 mg/day as per 0.55 mg/kg body weight) and an NSAID (loxoprofen sodium hydrate, 180 mg/day) because she was diagnosed with BCG-induced Reiter syndrome. She was administered steroid pulse therapy (methylprednisolone, 1000 mg/day) for three days because high WBC and CRP levels persisted, and the symptoms were prolonged. After the third day of administration, the symptoms and inflammation improved quickly. Subsequently, the dose of prednisolone was gradually reduced to a maintenance dose of 30 mg (as per 0.55 mg/kg body weight), and the symptoms did not recur.

2.3. Case 3. A 76-year-old man underwent 80 mg BCG intravesical instillation therapy for high-grade pTa bladder cancer. He presented with fever (>48 hours), knee and elbow joint pain, and conjunctival hyperemia after receiving four infusions. He was administered an NSAID (loxoprofen sodium hydrate, 180 mg/day) and steroid pulse therapy (methylprednisolone, 500 mg/day) for three days because of high WBC and CRP levels and a diagnosis of BCG-induced Reiter syndrome. After the tenth day of administration, the symptoms and inflammation improved. Subsequently, the dose of prednisolone was gradually reduced to a maintenance dose of 30 mg (as per 0.5 mg/kg body weight), and the symptoms did not recur.

2.4. Case 4. A 77-year-old woman underwent 40 mg BCG intravesical instillation therapy for high-grade pT1 bladder cancer. She presented with knee joint pain and urethritis after receiving three infusions. She was administered an NSAID (celecoxib, 200 mg/day) for a few days. Subsequently, she was administered steroid pulse therapy (methylprednisolone, 1000 mg/day) for three days because she presented with fever (>48 hours), joint pain, and urethritis. After the second day of administration, her symptoms and inflammation quickly improved. After that, the dose of prednisolone was gradually reduced from 50 mg (1 mg/kg), and the symptoms did not recur.

TABLE 2: Management options for treating the side effects of Bacillus Calmette-Guérin intravesical instillation therapy.

	Management options for local side effects
Symptomatic granulomatous prostatitis	Symptoms rarely present: perform urine culture. Administer quinolones. If quinolones are not effective, administer isoniazid (300 mg/day) and rifampicin (600 mg/day) for three months. Stop intravesical instillation therapy.
Epididymo-orchitis	Perform urine culture and administer quinolones. Stop intravesical instillation therapy. Perform orchidectomy if an abscess is present or if there is no response to treatment.
	Management options for systemic side effects
General malaise, fever	These generally resolve within 48 hours, with or without antipyretics.
Arthralgia and/or arthritis	This is a rare complication and is considered an autoimmune reaction. Arthralgia: treat with NSAIDs. Arthritis: treat with NSAIDs. If no/partial response, proceed to treatment with corticosteroids, high-dose quinolones, or antituberculosis drugs.
Persistent high-grade fever (>38.5°C for >48 h)	Permanently stop BCG instillation. Immediate evaluation: urine culture, blood tests, chest X-ray. Administer prompt treatment with more than two antimicrobial agents while a diagnostic evaluation is conducted. Consult with an infectious disease specialist.
BCG sepsis	Prevention: initiate BCG at least two weeks after transurethral resection of the bladder (if there are no signs and symptoms of hematuria). Stop BCG instillation. For severe infection: Administer high-dose quinolones or isoniazid, rifampicin, and ethambutol (1.2 g daily) for six months. Administer early, high-dose corticosteroids as long as symptoms persist. Consider administering an empirical nonspecific antibiotic to cover Gram-negative bacteria and/or *Enterococcus*.

BCG = Bacillus Calmette-Guérin; NSAIDs = nonsteroidal anti-inflammatory drugs.

TABLE 3: Patient characteristics.

	Age (y)	Sex	Bladder cancer stage/type	Number of BCG therapy sessions	Side effect	Antituberculosis drug	Steroid pulse therapy (type, dose; duration)	Outcome
Case 1	60	Female	pTa high-grade	4	Fever, knee joint pain, conjunctival hyperemia	INH, 300 mg/day; REP, 450 mg/day; EB, 750 mg/day	Methylprednisolone, 1000 mg/day; 3 days (1 course)	Alive
Case 2	66	Female	CIS	8	Knee joint pain, conjunctival hyperemia, urethritis	None	Methylprednisolone, 1000 mg/day; 3 days (1 course)	Alive
Case 3	76	Male	pTa high-grade	4	Fever, knee and elbow joint pain, conjunctival hyperemia	None	Methylprednisolone, 500 mg/day; 3 days (1 course)	Alive
Case 4	77	Female	pT1 high-grade	3	Fever, knee joint pain, urethritis	None	Methylprednisolone, 1000 mg/day; 3 days (1 course)	Alive
Case 5	73	Male	pT1 high-grade	14	Fever, impaired consciousness, BCG sepsis	INH, 300 mg/day; REP, 450 mg/day; EB, 750 mg/day	Methylprednisolone, 1000 mg/day; 6 days (2 courses)	Alive

BCG = Bacillus Calmette-Guérin; INH = isoniazid; REP = rifampicin; EB = ethambutol; CIS = carcinoma in situ.

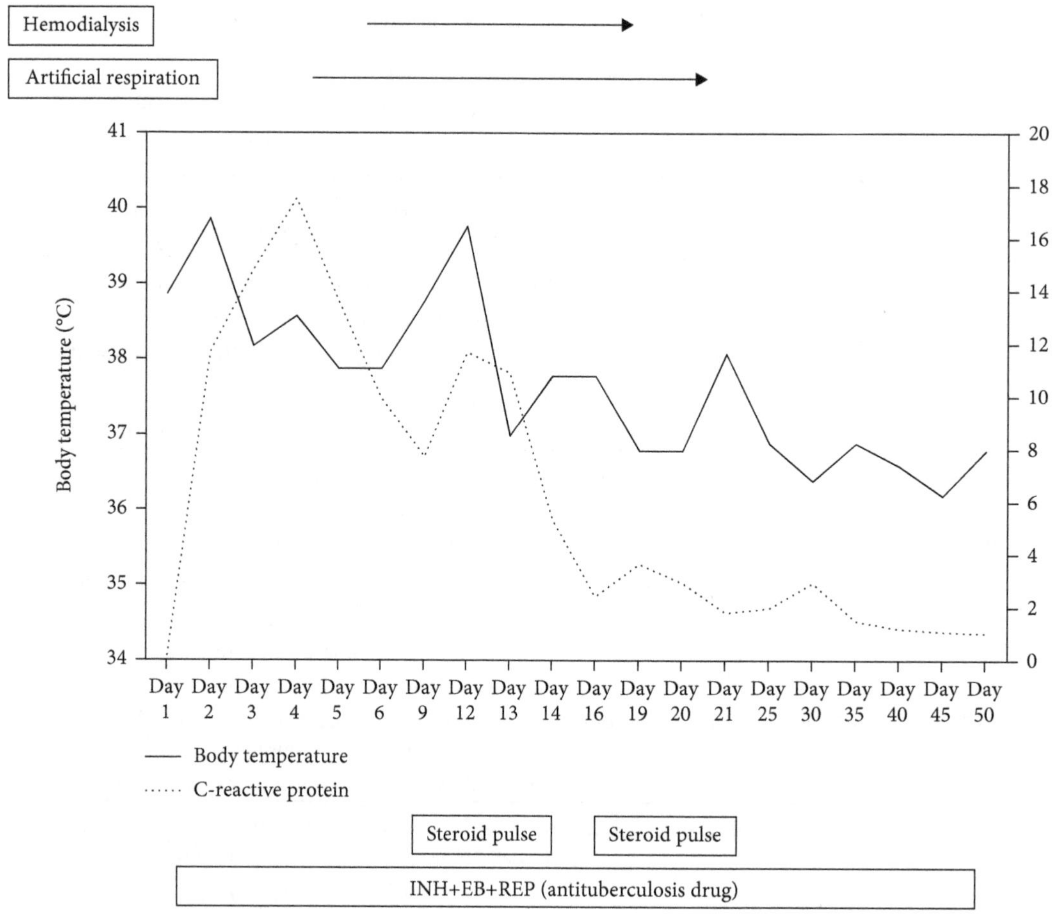

Figure 1: Treatment course of the patient with Bacillus Calmette-Guérin (case 5). EB = ethambutol; INH = isoniazid; REP = rifampicin.

2.5. Case 5. A 73-year-old man underwent 80 mg BCG intravesical instillation therapy for high-grade pT1 bladder cancer. In addition, after receiving six infusions, he underwent BCG maintenance therapy every three months for three weeks, which was administered after using a urethral bougie to dilate his urethral stricture. On the same day, he was referred to our hospital because of fever and impaired consciousness. Upon examination, fever and decreased blood pressure were noted and the infected area was unclear; however, computed tomography (CT) revealed an increase in the perirenal fat concentration. BCG sepsis was diagnosed based on these findings and the patient's medical history of BCG administration after receiving the urethral bougie. The progress of treatment after hospitalization is shown in Figure 1. He was administered antituberculosis drugs (INH, 300 mg/day; RFP, 450 mg/day; and EB, 750 mg/day), an empirical nonspecific antibiotic, and an antidisseminated intravascular coagulation drug (thrombomodulin alfa) for BCG sepsis and disseminated intravascular coagulation after various tuberculosis tests were performed. Steroids were not administered because of the possibility of *M. bovis* infection. Ventilator management was performed for airway obstruction caused by oral bleeding, and dialysis management was required because of acute renal failure. Steroid pulse therapy was started because the fever persisted. CT on day 12 revealed findings suggestive of interstitial pneumonia. A diagnosis of interstitial pneumonia due to BCG was established based on the patient's presentations as follows: fever, decreased oxygenation, and no history of imaging findings of interstitial pneumonia. Steroid pulse therapy was administered (methylprednisolone, 1000 mg/day) for three days, and prednisolone was administered at a maintenance dose of 80 mg/day (as per 1 mg/kg body weight). The fever and inflammatory response reduced, and dialysis was no longer required. Additional steroid pulse therapy (methylprednisolone, 1000 mg/day for three days) was administered on day 19, and mechanical ventilation was discontinued on day 20. The dose of prednisolone was gradually reduced from 80 mg, and the symptoms did not recur. He was discharged on day 51. EB was stopped on day 64, and INH and REP were stopped on day 322; the symptoms have not recurred since then.

3. Discussion

In cases 1–4, fever (>48 hours) and arthralgia symptoms were commonly observed; however, fortunately, no severe side effects, such as BCG sepsis, were observed. Reiter syndrome was diagnosed in cases 1 to 4, and urethritis, conjunctivitis, and arthritis are reportedly known as the classic triad [12]. Incomplete Reiter's syndrome, which is not characterized by all three symptoms, as in case 1, has similarly been observed and is currently regarded as a subtype of reactive arthritis [13]. NSAIDs are primarily used for treatment; however, steroids are recommended in severe cases or when NSAIDs are inadequate [14].

Case 5 developed BCG sepsis and was the most severe case we experienced. The cause of these BCG-related complications remains controversial, and it is believed that the cause is a hypersensitivity inflammatory reaction or active infection due to *M. bovis* [15, 16]. It is difficult to prove the presence of *M. bovis* infection, and Perez-Jacoiste et al. reported that the microbiological-based diagnosis of *M. bovis* infection was positive in only 118 of 246 patients [10]. In case 5, the results of tests, including polymerase chain reaction, staining for acid-fast bacilli, and culture, for *M. bovis* infection were negative. In clinical practice, BCG sepsis can rapidly become severe, and often, treatment should be performed even in situations wherein test results are not available. Therefore, it is important to classify and memorize the information about therapeutic agents and start treatment as soon as possible if BCG sepsis is suspected.

Cystitis is the most common local side effect associated with BCG administration (80%) and is the most frequently cited reason for the postponement of BCG administration. Other local side effects include gross hematuria, atrophic bladder, and ureteral obstruction [17]. As shown in Table 1, local BCG infections include infections of the bladder, kidney, renal pelvis, ureter, prostate, and epididymis. First, it is recommended to postpone BCG administration, and if there is no improvement, surgical treatment and antituberculosis drugs should be considered. Pyrazinamide is not effective against *M. bovis*; hence, INH, RFP, EB, and streptomycin are used. Three-month administration of INH+RFP is recommended for local infections. Next, the management of BCG sepsis requires the cessation of BCG administration and examinations for *M. bovis* infection, including polymerase chain reaction, staining for acid-fast bacilli, and culture. A whole-body examination should be performed using imaging tests, such as CT, to evaluate the presence or absence of interstitial pneumonia and local *M. bovis* infection. Antituberculosis drugs (INH, RFP, and EB), a high-dose fluoroquinolone antibiotic, an empirical nonspecific antibiotic, and high-dose steroid therapy should be considered if there is no local infection. When interstitial pneumonia is observed, combination therapy with antituberculosis drugs and steroid therapy is often administered, and there are many reports of using pulse therapy as a steroid administration method [18]. The reason for the delay in the administration of steroid pulse therapy in case 5 was that there was a dissenting opinion that administration in a situation wherein the possibility of *M. bovis* infection could not be excluded was highly risky.

If steroid pulse therapy can be performed early, it is undeniable that it may have been relieved without becoming so severe. For urologists, steroid pulse therapy is not a routine treatment, and they may be hesitant to administer it owing to the associated side effects. According to a report on the side effects of steroid pulse therapy in other diseases, side effects (diabetes mellitus, moon face, hypertension, peptic ulcer, urinary tract infection, psychiatric symptoms, and susceptibility to infection, among others) are fewer with intravenous administration than with oral administration; however, severe liver damage may occur in 0.8% of the patients, and deaths were reported in 0.3%. The total recommended dose of methylprednisolone should be 8 g or less to reduce the risk of serious side effects [19–21]. Although high-dose steroids are described as one of the treatments for BCG sepsis, the dose and duration have not been clarified. Therefore, it seems that there are many cases wherein the effect is remarkable, as in our case; therefore, we think that early steroid pulse therapy for systemic side effects of BCG instillation is effective after monitoring for potential side effects.

BCG intravesical instillation therapy is one of the daily treatments for CIS of the bladder, and it is necessary to understand the associated side effects and be familiar with their management. To prevent side effects, the administration should be performed at least two weeks after TURBT and postponed for patients with gross hematuria, trauma due to catheter insertion, or urinary tract infection [22]. In case 5, the patient was administered BCG therapy after using a urethral bougie to dilate the urethral stricture. Since the patient developed an iatrogenic side effect caused by injecting BCG on the same day, we think that sufficient caution and consideration were required. BCG is thought to elicit a cell-mediated immune response and induce an attack on malignant cells [8]. The cause of BCG-related systemic side effects is supposedly a hypersensitivity inflammatory reaction or active infection due to *M. bovis* [16, 17]. One of the causes of Reiter syndrome after BCG administration is considered to be mediated by an immune response, including a lymphocyte T cell response [23]. Therefore, steroid administration, especially pulse therapy, is considered effective to strongly suppress the immune response. Steroid pulse therapy should be performed for Reiter syndrome or Reiter syndrome with fever when there are no locally infected lesions and in cases without sepsis or organ damage. Therefore, high-dose fluoroquinolones, antituberculosis drugs, an empirical nonspecific antibiotic, and early steroid pulse therapy should be considered for BCG sepsis.

4. Conclusions

We described five cases wherein steroid pulse therapy was used to treat systemic side effects after BCG intravesical instillation therapy. Our cases suggest that steroid pulse therapy may be important for early recovery from the systemic side effects after BCG intravesical instillation therapy in the absence of local infection. Additionally, in BCG sepsis, it is important to always consider not only antituberculosis drugs but also steroid pulse therapy as a treatment option.

Consent

Written informed consent was obtained from the patients for publication of this case series.

References

[1] H. W. Herr, C. M. Pinsky, W. F. Whitmore Jr., H. F. Oettgen, and M. R. Melamed, "Effect of intravesical bacillus Calmette-Guerin (BCG) on carcinoma in situ of the bladder," *Cancer*, vol. 51, no. 7, pp. 1323–1326, 1983.

[2] A. Morales, D. Eidinger, and A. W. Bruce, "Intracavitary bacillus Calmette-Guerin in the treatment of superficial bladder tumors," *The Journal of Urology*, vol. 116, no. 2, pp. 180–182, 1976.

[3] P. U. Malmström, R. J. Sylvester, D. E. Crawford et al., "An individual patient data meta-analysis of the long-term outcome of randomised studies comparing intravesical mitomycin C versus bacillus Calmette-Guerin for non-muscle-invasive bladder cancer," *European Urology*, vol. 56, no. 2, pp. 247–256, 2009.

[4] M. D. Shelley, H. Kynaston, J. Court et al., "A systematic review of intravesical bacillus Calmette-Guérin plus transurethral resection vs transurethral resection alone in Ta and T1 bladder cancer," *BJU International*, vol. 88, no. 3, pp. 209–216, 2001.

[5] R. F. Han and J. G. Pan, "Can intravesical bacillus Calmette-Guerin reduce recurrence in patients with superficial bladder cancer? A meta-analysis of randomized trials," *Urology*, vol. 67, no. 6, pp. 1216–1223, 2006.

[6] M. D. Shelley, T. J. Wilt, J. Court, B. Coles, H. Kynaston, and M. D. Mason, "Intravesical bacillus Calmette-Guerin is superior to mitomycin C in reducing tumour recurrence in high-risk superficial bladder cancer: a meta-analysis of randomized trials," *BJU International*, vol. 93, no. 4, pp. 485–490, 2004.

[7] A. Böhle, D. Jocham, and P. R. Bock, "Intravesical bacillus Calmette-Guerin versus mitomycin C for superficial bladder cancer: a formal meta-analysis of comparative studies on recurrence and toxicity," *The Journal of Urology*, vol. 169, no. 1, pp. 90–95, 2003.

[8] O. Y. Gonzalez, D. M. Musher, I. Brar et al., "Spectrum of bacille Calmette-Guerin (BCG) infection after intravesical BCG immunotherapy," *Clinical Infectious Diseases*, vol. 36, no. 2, pp. 140–148, 2003.

[9] D. L. Lamm, A. P. M. Van Der Meijden, A. Morales et al., "Incidence and treatment of complications of bacillus Calmette-Guerin intravesical therapy in superficial bladder cancer," *The Journal of Urology*, vol. 147, 3 Part 1, pp. 596–600, 1992.

[10] M. A. P.-J. Asín, M. Fernández-Ruiz, F. López-Medrano et al., "Bacillus Calmette-Guérin (BCG) infection following intravesical BCG administration as adjunctive therapy for bladder cancer," *Medicine (Baltimore)*, vol. 93, no. 17, pp. 236–254, 2014.

[11] G. E. J. Harding and D. K. Lawlor, "Ruptured mycotic abdominal aortic aneurysm secondary to Mycobacterium bovis after intravesical treatment with bacillus Calmette-Guerin," *Journal of Vascular Surgery*, vol. 46, no. 1, pp. 131–134, 2007.

[12] H. Reiter, "Ueber eine bisher unerkannte spirochäteninfektion (Spirochaetosis arthritica)," *DMW - Deutsche Medizinische Wochenschrift*, vol. 42, no. 50, pp. 1535-1536, 1916.

[13] N. Hatano, H. Hikiji, M. Matsubara et al., "Reiter's syndrome (reactive arthritis) with trismus after intravesical BCG immunotherapy: a case report," *Asian Journal of Oral and Maxillofacial Surgery*, vol. 23, no. 1, pp. 25–27, 2011.

[14] J. Sieper and D. Poddubnyy, "New evidence on the management of spondyloarthritis," *Nature Reviews Rheumatology*, vol. 12, no. 5, pp. 282–295, 2016.

[15] K. A. Nadasy, R. S. Patel, M. Emmett et al., "Four cases of disseminated mycobacterium bovis infection following intravesical BCG instillation for treatment of bladder carcinoma," *Southern Medical Journal*, vol. 101, no. 1, pp. 91–95, 2008.

[16] M. Elkabani, J. N. Greene, A. L. Vincent, S. VanHook, and R. L. Sandin, "Disseminated mycobacterium bovis after intravesicular bacillus Calmette-Guérin treatments for bladder cancer," *Cancer Control*, vol. 7, no. 5, pp. 476–481, 2000.

[17] D. Lamm, R. Persad, M. Colombel, and M. Braiso, "Maintenance Bacillus Calmette-Guérin: The Standard of Care for the Prophylaxis and Management of Intermediate- and High-Risk Non–Muscle-Invasive Bladder Cancer," *Eureopean Urology Supplements*, vol. 9, no. 9, pp. 715–734, 2010.

[18] G. Shimizu, R. Amano, I. Nakamura, A. Wada, M. Kitagawa, and S. Toru, "Disseminated bacillus Calmette–Guérin (BCG) infection and acute exacerbation of interstitial pneumonitis: an autopsy case report and literature review," *BMC Infectious Diseases*, vol. 20, no. 1, p. 708, 2020.

[19] H. Stiebel-Kalish, E. Robenshtok, M. Hasanreisoglu, D. Ezrachi, I. Shimon, and L. Leibovici, "Treatment modalities for Graves' ophthalmopathy: systematic review and metaanalysis," *The Journal of Clinical Endocrinology and Metabolism*, vol. 94, no. 8, pp. 2708–2716, 2009.

[20] L. Bartalena, L. Baldeschi, A. Dickinson et al., "Consensus statement of the European Group on Graves' orbitopathy (EUGOGO) on management of GO," *European Journal of Endocrinology*, vol. 158, no. 3, pp. 273–285, 2008.

[21] M. Marinó, E. Morabito, M. R. Brunetto, L. Bartalena, A. Pinchera, and C. Marocci, "Acute and severe liver damage associated with intravenous glucocorticoid pulse therapy in patients with Graves' ophthalmopathy," *Thyroid*, vol. 14, no. 5, pp. 403–406, 2004.

[22] European Association of Urology, *Guidelines on non-muscle-invasive bladder cancer (TaT1 and CIS)*, European Association of Urology Guidelines, 2018.

[23] D. C. Cheung, A. L. Millman, and R. J. Hamilton, "Case: bacillus Calmette-Guerin (BCG)-induced Reiter syndrome with an attempt at repeat BCG induction," *Canadian Urological Association Journal*, vol. 12, no. 1, pp. E37–E39, 2018.

35

Squamous Cell Carcinoma Developing in a Buccal Mucosa Graft after Urethroplasty: A Report of 2 Cases of Malignant Degeneration

Catti Massimo,[1] Nappo Gerocarni Simona,[1] Tadini Barbara,[1] Cerchia Elisa,[1] Ferrero Luisa,[1] Gambella Alessandro,[2] Pacchioni Donatella,[3] Elisabetta Teruzzi,[1] Marco Falcone,[4] Sedigh Omidreza,[4] and Gontero Paolo[4]

[1]*Paediatric Urology, Città Della Salute e Della Scienza Torino, Italy*
[2]*Pathology Unit, Department of Medical Sciences, Città Della Salute e Della Scienza Torino, Italy*
[3]*Pathology Unit, Città Della Salute e Della Scienza Torino, Italy*
[4]*Urology Department, Città Della Salute e Della Scienza Torino, Italy*

Correspondence should be addressed to Catti Massimo; massimocatti@libero.it

Academic Editor: Fumitaka Koga

Buccal mucosa graft (BMG) was originally described in 1992 for the treatment of challenging cases of hypospadias (proximal or redo cases) and has gained increasingly popularity also when dealing with complicated urethral stenosis, as it is associated with a good outcome. The development of a malignancy in a BMG urethroplasty was reported for the first time in 2017. We report two more cases of a malignant degeneration of a BMG used in a urethroplasty to treat recurrent urethral stricture.

1. Introduction

AUA guidelines for the management of male urethral strictures include urethral dilation, direct visual internal urethrotomy, and urethroplasty. According to AUA and SIU recommendations, urethroplasty is the gold standard to treat long or recurrent urethral strictures. BMG, since its original description in 1992 [1], is considered the graft of choice in urethral surgery when dealing with challenging hypospadias and urethral strictures, as it provides good results. Only one case of tumor developing in a BMG urethroplasty was previously reported [2]; we describe the 2nd and 3rd cases.

2. Case Presentation

(1) A male smoker patient developed a postinfectious HPV-related bulbar urethral stricture which was unsuccessfully treated with 2 internal urethrotomies. He underwent ventral urethroplasty with BMG in 2008, at the age of 46 years. In 2011, he developed an HPV-related squamous papilloma of the tongue and genital condyloma. In 2013, he presented urethral discharge with dysuria and developed a bulbar nodule and inguinal adenopathy. A nodular, hard, nonstenotic lesion was detected at cystoscopy on the site of previous BMG implantation (bulbar urethra) and biopsied, showing poorly differentiated SCC (Figure 1). Normal buccal mucosa was found at oral exploration. Considering the presence of inguinal nodal diffusion and the absence of urethral stricture, chemotherapy with paclitaxel, cisplatin, and ifosfamide was completed. In 2014, obturator-iliac laparoscopic lymphadenectomy was performed for locoregional diffusion together with a new biopsy of the persisting bulbar lesion. Histology confirmed poorly differentiated SCC pT2N2 in the bulbar urethra (Figure 2). Despite new chemotherapy treatment with docetaxel and cetuximab, the disease rapidly progressed to metastatic diffusion and the patient passed away

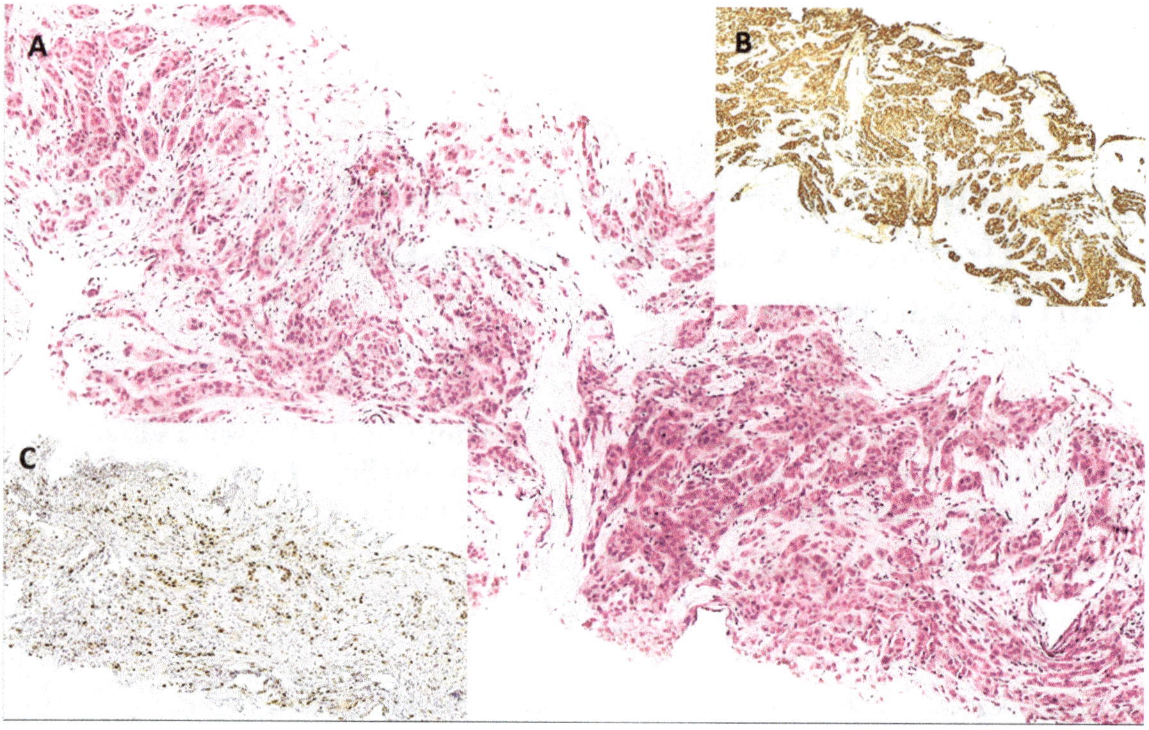

FIGURE 1: Diagnostic biopsy in case 1 (a) staining with hematoxylin and eosin; the epithelial origin is confirmed by the positivity to high MW cytokeratin (b); the proliferative index, evaluated with the MIB-1 clone of the Ki-67 antibody, highlights the malignant nature of the lesion with high proliferation (c).

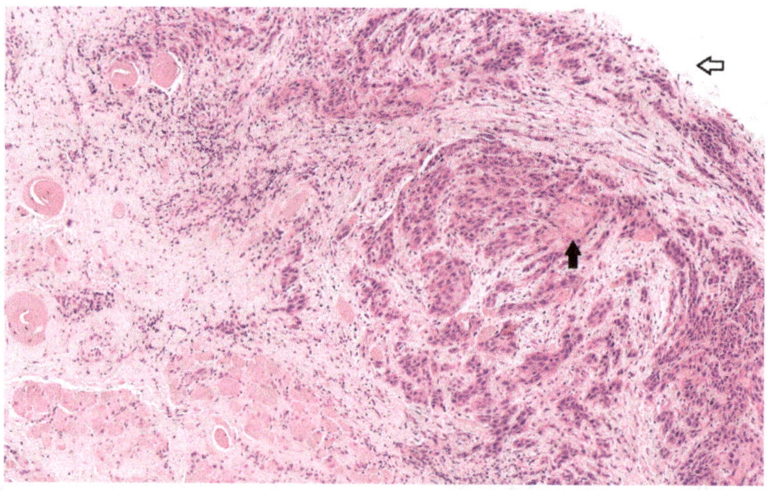

FIGURE 2: Representative sections of the surgical specimen of case 1 (surgical biopsy of bulbar urethra). Well-differentiated squamous cell carcinoma with a horn-like appearance of pearls (full arrow) and surface erosion (empty arrow). The lesion invades the dermis and muscle tissue (staining with hematoxylin and eosin).

(2) A male smoker patient with a posttraumatic stricture of the bulbar urethra, after unsuccessful internal urethrotomies, underwent ventral BMG urethroplasty at the age of 45 years. After 6 months, he presented with hematuria, inguinal adenopathy, and a hard, nodular mass of the posterior urethra; endoscopy showed thickening of the perineal and bulbar urethra and histology showed infiltrating, poorly differentiated keratinizing SCC. Biopsy of the ulcerated oral site of BMG harvest showed hyperplasia and fibrosis of the chorion with no malignancy. The patient then developed major psychiatric disorders with suicidal and uxoricidal tendencies, refused the proposed radical surgery, and underwent excision of the perineal, bulbar, and penile urethra with suprapubic cystostomy. Histology showed poorly differentiated SCC of the urethra,

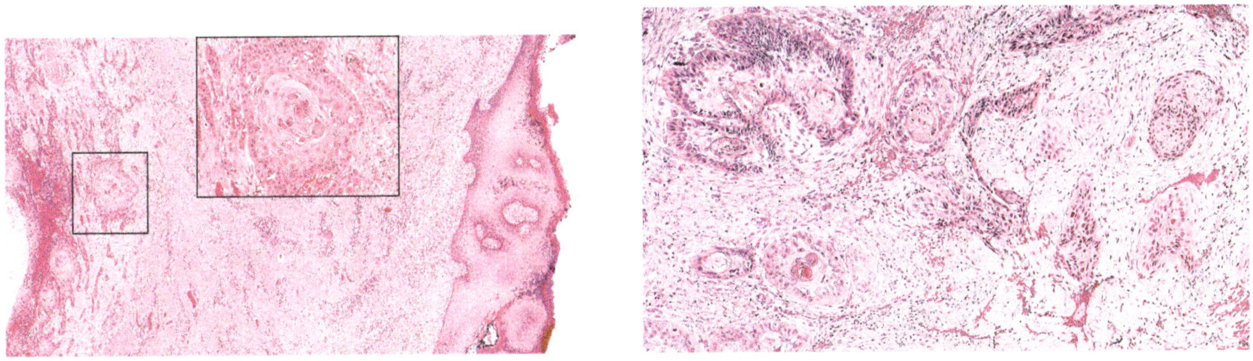

(a) (b)

FIGURE 3: Representative sections of the surgical specimen of case 2 (hematoxylin and eosin staining): surgical resection specimen of the buccal patch (a; original magnification ×50); keratinized epithelium on the right side of the image on the left side lies the infiltrating carcinoma (inset: detail at higher magnification of squamous nature consisting in keratin pearl). Aggregates and nests of intensely eosinophilic neoplastic cells with densely, hyperchromatic nuclei and keratinizing features are widely identified all over the specimen, confirming the carcinoma's squamous nature (b; original magnification ×100).

diffusely infiltrating the corpora cavernosa (Figure 3). The patient refused any other treatment including chemotherapy and eventually died

3. Discussion

Primitive tumor of the urethra is rare, accounting for 1% of urinary malignancies [3]. It affects mainly males, with a reported incidence of 4.3 males and 1.5 females per million. According to the literature [3], the most frequent histological type is urothelial carcinoma (54-65% of the cases), followed by squamous cell carcinoma (16-22%). Major risk factors are represented by urethral stenosis, chronic irritation after intermittent catheterization or urethroplasty, external beam irradiation therapy, radioactive seed implantation, chronic urethral inflammation or urethritis following sexually transmitted diseases (STD) (i.e. condylomata associated with human papillomavirus 16), and lichen sclerosus [3].

Diagnosis is made in most cases by endoscopic biopsy in patients presenting with urethral bleeding and discharge, hematuria, obstructive, and irritative urinary symptoms. Treatment is multidisciplinary, including surgery, chemo, and radiotherapy, and is not standardized [4], especially in advanced disease. It is aimed at preventing and stopping local and regional lymphatic diffusion, since the prognosis is mainly influenced by nodal stage [3].

Tumors of the oral cavity account for 2% of all malignancies, with a male/female ratio of 2/1. In most cases (90%), histotype is SCC[5]. Major risk factors are smoking, alcohol assumption, and HPV-related oral infection [5].

We speculated about the origin of the urethral tumor in these 2 patients, debating whether they were primitive tumors of the bulbar urethra or malignant transformations of the implanted BMG. Furthermore, we focused our attention on trying to determine whether the tumors originally developed in the buccal cavity or if the oral mucosa grafts underwent malignant transformation after implantation in the urethra.

Consider that

(1) the histological type was SCC, being the most frequent oral malignancy and less frequently insurging in the urethra

(2) the tumors developed in the bulbar urethra, precisely at the site of implantation of the BMG

(3) these patients presented with typical risk factors for oral SCC, such as smoking, and, in case 1, confirmed oral HPV+ papilloma

(4) both patients had no evidence of other SCC localization in the oral cavity

We came to the conclusion that, most probably, these tumors originated from the implanted BMG as a result of these main oncological predisposing factors: chronic inflammation after urethroplasty and progression of chronical HPV infection in case 1.

This report underlines the importance of extensive endoscopic and histological evaluation of all urinary symptoms presenting in patients after urethral reconstruction, to early detect complications and the development of malignancy.

Furthermore, these reports of malignant transformation challenge the assumption that BMG urethroplasty is a totally safe procedure. In case 1, sexually transmitted HPV infection most probably played a crucial role in oncological transformation, and for this reason, it is mandatory to inform the patient about STD-related risks and to prevent HPV or other sexually transmitted infections.

4. Conclusion

We report the second and third cases of malignancy developing in a BMG used for urethroplasty. BMG is largely used in children and adults, when a challenging urethral surgery is needed for long or persistent urethral strictures or for proximal/redo hypospadias. This complication, although very rare, should be kept in mind when informing the patient about the potential risks of the procedure and when obtaining informed consent. Prevention of STD is mandatory in these patients, as it associates with an augmented oncological risk.

Abbreviations

BMG: Buccal mucosa graft
SCC: Squamous cell carcinoma
STD: Sexually transmitted disease.

References

[1] A. Dessanti, W. Rigamonti, V. Merulla, D. Falchetti, and G. Caccia, "Autologous buccal mucosa graft for hypospadias repair: an initial report," *The Journal of Urology*, vol. 147, no. 4, pp. 1081–1083, 1992.

[2] P. M. Domino, J. T. Kim, and L. L. Yeung, "Development of squamous cell carcinoma of buccal mucosa graft used for urethroplasty: a case report," *Urology Case Reports*, vol. 10, pp. 60–62, 2016.

[3] G. Gakis, J. A. Witjes, E. Compérat et al., "EAU Guidelines on primary urethral carcinoma," *European Urology*, vol. 64, no. 5, pp. 823–830, 2013.

[4] F. Janisch, M. Abufaraj, H. Fajkovic et al., "Current disease management of primary urethral carcinoma," *European Urology Focus*, vol. 5, no. 5, pp. 722–734, 2019.

[5] P. H. Montero and S. G. Patel, "Cancer of the oral cavity," *Surgical Oncology Clinics of North America*, vol. 24, no. 3, pp. 491–508, 2015.

36

Clear Cell Adenocarcinoma of the Ureter Similar to Clear Cell Renal Cell Carcinoma Histology

Kazuhiro Watanabe,[1] Go Hasegawa,[2] Yohei Ikeda,[3] Noboru Hara,[1] and Tsutomu Nishiyama[1]

[1]*Department of Urology, Uonuma Institute of Community Medicine, Niigata University Medical and Dental Hospital, Urasa 4132, Minamiuonumashi, Niigata 949-7302, Japan*
[2]*Department of Pathology, Uonuma Institute of Community Medicine, Niigata University Medical and Dental Hospital, Minamiuonumashi, Niigata 949-7302, Japan*
[3]*Department of Diagnostic Radiology, Uonuma Institute of Community Medicine, Niigata University Medical and Dental Hospital, Minamiuonuma, Niigata, Japan*

Correspondence should be addressed to Tsutomu Nishiyama; nisiyama@med.niigata-u.ac.jp

Academic Editor: Fumitaka Koga

A 70-year-old woman was referred to our hospital with gross hematuria and diagnosed with right invasive ureteral cancer and bladder urothelial carcinoma in situ. Intravesical BCG therapy and neoadjuvant chemotherapy with carboplatin and gemcitabine were performed at the same time. Subsequently, laparoscopic right nephroureterectomy was performed. Urothelial carcinoma in situ persisted; however, most of the tumor was clear cell carcinoma. The clear cell carcinoma lesion had clear cytoplasm with round nuclei and visible nucleoli in an insular arrangement as is the case with clear cell renal cell carcinoma. No transitional lesion between clear cell adenocarcinoma and urothelial carcinoma was presented. The clear cell carcinoma lesion was GATA3 negative and HNF4α positive; however, the urothelial cancer lesion was GATA3 positive and HNF4α negative. Clear cell carcinoma was diagnosed as clear cell adenocarcinoma similar to clear cell renal cell carcinoma histology.

1. Introduction

Clear cell adenocarcinoma of the urinary tract, that is a subtype of tumors of Müllerian type, is a rare genitourinary malignancy occurring predominantly in the bladder or urethra; however, it rarely occurs in the ureter [1]. Clear cell renal cell carcinoma is the most common histology of renal cell carcinoma. However, metastases to the urinary tract are extremely rare. Furthermore, clear cell adenocarcinoma of the ureter similar to clear cell renal cell carcinomas in an extrarenal location is extremely rare.

2. Case Report

In December 2019, a 70-year-old woman was referred to our hospital with awareness of gross hematuria. Abdominal ultrasonography showed dilatation of the right renal pelvis and calyces. Cystoscopy showed a reddish abnormal mucosa including papillary tumors on the posterior and dome of the bladder wall. Because of her severe renal function, she could not use the administration of contrast media while computed tomography (CT) examination. Plain CT showed a right invasive ureteral tumor and no renal tumors and no metastatic findings (Figure 1(a)). Urine cytology was class V in five classes (negative, suspicious, and positive corresponding to classes I–II, III, and IV–V, respectively). In January 2020, transurethral resection of the bladder tumor (TUR-BT) was performed. Histopathological findings were urothelial carcinoma in situ. The patient was diagnosed with right invasive ureteral cancer and bladder urothelial carcinoma in situ. We made a treatment proposal to the patient: intravesical Bacillus Calmette-Guerin (BCG) therapy for preservation of urinary bladder and neoadjuvant chemotherapy for right invasive ureteral cancer, thereafter laparoscopic right nephroureterectomy. The patient was consented for the treatment. Intravesical BCG therapy, 80 mg/40 ml

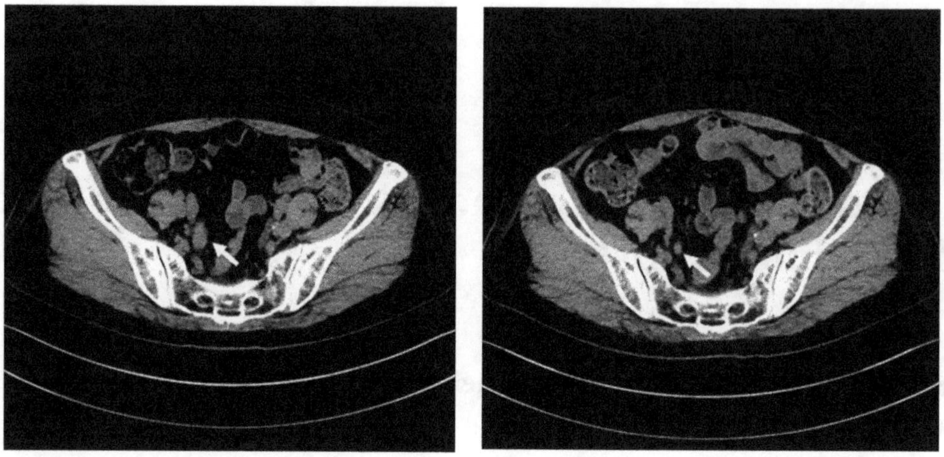

(a) (b)

Figure 1: CT findings. (a) Plain CT at diagnosis shows a right invasive ureteral tumor and no metastatic findings ((a) arrow). (b) Plain CT after four course of chemotherapy shows the right ureteral tumor diminished in size after the therapy ((b) arrow).

normal saline solution, once a week, was performed 8 times. She could not use cisplatin for standard anticancer drug because of her severe renal function. Creatinine clearance (eGFR) was determined by using serum creatinine and the Cockcroft and Gault formula. Her eGFR was 20.9 ml/min/1.73 m^2. Four courses of neoadjuvant chemotherapy with carboplatin instead of cisplatin and gemcitabine were performed at the same time of BCG therapy. The patient was design to be treated on an outpatient basis. Gemcitabine 1100 mg/body was design to be given by intravenous infusion over 30 minutes on day 1, 8 and 15 of a 28-day cycle; however, day 15, gemcitabine was omitted because of thrombopenia. Carboplatin dosed to an AUC of 5 (250 mg/body) was given as an intravenous infusion over one hour on day 1 of a 28-day cycle. The cancer cells in urine were disappeared, and the right ureteral tumor diminished in size after the therapy (Figure 1(b)). In May 2020, laparoscopic right nephroureterectomy was performed. Histopathological findings of the lesion revealed that urothelial carcinoma in situ persisted in part; however, most of the tumor was clear cell carcinoma similar to clear-cell renal cell carcinomas, pT1, and margin negative. The clear cell carcinoma lesion of the present case had clear cytoplasm with round nuclei and visible nucleoli in an insular arrangement as is the case with clear cell renal cell carcinoma. The clear cell carcinoma lesion was CK5/6 negative, CK20 negative, GATA3 negative, CK7 negative, 34β-E12 negative, CD10 positive, EMA weak positive, vimentin negative, HNF4α positive, Uroplakin negative, PAX8 negative, and CEA weak positive; however, the urothelial cancer lesion was CK7 positive, CK5/6 weak positive, CK20 positive, GATA3 positive, 34β-E12 negative, CD10 weak positive, EMA weak positive, vimentin negative, HNF4α negative, Uroplakin weak positive, PAX8 weak positive, and CEA negative (Table 1, Figure 2). No transitional lesion between clear cell carcinoma and urothelial carcinoma was presented in the ureteral lesion in the present case. HNF1B was negative for both clear cell adenocarcinoma lesion and urothelial cancer lesion. Therefore, clear cell carcinoma in the present case was diagnosed with clear cell adenocarcinoma

Table 1: Immunohistochemical results.

(a)

	CK7	CK20	CK5/6	Uroplakin	GATA3	CD10	34β-E12
UC	(+)	(+)	(+/-)	(+/-)	(+)	(+/-)	(-)
CCC	(-)	(-)	(-)	(-)	(-)	(+)	(-)

(b)

	EMA	Vimentin	PAX8	CEA	HNF4α	HNF1β
UC	(+/-)	(-)	(+/-)	(-)	(-)	(-)
CCC	(+/-)	(-)	(-)	(+/-)	(+)	(-)

UC: urothelial carcinoma; CCC: clear cell adenocarcinoma; (+): positive; (+/-): weak positive; (-): negative.

similar to clear cell renal cell carcinoma histology rather than clear cell urothelial carcinoma of a variant of urothelial carcinoma. No clear cell renal cell carcinoma lesion was found in the kidney of the nephroureterectomy specimen. For these reasons, the pathological diagnosis of the present case was clear cell adenocarcinoma of the ureter similar to clear cell renal cell carcinoma histology.

The patient is being followed up for nine months without postoperative adjuvant therapy and without tumor recurrence.

3. Discussion

Clear cell carcinoma that occurs in the urinary tract is rare and generally clear cell urothelial carcinoma or clear cell carcinoma of the Müllerian type [1]. Renal-type clear cell carcinoma occurring as a primary tumor in an extrarenal location is extremely rare, and there are several case reports of renal-type clear cell carcinoma occurring in the prostate [2]. We described a case of a clear cell adenocarcinoma of the ureter with the histologic and immunohistochemical

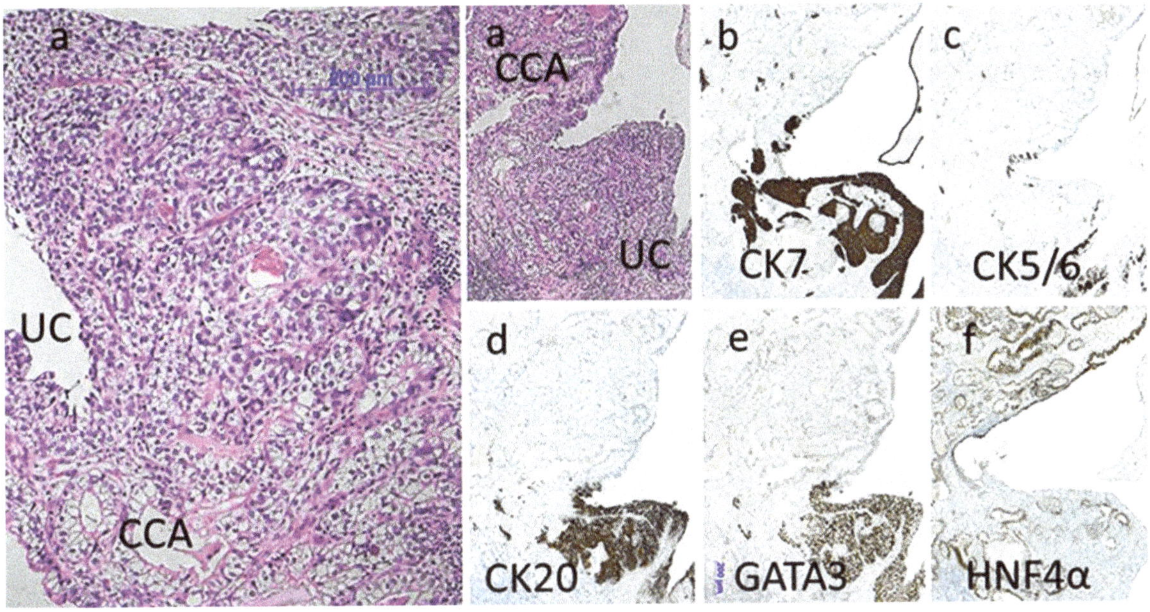

Figure 2: Pathological findings. Histopathological findings reveal that urothelial carcinoma in situ ((a) UC) persisted in part; however, most of the tumor is clear cell adenocarcinoma ((a) CCA) ((a) hematoxylin and eosin). The clear cell adenocarcinoma lesion has clear cytoplasm with round nuclei and visible nucleoli in an insular arrangement. No transitional lesion between clear cell adenocarcinoma and urothelial carcinoma can be presented in this lesion. The clear cell adenocarcinoma lesion is CK7 negative (b), CK5/6 negative (c), CK20 negative (d), GATA3 negative (e), and HNF4α positive (f). The urothelial cancer lesion is CK7 positive (b), CK5/6 weak positive (c), CK20 positive (d), GATA3 positive (e), and HNF4α negative (f). CCA: clear cell adenocarcinoma; UC: urothelial carcinoma.

features identical to that of clear cell carcinoma occurring in the kidney. In 2016, the *WHO Classification of Tumours of the Urinary System and Male Genital Organs* was revised [1]. With this revision, clear cell adenocarcinoma is classified as tumor of Müllerian type. Urinary tract clear cell adenocarcinoma occurs primarily in women and is thought to originate from Müllerian progenitor cells present in the bladder wall or adjacent soft tissues. On the other hand, reported cases of clear cell urothelial carcinoma were male [3]. Müllerian type clear cell adenocarcinoma is said to be immunoreactive to PAX8, HNF1B, CA125, and p53 [1]. On the other hand, clear cell urothelial carcinoma is a variant of urothelial carcinoma and is said to show positive findings of CK5/CD44, CK20, PAX8, and GATA3/CK7 [1]. In the present case, histopathological findings revealed that urothelial carcinoma in situ persisted in part; however, most of the tumor was clear cell adenocarcinoma, pT1, and margin negative. The clear cell adenocarcinoma lesion of the present case had clear cytoplasm with round nuclei and visible nucleoli in an insular arrangement as is the case with clear cell renal cell carcinoma. The clear cell adenocarcinoma lesion of the present case was CK5/6 negative, CK20 negative, GATA3 negative, CK7 negative, and HNF4α positive; however, the urothelial cancer lesion was CK5/6 weak positive, CK20 positive, GATA3 positive, and HNF4α negative (Figure 2). Müllerian type clear cell adenocarcinomas should be characterized by the usual tubulocystic, papillary, or diffuse growth patterns and should have hobnail cells with scant cytoplasm and hyperchromatic dense nuclei but were not observed in the present case [1]. No transitional lesion between clear cell adenocarcinoma and urothelial carcinoma was presented in the ureteral lesion in the present case. Immunohistochemically in the present case, HNF1B classified as tumor of Müllerian type was negative for both clear cell adenocarcinoma lesion and urothelial cancer lesion; however, HNF4α was positive for clear cell adenocarcinoma lesion similar to clear cell renal cell carcinomas [4]. Based on the above results, clear cell carcinoma in the present case was diagnosed as clear cell adenocarcinoma similar to clear cell renal cell carcinoma histology. Clear cell carcinomas that occur in the urinary tract have been reported in various articles; however, a clear cell adenocarcinoma of the ureter similar to clear cell renal cell carcinoma histology has not been confirmed in the reported articles.

4. Conclusion

We reported an extremely rare clear cell adenocarcinoma of the ureter that showed histology similar to clear cell renal cell carcinomas other than urothelial carcinoma variant or clear cell carcinoma of the Müllerian type.

References

[1] P. A. Humphrey, H. Moch, A. L. Cubilla, T. M. Ulbright, and V. E. Reuter, "The 2016 WHO classification of tumours of the urinary system and male genital organs–part B: prostate and bladder tumours," *European Urology*, vol. 70, no. 1, pp. 106–119, 2016.

[2] H. Singh, N. Flores-Sandoval, and J. Abrams, "Renal-type clear cell carcinoma occurring in the prostate," *The American Journal of Surgical Pathology*, vol. 27, no. 3, pp. 407–410, 2003.

[3] K. T. Mai, J. Bateman, B. Djordjevic, T. A. Flood, and E. C. Belanger, "Clear cell urothelial carcinoma," *International Journal of Surgical Pathology*, vol. 25, no. 1, pp. 18–25, 2017.

[4] Y. H. Gao, Z. X. Wu, L. Q. Xie et al., "VHL deficiency augments anthracycline sensitivity of clear cell renal cell carcinomas by down-regulating ALDH2," *Nature Communications*, vol. 8, no. 1, article 15337, 2017.

37

Leptomeningeal Metastases in a Patient with Castration-Resistant Prostate Cancer

Takuya Koie,[1] Yasuhiro Hashimoto,[2] Yuichiro Suzuki,[2] Yoshiomi Hatayama,[3] and Futoshi Kimura[4]

[1]*Department of Urology, Gifu University Graduate School of Medicine, Gifu, Japan*
[2]*Department of Urology, Hirosaki University Graduate School of Medicine, Aomori, Japan*
[3]*Department of Radiation Oncology, Hirosaki University Graduate School of Medicine, Aomori, Japan*
[4]*Department of Anesthesiology, Hirosaki University Graduate School of Medicine, Aomori, Japan*

Correspondence should be addressed to Takuya Koie; goodwin@gifu-u.ac.jp

Academic Editor: Giorgio Carmignani

A 42-year-old man visited a community hospital with chief complaints of lumbago and dyschesia. Computed tomography (CT) showed multiple lung, lymph node, and bone metastases and the irregular enlarged prostate with urinary bladder invasion. Serum prostate-specific antigen (PSA) was 544.0 ng/mL. Histological evaluation showed adenocarcinoma with the Gleason score 5 + 4, and the clinical stage was T4N1M1c as an initial diagnosis. Although androgen deprivation therapy was performed immediately, he had castration-resistant PCa after 3 months. Therefore, he received 6 courses of docetaxel chemotherapy every 3 weeks. Serum PSA was decreased to 0.2 ng/mL, and multiple metastases and prostate size were obviously reduced based on CT. He underwent robot-assisted radical prostatectomy and radiation therapy for prostatic fossa and multiple metastases. Although serum PSA level remained low, CT showed multiple liver metastases after 3 years from surgery. He received the combination therapy of cisplatin and etoposide (PE) every 4 weeks. Liver metastases had complete response. However, he visited our hospital with complaint of vomiting and a right drooping eyelid after 6 weeks from withdrawal of PE therapy. T2-weighted magnetic resonance imaging revealed multiple leptomeningeal metastases (LM). He received RT for the brain and was administered amrubicin. However, he died of PCa after 6 weeks from the diagnosis of LM.

1. Introduction

Prostate cancer (PCa) is the most commonly diagnosed neoplasm in male worldwide, and the vast majority of patients with PCa developed bone and/or lymph node metastases [1]. Conversely, leptomeningeal metastasis (LM) from genitourinary cancer is rare, especially from PCa [1, 2]. Herein, we report a patient with castration-resistant PCa (CRPC) who developed LM after multidisciplinary therapy.

2. Case Reports

A 42-year-old man visited a community hospital with chief complaints of lumbago and dyschesia. Computed tomography (CT) showed multiple lung, lymph node, and bone metastases and the irregular enlarged prostate with urinary bladder invasion (Figure 1). Serum prostate-specific antigen (PSA) was 544.0 ng/mL (normal range: <4.0 ng/mL), so that he underwent transrectal prostate biopsy. Histological evaluation showed adenocarcinoma with the Gleason score 5 + 4, and the clinical stage was T4N1M1c as an initial diagnosis. Although androgen deprivation therapy (ADT) was performed immediately, he had CRPC after 3 months. Therefore, he received 6 courses of docetaxel (70 mg/m^2) chemotherapy every 3 weeks. Serum PSA was decreased to 0.2 ng/mL, and multiple metastases and prostate size were obviously reduced based on CT (Figure 2). He underwent robot-assisted radical prostatectomy after 10 months from ADT. Pathological diagnosis was PCa with a positive surgical margin. One month later, radiation therapy (RT) was

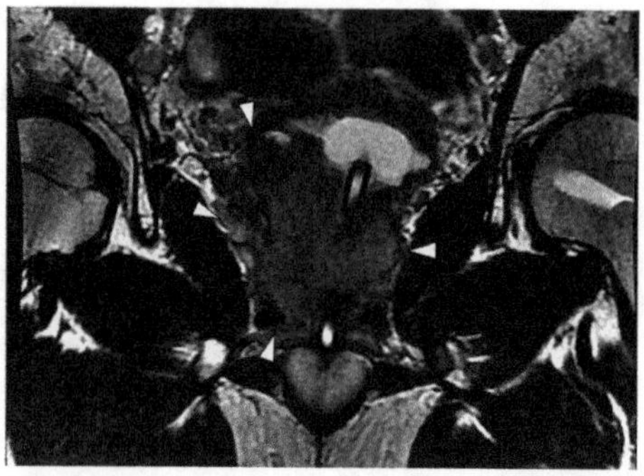

FIGURE 1: The irregular enlarged prostate with urinary bladder invasion (arrows).

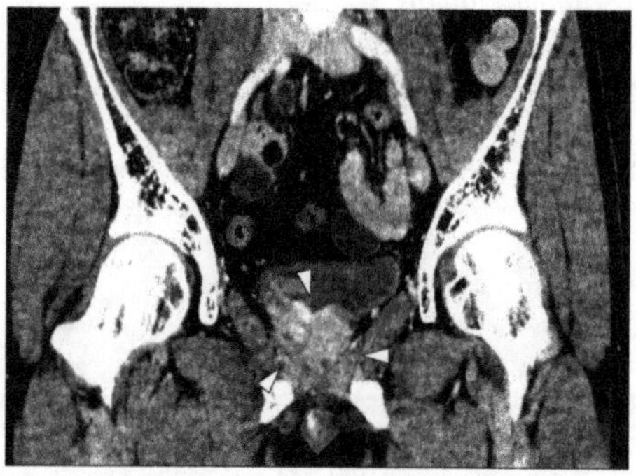

FIGURE 2: Prostate size was obviously reduced based on computed tomography after the administration of docetaxel (arrows).

performed for prostatic fossa (total 60 Gy), iliac lymph nodes (total 54 Gy), and lung metastases (total 72 Gy). Nadir PSA level was 0.09 ng/mL after surgery and RT. However, serum PSA level gradually increased. Therefore, he received several treatment modalities for PCa, including enzalutamide, abiraterone, cabazitaxel, and rechallenge of docetaxel. Although serum PSA level remained low (0.75 ng/mL), CT showed multiple liver metastases after 3 years from surgery (Figure 3(a)). At the time of liver metastases, several tumor markers showed: PSA 3.01 ng/mL, neuron-specific enolase 8.9 ng/mL (normal range: <16.3 ng/mL), and pro-gastrin-releasing peptide 58.1 pg/mL (normal range: <81 pg/mL). The patient did not undergo biopsy for liver metastases. However, we consider that his cancer cells might increase aggressiveness by stimulating angiogenesis even though tumor markers were normal. Therefore, we selected the regimen of cisplatin-based combination chemotherapy. He received 6 courses of combination therapy of cisplatin (80 mg/m^2) and etoposide (100 mg/m^2) (PE) every 4 weeks. Liver metastases had complete response (Figure 3(b)). Therefore, chemotherapy was discontinued temporarily despite continuous ADT. However, he visited our hospital with complaint of vomiting and a right drooping eyelid after 6 weeks from withdrawal of PE therapy. T2-weighted magnetic resonance imaging (MRI) revealed multiple LM at bilateral trigeminal, facial, and abductor nerves and surrounding tissues of the brain stem and cervical spinal cord (Figure 4). He received RT for the brain (total 30 Gy) and was administered amrubicin (30 mg/m^2). However, he died of PCa after 6 weeks from the diagnosis of LM.

3. Discussion

LM results from the dissemination of cancer cells to both the leptomeninges and cerebrospinal fluid compartment [3]. LM is diagnosed in 4-15% of patients with solid tumors [3]. Adenocarcinoma is the most frequent histological finding, and the breast (5%), lung (11%), and skin (melanoma) (20%) are the most common primary sites to LM [2, 3]. Conversely, LM from genitourinary tract cancer is very rare, especially in PCa. The vast majority of PCa patients with metastases will eventually die from bone metastases, while spread to the lungs, liver, and brain is a later and less common event [2]. Clinical reviews report the incidence of central nervous system (CNS) metastasis from PCa to be less than 1%, while on autopsy, it ranges from 1 to 11% [2].

LM is usually a late manifestation of systemic disease and most often occurs in patients after multidisciplinary therapies [2]. Cancer cells spread to the leptomeninges by several reasons: (1) arterial or venous circulation, (2) initiation of contact of leptomeninges with the tumor, and (3) centripetal progression along perineural or perivascular spaces [3]. Once in the subarachnoid space, tumor cells can seed multiple areas of the CSF circulation [3]. In this case, multiple liver metastases were identified before LM. Therefore, the authors consider that PCa cells may disseminate to the leptomeninges through hematogenous spread. In this case, we opted to perform RARP for the prostate even though he had multiple metastases. Faiena et al. reported that patients with metastatic disease who received definitive local therapy had greater survival than patients who received no treatment [4]. In addition, a recent Surveillance, Epidemiology, and End Results database study analyzed the cancer-specific survival (CSS) in patients with metastatic PCa who received definitive local therapy or observation [5]. The 5-year OS and predicted cancer-specific survival were significantly higher in patients who underwent RP (67.4 and 75.8%, respectively) or brachytherapy (52.6 and 61.3%, respectively) compared with patients with no treatment (22.5 and 48.7%, respectively) ($P < 0.001$) [5]. Furthermore, definitive therapy for the prostate was significantly associated with decreased cancer-specific mortality ($P < 0.01$) [5]. Therefore, we performed RARP for the patient in spite of multiple metastases.

The diagnosis of LM is made either by identifying malignant cells in CSF or by gadolinium-enhanced MRI, although there are high rates of false-negative results with both methods [6]. To date, gadolinium-enhanced MRI represents the best imaging modality for the detection of LM [6].

There is no standard treatment for LM [2]. The typical treatment for LM includes RT and systemic chemotherapy. However, chemotherapy is of limited value because of the blood brain barrier. Therefore, prognosis for PCa patients with LM is poor, and these patients do not survive more than a few weeks to months following the diagnosis of LM [6]. In

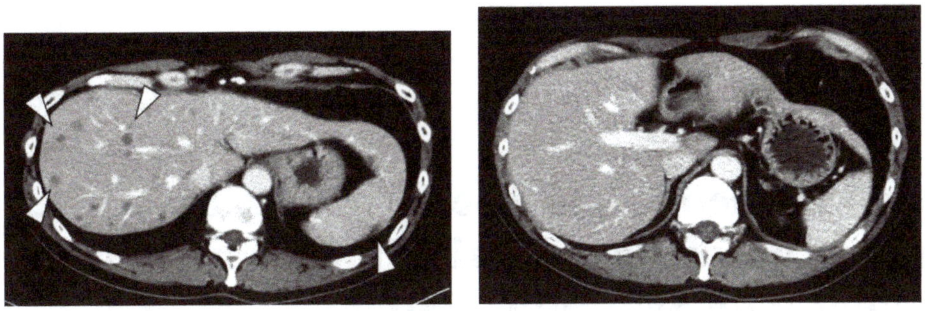

(a) (b)

FIGURE 3: Liver metastases before and after the combination chemotherapy of cisplatin and etoposide: (a) computed tomography showed multiple liver metastases (arrows); (b) liver metastases had achieved complete response in a patient who received combination chemotherapy of cisplatin and etoposide.

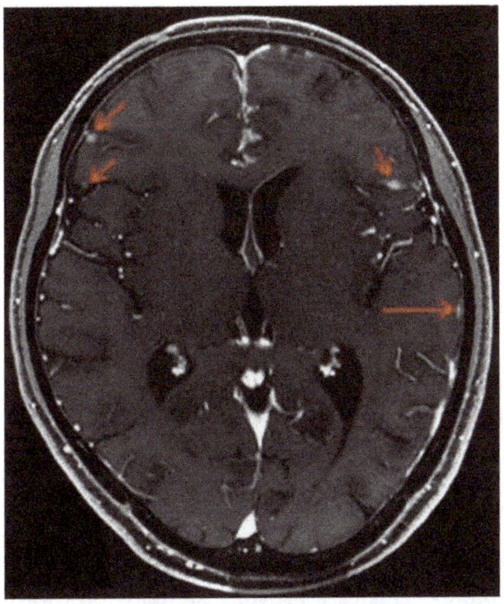

FIGURE 4: T2-weighted magnetic resonance imaging revealed multiple leptomeningeal metastases at bilateral trigeminal, facial, and abductor nerves and surrounding tissues of the brain stem and cervical spinal cord (arrows).

this case, the patient died of PCa after 6 weeks from the diagnosis of LM. Although LM is rare, early neurological symptoms may help the oncologists to make an early diagnosis of LM.

Acknowledgments

This study was supported by the grants-in-aid for scientific research from the Japan Society for the Promotion of Science (17K11118). We thank Yuki Fujita for the invaluable help with data collection. We also thank all nurses of the urological ward for providing utmost nursing for this patient.

References

[1] L. Bubendorf, A. Schöpfer, U. Wagner et al., "Metastatic patterns of prostate cancer: an autopsy study of 1,589 patients," *Human Pathology*, vol. 31, no. 5, pp. 578–583, 2000.

[2] W. R. Wasserstrom, J. P. Glass, and J. B. Posner, "Diagnosis and treatment of leptomeningeal metastases from solid tumors: experience with 90 patients," *Cancer*, vol. 49, no. 4, pp. 759–772, 1982.

[3] S. Taillibert and M. C. Chamberlain, "Leptomeningeal metastasis," *Handbook of Clinical Neurology*, vol. 149, pp. 169–204, 2018.

[4] I. Z. A. K. Faiena, E. A. Singer, C. Pumill, and I. Y. Kim, "Cytoreductive prostatectomy: evidence in support of a new surgical paradigm (review)," *International Journal of Oncology*, vol. 45, no. 6, pp. 2193–2198, 2014.

[5] S. H. Culp, P. F. Schellhammer, and M. B. Williams, "Might men diagnosed with metastatic prostate cancer benefit from definitive treatment of the primary tumor? A SEER-based study," *European Urology*, vol. 65, no. 6, pp. 1058–1066, 2014.

[6] G. Orphanos and A. Ardavanis, "Leptomeningeal metastases from prostate cancer: an emerging clinical conundrum," *Clinical & Experimental Metastasis*, vol. 27, no. 1, pp. 19–23, 2010.

38

Pulsed Electromagnetic Field Therapy as a Complementary Alternative for Chronic Pelvic Pain Management in an Interstitial Cystitis/Bladder Pain Syndrome Patient

Tyler L. Overholt[1], **Christina Ross**[2], **Robert J. Evans**[1] **and Stephen J. Walker**[1,2]

[1]*Department of Urology, Wake Forest Baptist Health, USA*
[2]*Wake Forest Institute for Regenerative Medicine, USA*

Correspondence should be addressed to Tyler L. Overholt; toverhol@mix.wvu.edu

Academic Editor: Tun-Chieh Chen

Interstitial cystitis/bladder pain syndrome is a chronic pelvic pain condition with no known etiology that affects millions of women and men in the United States. Current management can be aggressive for individuals who are refractory to less invasive options, often resulting in the use of opioid narcotics and/or surgical procedures under general anesthesia, with higher risks and side effects to patients. Pulsed electromagnetic field therapy is a noninvasive therapeutic strategy that is thought to reduce inflammation and pain via alteration of cellular function and microcirculation. This therapy has demonstrated efficacy in management of other chronic pain syndromes including fibromyalgia and chronic low back pain. Herein, we describe a case of pulsed electromagnetic field therapy for management of interstitial cystitis/bladder pain syndrome that resulted in decreases in pelvic pain, burning with bladder filling, and other nonpelvic pain symptoms. This case provides support for a formal clinical trial to evaluate the efficacy of pulsed electromagnetic field therapy for the management of chronic pelvic pain in interstitial cystitis/bladder pain syndrome.

1. Introduction

Interstitial cystitis/bladder pain syndrome (IC/BPS) is a chronic pelvic pain condition that affects millions of women and men in the United States [1, 2]. This disease is vastly heterogeneous across the affected population, and there is no clearly defined etiology of the underlying disease pathophysiology. Given the widespread variety of disease presentation, finding an effective management strategy is often difficult. This commonly leads to the utilization of more invasive options including long-term opioid narcotic use and aggressive surgical procedures under general anesthesia, resulting in billions of dollars in healthcare costs for management of these patients' symptoms [2, 3]. A minimally invasive therapeutic option for IC/BPS and related symptoms is critically needed for this patient population. Herein, we describe a case of the use of pulsed electromagnetic field (PEMF) therapy for management of chronic pelvic pain in an IC/BPS patient.

2. Case Presentation

This is a 29-year-old female who was first diagnosed with IC/BPS in 2011. Her past medical history includes chronic pelvic pain for more than ten years, dyspareunia, migraine headaches, depression, anxiety, panic attacks, and asthma. Since her diagnosis, management across the spectrum of the American Urological Association (AUA) guidelines for IC/BPS has been attempted, spanning from minimally invasive to invasive strategies. These include pelvic floor physical therapy, topical lidocaine injections, several oral pharmacological therapies such as opioid narcotics, and surgical procedures such as cystoscopic hydrodistention. Almost all AUA recommendations have been tried in this patient with limited success. In addition, she has undergone detailed gynecological and gastrointestinal evaluations including an exploratory laparotomy with little success in finding additional causes for her pelvic pain in addition to IC/BPS and/or relief for her symptoms.

During the summer of 2018, she was first introduced, through a medical professional outside of our institution's health network, to a pulsed electromagnetic field (PEMF) device as an alternative therapeutic strategy for pain management. PEMF is administered via an FDA-registered device that is thought to function by affecting cellular interactions and the microvascular circulation of targeted organs to reduce overall inflammation and pain. The PEMF device consisted of a mat designed to target the entire body, as well as a belt that was laid specifically over the pelvis to provide generalized exposure as well as targeted therapy (Figure 1). This device was programmed as per standard device protocols to a frequency of 33 Hz, a sinusoidal waveform, and to an intensity setting ranging from 3.5 to 35 microtesla. Each treatment session was eight minutes total in duration [4, 5].

For several months, the patient reported using this device at least one or two times weekly. She specifically described a two-week period where she used this device every morning and evening and reported a significant, continuous relief of many of her pelvic pain-related symptoms. Most notably, she reported experiencing reductions in bloating, burning with bladder filling, and her overall pelvic pain. She additionally reported improvements in her energy level and her ability to participate in regular physical exercise as well as a reduction in migraine headache episodes. Symptoms that were not changed with the use of this device were urgency and frequency of urination.

During the entire duration of use, the patient reported no apparent side effects to this therapy and found it to be a minimally invasive and easy to use therapeutic strategy for symptom relief. Due to the inability of the patient to purchase her own device, given the very expensive out-of-pocket price, the patient was not able to continue use for this reason alone. Following discontinuation of use, the patient reported a return of symptoms to her baseline level within 12-24 hours.

3. Discussion

Interstitial cystitis/bladder pain syndrome (IC/BPS) is a chronic pelvic pain disorder that is thought to affect 3-8 million women and ~4 million men in the United States [1, 2]. While this disease is vastly heterogeneous in presentation, the most common clinical presentations include lower urinary tract symptoms such as urgency, frequency, and dysuria, as well as bladder/pelvic pain most notably with bladder filling [1, 2]. Additionally, many IC/BPS patients experience nonbladder symptoms that are closely related to their pelvic symptoms including fibromyalgia, irritable bowel syndrome, endometriosis, and mental health disorders [1, 2].

There are several hypotheses regarding the etiology of IC/BPS. One theory with a large and growing body of research involves the structure and function of the urothelial cell layer of the bladder [6]. Studies have shown that urothelial cells from IC/BPS patients proliferate slower and enable an increased amount of leaking across cell-cell tight junctions when compared to non-IC/BPS controls [6]. Other theories involve detrusor mastocytosis with infiltration of inflammatory cells and subsequent pain [7], nerve fiber overproliferation and neurogenic inflammation [8], and central nervous system (CNS) involvement through central sensitization and amplification of the pain response [9]. While there are many different hypotheses, it is thought that multiple pathophysiologic mechanisms may be occurring simultaneously, indicating a likely multicomplex etiology of IC/BPS in affected patients.

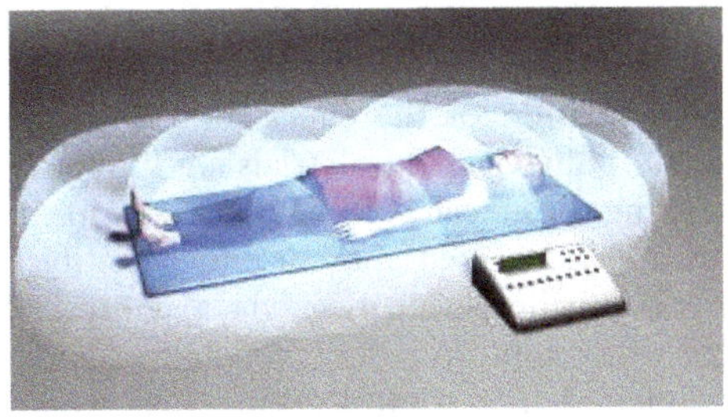

Figure 1: A pulsed electromagnetic field device. PEMF devices consist of a mat designed to target the entire body for generalized exposure, as well as a belt that can be specifically laid over the pelvis to provide targeted therapy to specific areas.

Given the unclear underlying pathophysiology, management strategies are predominantly centered around pain control and symptom reduction [1, 2]. The American Urological Association (AUA) most recently amended guidelines for IC/BPS management in 2014 that present potential treatment strategies as first through sixth line options [2]. Minimally invasive strategies such as pelvic floor physical therapy and stress/behavior modifications have the highest grade evidence for efficacy, but many patients require more aggressive management strategies [2]. These include multimodal, oral pharmacological therapy including opioid narcotics and surgical therapies under general anesthesia such as cystoscopic hydrodistention and cystectomy [2]. Even for the guidelines considered first line, the data supporting these strategies are mostly based on observational, retrospective studies, and demonstration of efficacy is often weak [2].

Pulsed electromagnetic field (PEMF) therapy, based on Faraday's Law of electromagnetism, is a combination of frequency, intensity, and time duration used to alter cellular function and restore the cells to normal rhythms [10]. Modulation of cellular function via the electromagnetic field has been reported to improve overall cell-cell interactions and microvascular circulation of targeted organs to improve inflammation and pain [10]. PEMF devices have been clinically studied in other patient subgroups with successful demonstration of symptom resolution. For example, randomized, controlled trials have showed that PEMF device therapy resulted in improved mobility, pain scores, and energy level in fibromyalgia and chronic musculoskeletal pain patients [11, 12]. Another randomized, controlled trial has shown that PEMF therapy resulted in significantly improved scores on validated pain assessment questionnaires and a reduction in disability in patients with chronic low back pain [13].

Pelvic pain reduction in a difficult patient through the use of PEMF therapy demonstrates clinical usefulness and argues for further evaluation of the effects of PEMF therapy on chronic pelvic pain via clinical trials. A limitation of this report regarding the efficacy of PEMF therapy in this patient is a lack of a standardized approach to quantify symptom improvement. Further evaluation via a controlled trial is needed to assess symptom relief through standardized measures as compared to a control group. This would include validated instruments for quantifying symptom reduction/-resolution such as IC/BPS questionnaires and depression and anxiety questionnaires. Additionally, a controlled trial would be necessary for assessment of optimal dosing and duration of treatment parameters. In summary, PEMF therapy is a minimally invasive therapeutic strategy for treating chronic pain, with no reported side effects, that provided benefit to an IC/BPS patient who experienced chronic pelvic pain refractory to almost all standard therapeutic strategies for pelvic pain relief.

References

[1] A. J. Wein, L. R. Kavoussi, A. W. Partin, and C. A. Peters, *Campbell-Walsh Urology*, Elsevier, Pennsylvania, PA, 10th edition, 2012.

[2] P. M. Hanno, D. A. Burks, J. Q. Clemens et al., "AUA guideline for the diagnosis and treatment of interstitial cystitis/bladder pain syndrome," *The Journal of Urology*, vol. 185, no. 6, pp. 2162–2170, 2011.

[3] A. Tung, Z. Hepp, A. Bansal, and E. B. Devine, "Characterizing health care utilization, direct costs, and comorbidities associated with interstitial cystitis: a retrospective claims analysis," *Journal of Managed Care & Specialty Pharmacy*, vol. 23, no. 4, pp. 474–482, 2017.

[4] L. A. Fergany, H. Shaker, M. Arafa, and M. S. Elbadry, "Does sacral pulsed electromagnetic field therapy have a better effect than transcutaneous electrical nerve stimulation in patients with neurogenic overactive bladder?" *Arab Journal of Urology*, vol. 15, no. 2, pp. 148–152, 2017.

[5] W. Jorgensen, B. M. Frome, and C. Wallach, "Electrochemical therapy of pelvic pain: effects of pulsed electromagnetic fields (PEMF) on tissue trauma," *The European Journal of Surgery. Supplement*, vol. 574, pp. 83–86, 1994.

[6] S. K. Keay, L. A. Birder, and T. C. Chai, "Evidence for bladder urothelial pathophysiology in functional bladder disorders," *BioMed Research International*, vol. 2014, Article ID 865463, 15 pages, 2014.

[7] Y. Luo, "A potential modality for interstitial cystitis: intravesical use of anti-inflammatory peptide RDP58," *The Journal of Urology*, vol. 173, no. 2, p. 340, 2005.

[8] T. J. Christmas, J. Rode, C. R. Chapple, E. J. Milroy, and R. T. Turner-Warwick, "Nerve fibre proliferation in interstitial cystitis," *Virchows Archiv. A, Pathological Anatomy and Histopathology*, vol. 416, no. 5, pp. 447–451, 1990.

[9] J. J. Kutch, E. Ichesco, J. P. Hampson et al., "Brain signature and functional impact of centralized pain: a multidisciplinary approach to the study of chronic pelvic pain (MAPP) network study," *Pain*, vol. 158, no. 10, pp. 1979–1991, 2017.

[10] C. Ross and B. S. Harrison, "An introduction to electromagnetic field therapy and immune function: a brief history and current status," *Journal of Science and Applications: Biomedicine*, vol. 3, no. 2, pp. 17–28, 2015.

[11] S. T. Sutbeyaz, N. Sezer, F. Koseoglu, and S. Kibar, "Low-frequency pulsed electromagnetic field therapy in Fibromyalgia," *The Clinical Journal of Pain*, vol. 25, no. 8, pp. 722–728, 2009.

[12] A. Thomas, K. Graham, F. S. Prato et al., "A randomized, double-blind, placebo-controlled clinical trial using a low-frequency magnetic field in the treatment of musculoskeletal chronic pain," *Pain Research & Management*, vol. 12, no. 4, pp. 249–258, 2007.

[13] K. A. Alzayed and S. M. Alsaadi, "Efficacy of pulsed low-frequency magnetic field therapy on patients with chronic low back pain: a randomized double-blind placebo-controlled trial," *Asian Spine Journal*, vol. 43, 2019.

39

New Methods of Reconstruction for Old Challenges: The Use of the Integra Graft in Necrotizing Soft Tissue Infections of the Male Genitalia

Katharina Mitchell,[1] Chad Crigger,[1] Chad Morley,[1] John Barnard,[1] and Vidas Dumasius[2]

[1]*West Virginia University Department of Urology, USA*
[2]*Marietta Memorial Hospital Department of Cosmetic, Plastic and Reconstructive Surgery, USA*

Correspondence should be addressed to Katharina Mitchell; kmm0051@mix.wvu.edu

Academic Editor: Apul Goel

In this paper, we describe two cases of Fournier's gangrene (FG) in which Integra grafting was used for reconstruction. FG is a progressive necrotizing infection occurring in the perineal region and on the external genitalia. Reconstructive options using local tissue are limited due to the destruction this infection imposes on the soft tissue. Integra graft is a bilaminate artificial dermis made of shark chondroitin 6-sulfate and bovine collagen. It is applied to the wound bed after debridement and establishment of a healthy, well-vascularized wound base. The patients in this case series had large defects which could not be closed primarily with tissue beds and would not have been appropriate for skin grafting. Therefore, an Integra graft was placed. In both patients, the wound beds were appropriate for skin grafting after three weeks. Without the Integra graft, both of our patients would have needed to wait a considerable amount of time prior to reconstruction. Our case series further illustrates and supports the use of Integra grafts in such a scenario following Fournier's gangrene which has only previously been published on three occasions, all of which demonstrated successful outcomes.

1. Introduction

Fournier's gangrene (FG), often also referred to as necrotizing fasciitis, is a progressive necrotizing infection occurring in the perineal region and on the external genitalia [1]. The underlying pathology of FG is an obliterative endarteritis of the subcutaneous arteries which leads to ischemia, destruction, and subsequent gangrene of the overlying skin and subcutaneous tissues. It is a rare, but highly lethal, process due to severe multiple organ failure. The incidence is more common in men, persons over 50 years, those with diabetes mellitus, long-term alcoholics, and people with malignant neoplasms [1, 2].

Often the nidus for this synergistic polymicrobial infection is found in the genitourinary tract, lower gastrointestinal tract, and/or skin [1]. Though often polymicrobial, *Proteus mirabilis* has been found to be the predominant pathogen [3]. Standard of care in treating this disease process begins with rapid and aggressive surgical debridement of necrotic tissue, hemodynamic support, and broad-spectrum parental antibiotics. Following radical debridement, sterile dressings and negative pressure wound therapy (wound vacuum devices) are typically used to treat open wounds [1].

Reconstructive options using local tissue are limited due to the destruction this infection imposes on the soft tissue, which is often too inflamed or lacking altogether due to the extensive surgical debridement required. These factors limit reconstructive options based on local tissue transfers or utilization of adjacent fasciocutaneous flaps. Tissue flaps in turn can also be problematic—either too bulky or insufficient coverage if skin grafting alone is utilized [3]. A new use for existing technologies may fill the void. The Integra graft

(Integra LifeSciences, Plainsboro, NJ) is a bilaminate artificial dermis made of shark chondroitin 6-sulfate and bovine collagen. It is applied to the wound bed after debridement and establishment of a healthy, well-vascularized wound base. Vascularization occurs in approximately two or three weeks after application, which creates a neodermis which can be skin grafted [3]. An Integra bilayer has been used in many other reconstructive modalities since it first was approved in 2004. However, there are very few cases which report using Integra for scrotal and/or penile reconstruction following Fournier's gangrene. We present two cases which highlight the use of the Integra graft to initiate scrotal and penile reconstruction following extensive debridement of Fournier's gangrene.

2. Case Reports

2.1. Case 1. A 43-year-old Caucasian male with a past medical history of poorly controlled diabetes mellitus type 2 confirmed by most recent hemoglobin A1C of 13%, history of obstructive sleep apnea (OSA), and remission of polycythemia vera presented with scrotal pain, edema, and rash, after noticing what he believed was a yeast infection of his skin. A necrotic eschar was noted on his scrotum. Computed tomography (CT) revealed gas gangrene concerning necrotizing soft tissue infection. He was started on vancomycin, Zosyn, and clindamycin and then underwent emergent scrotal and penile skin subcutaneous tissue incision and drainage. Subcutaneous tissue was noted to be edematous and skin without blood flow. The necrotic skin was sharply excised until the edges bled; this resulted in a large portion of the scrotal skin being removed. He was admitted to the surgical intensive care unit (SICU) in stable condition. On hospital day three, he returned to the operative suite for a second exploration of the wounds with washout and further debridement (Figure 1). Patient treatment continued with broad antimicrobial coverage along with local wound care. After coordinating with our plastic surgery colleagues, he was taken back to the operating room on hospital day eight for further sharp debridement of open scrotal and perineal wounds, complex perineal wound closure, and placement of an Integra graft covering the scrotal wound measuring 11×9 cm (Figure 2). An additional Integra graft measuring 10×12.5 cm was used to cover the perineal wound followed by placement of wound vac in place for 72 hours.

Twenty-one days after his last surgery with urology, he returned to the operating theater with plastic surgery. At this time, he underwent a 13×14 cm full-thickness skin graft which was obtained from the patient's suprapubic region which was then thinned out, and fibrous tissue was removed. Next, the scrotal area was debrided with a curette and scraping pad; once bleeding was observed, both the scrotal area tissue and harvested tissue were copiously irrigated with sterile saline; the skin graft was sutured to the scrotal defect with openings made for drainage of the serous fluid. Finally, a wound vacuum device was placed over top. He was discharged home on a two-week course of oral antibiotics, and at his 1-month follow-up, his scrotal wound with a skin graft was well healed.

2.2. Case 2. A 59-year-old male with a past medical history of chronic obstructive pulmonary disease (COPD), hyperlipidemia, diabetes mellitus type 2, and coronary artery disease (CAD) requiring multiple coronary stents and on Plavix presented with a giant condyloma involving his penis and perineum for greater than twelve years (see Figure 2). He arrived as a transfer from the outside facility with Fournier's gangrene. On presentation, his Fournier's gangrene severity index (FGSI) was 10. Preoperatively, he carried several diagnoses including Fournier's gangrene, sepsis, giant genital condyloma, and left inguinal hernia (Figure 3). Prior to surgical debridement, he was placed on broad-spectrum antibiotics.

Intraoperatively, he underwent incision and drainage of the penis and scrotum, complete scrotectomy, right orchiectomy, left orchiectomy, and penile circumcision. With exploration, the patient had extensive genital condyloma covering his suprapubic region, penis, scrotum, perineum, and perianal area with Fournier's gangrene of the scrotum extending proximally and involving the suprapubic region. All necrotic tissue was excised down to the abdominal fascia which was inspected and uninvolved. Bilateral testicles were necrotic, and bilateral orchiectomy was performed as a result. General surgery was consulted and evaluated the perineum, rectum, and left inguinal hernia. Postoperatively, he was taken to the SICU in stable condition for medical optimization and management of his complex wounds.

Six days after his initial surgery, he returned to the operating room with general surgery and plastic surgery. General surgery performed laparoscopic inguinal hernia repair for his left inguinal hernia, laparoscopic transverse loop colostomy, and open excision of bilateral thigh and groin condyloma. Simultaneously, plastic surgery performed sharp debridement of the lower abdominal wall and genital area with application of an Integra graft in addition to a traditional wound vacuum device (Figure 4). Fourteen days after surgery, he was discharged home. At his postoperative visit at 5 weeks, the Integra graft was noted to be well incorporated to the lower abdomen and penis.

Final pathology from the patient's bilateral thigh condylomas and scrotal sac was significant for condyloma acuminata with focus of high-grade intraepithelial carcinoma in the scrotal sac (with negative margins). Despite review of pathology and further reconstructive options offered to the patient at that point, such as full-thickness skin graft, the patient declined any further surgical intervention. The patient passed away shortly after.

3. Discussion

Fournier's gangrene is an ominous diagnosis associated with a high mortality and even greater morbidity that is often prolonged. In the cases provided, our patients shared similar characteristics—obese males with poorly controlled type 2 diabetes mellitus. While these characteristics are often found in the "index patient" with Fournier's gangrene, the disease has an incidence of just 1.6 cases per 100,000 men per year. Demographically, the mean age is 50.9 years with the disease substantially more common in men with a male-to-female ratio of 10 : 1 [2]. Additionally, diabetes mellitus is present

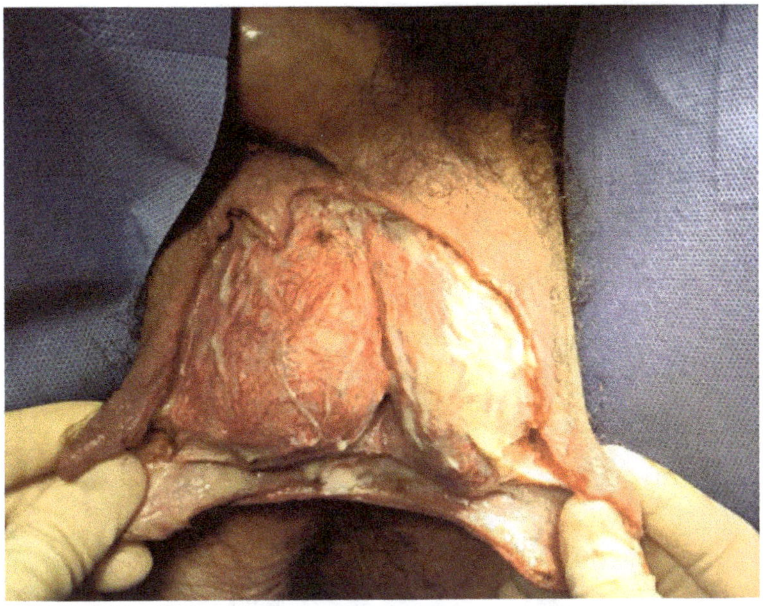

FIGURE 1: Scrotal wall wound measurement 12 cm (width) × 11 cm (length). Right base of penis wound measuring 3 cm (width) × 4 cm (length) × 3 cm (depth). Intraoperative during debridement.

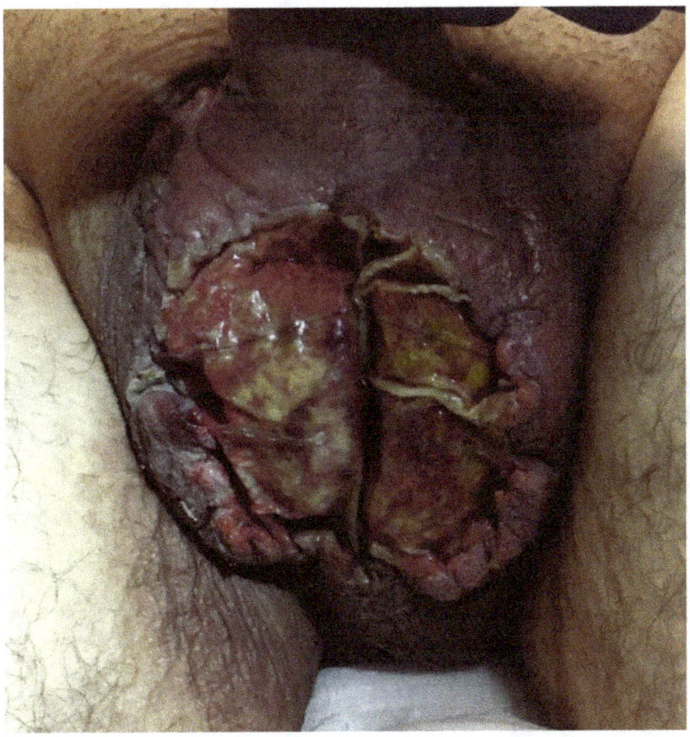

FIGURE 2: POD 3 after wound vac was removed. Integra graft seen to have taken well.

in 20–70% of the patients who present with Fournier's gangrene [3]. It is worth mentioning that both our cases were diagnosed clinically, which is the mainstay of diagnosis, with imaging being reserved during instances of clinical uncertainty [3]. While reconstructive options are often limited due to lack of available healthy tissue, both our cases demonstrate stable wound coverage using Integra grafting. Furthermore, coverage with the Integra bilayer minimizes patient discomfort due to repeat dressing changes, while avoiding immediate reconstruction with possibly compromised patient tissue and recovering from major surgical insult. Additionally, the Integra bilayer allows for the necessary time to optimize patient nutritional-metabolic status prior to final reconstruction.

While our case series focuses on the use of Integra grafts in the reconstruction of Fournier's gangrene, many other

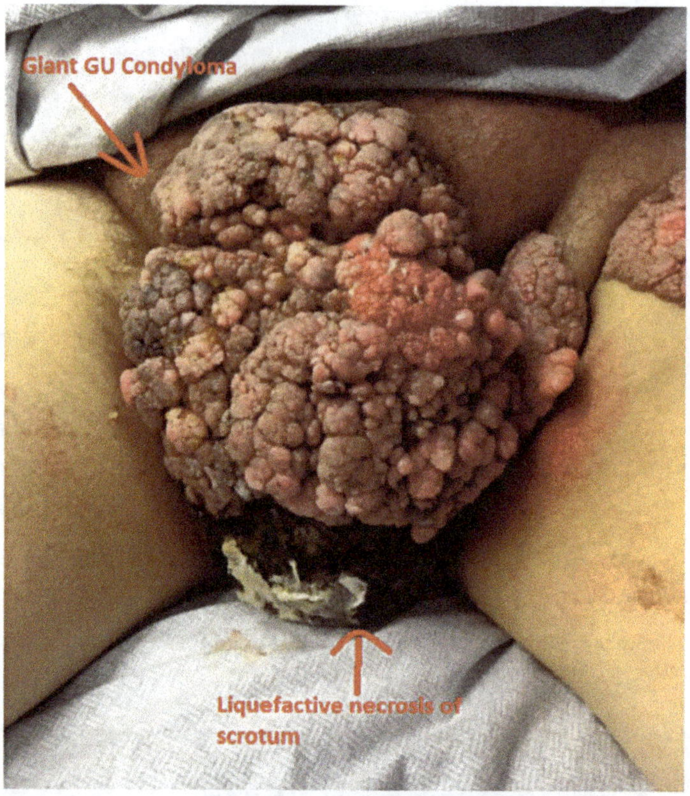

FIGURE 3: A patient's presentation with giant GU condyloma and liquefactive necrosis of the scrotum.

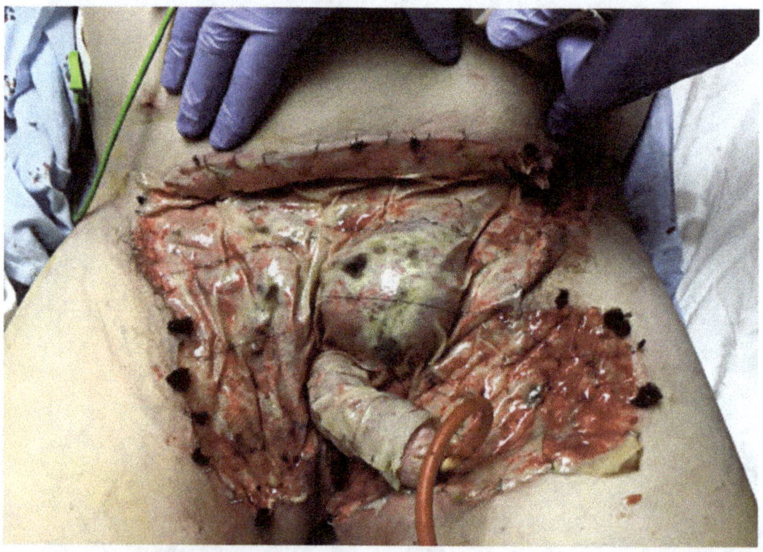

FIGURE 4: POD 7 from incision and debridement of the penis and scrotum, scrotectomy, and bilateral orchiectomy. POD 2 from colostomy creation, excision of condyloma, sharp debridement with Integra graft application, and wound vac placement. Photo taken after wound vac was removed.

methods have been more frequently used for reconstruction. A study analyzing aggregate data from 16 studies regarding Fournier's gangrene reconstruction found the following methods to be implemented with these corresponding frequencies: secondary intention with delayed primary closure 10.4%, implantation of the testicle in a medial thigh pocket 8.5%, loose wound approximation 1.4%, skin grafts 22.6%, scrotal advancement flaps 16.0%, flaps 30.1%, and flaps or grafts in combination with tissue adhesives 5.2% [4]. Each method of reconstruction has different implications as well as demands on the healthcare system and patient. For example, healing by secondary intention is used in patients with a small postsurgical defect confined to the scrotum. In the case of Fournier's gangrene, inflammation and infection of the surrounding tissue limit the reconstruction techniques possibly—our patients had large defects which could not be closed primarily with tissue beds which would not have been appropriate for skin grafting. Therefore, an Integra graft was placed. In both patients, the wound beds were appropriate for skin grafting after three weeks. Without the Integra graft, both of our patients would have needed to wait a considerable amount of time prior to reconstruction.

Our case series further illustrates and supports the use of Integra grafts in such a scenario following Fournier's gangrene which has only previously been published on three occasions, all of which demonstrated successful outcomes [3, 5, 6]. Successful outcomes were determined based on a follow-up at 1-3 months postop with patients demonstrating complete wound healing with good functional and aesthetic results. Indeed, larger aggregate studies following patients who have undergone scrotal reconstruction using Integra grafts in the setting of Fournier's gangrene are needed to better understand the long-term outcomes associated with the use of Integra grafting for genitourinary reconstruction.

References

[1] A. Chennamsetty, I. Khourdaji, F. Burks, and K. A. Killinger, "Contemporary diagnosis and management of Fournier's gangrene," *Therapeutic Advances in Urology*, vol. 7, no. 4, pp. 203–215, 2015.

[2] S. A. Chernyadyev, M. A. Ufimtseva, I. F. Vishnevskaya et al., "Fournier's gangrene: literature review and clinical cases," *Urologia Internationalis*, vol. 101, no. 1, pp. 91–97, 2018.

[3] B. L. Dent, A. Dinesh, K. Khan, and R. Engdahl, "Scrotal reconstruction with Integra following necrotizing fasciitis," *Journal of Emergencies, Trauma, and Shock*, vol. 11, no. 1, pp. 57–59, 2018.

[4] L. S. Karian, S. Y. Chung, and E. S. Lee, "Reconstruction of defects after Fournier gangrene: a systematic review," *Eplasty*, vol. 15, 2015.

[5] T. Agostini, F. Mori, R. Perello, M. Dini, and G. L. Russo, "Successful combined approach to a severe Fournier's gangrene," *Indian Journal of Plastic Surgery: official publication of the Association of Plastic Surgeons of India*, vol. 47, no. 1, pp. 132–136, 2014.

[6] D. W. Barham, M. Y. Lee, and D. A. Stackhouse, "Novel scrotal reconstruction after Fournier's gangrene using the Integra™ dermal regeneration template," *Urology*, vol. 128, pp. e3–e4, 2019.

Simultaneous Laparoscopic Surgery for Bladder Diverticulum and Urachal Remnant: A Case Report

Masaki Murata,[1] Kohei Inui,[1] Moto Hasegawa,[1] Yohei Ikeda,[2] Yuki Nakagawa,[1] Noboru Hara,[1] and Tsutomu Nishiyama[1]

[1]*Department of Urology, Uonuma Institute of Community Medicine, Niigata University Medical and Dental Hospital, Niigata, Japan*
[2]*Department of Diagnostic Radiology, Uonuma Institute of Community Medicine, Niigata University Medical and Dental Hospital, Niigata, Japan*

Correspondence should be addressed to Tsutomu Nishiyama; nisiyama@med.niigata-u.ac.jp

Academic Editor: Nicola Zampieri

A 44-year-old woman visited a hospital with microscopic hematuria in June 2009. Computed tomography showed a large bladder diverticulum at right lateral wall and urachal remnant. Cystoscopic examination showed a large diverticulum at the right lateral wall that closes to the dome. She was followed up closely without therapeutic intervention; however, the residual urine increased gradually and frequent bladder diverticulitis developed. She underwent laparoscopic bladder diverticulectomy and excision of the urachal remnant simultaneously without any complications in August 2017. Laparoscopic approach for a large bladder diverticulum and urachal remnant is useful with safe, effective, and minimally invasive.

1. Introduction

Bladder diverticulum is a bladder abnormality that mainly acquired, forms by the herniation of bladder mucosa through the muscle layers [1]. It can cause lower urinary tract symptoms (LUTS), urinary tract infections (UTIs), residual urine, bladder stones, and malignancy [1]. Urachal remnant is a rare congenital anomaly that is caused by a failure in the obliteration of the allantois [2]. A surgical approach for these diseases is not necessary in many cases. On the other hand, surgical treatment is performed when symptomatic or malignant [1–4]. Recently, a minimally invasive procedure is required, and the laparoscopic approach is useful in this regard [3]. We report a laparoscopic surgery for a patient with simultaneous occurrence of bladder diverticulum and urachal remnant.

2. A Case Report

A 44-year-old woman visited a nearby hospital with microscopic hematuria in June 2009. Her past medical history is tetralogy of Fallot. She had no medications at the time of the visit. There was no abnormality on physical examination. Computed tomography (CT) showed urachal remnant (urachal diverticulum at the dome of the bladder) and a large bladder diverticulum at the right lateral wall (Figures 1(a)– 1(e)). Urine cytology was negative. Since she did not have any symptoms, she was followed up without therapeutic intervention. However, the residual urine had been increasing gradually, and she was referred to our hospital for continuous follow-up in February 2016. The postvoid residual urine was 150 ml at the time. After six months, she complained of severe dysuria and repeated urinary tract infection possibly caused by bladder diverticulitis. Cystoscopic examination showed a large diverticulum at the right wall, and diverticular mucosa was reddish and erosive (Figures 2(a) and 2(c)). Urachal diverticulum was small and without inflammation (Figure 2(b)). Antibiotic therapy with Levofloxacin was effective for UTI. She was started treatment with Urapidil of 30 mg/day simultaneously; however, the postvoid residual urine and dysuria did not improve.

We performed bladder diverticulectomy and excision of urachal remnant simultaneously with the laparoscopic approach in August 2017. We cut out the umbilicus circumferentially with the umbilical ligament connected and then

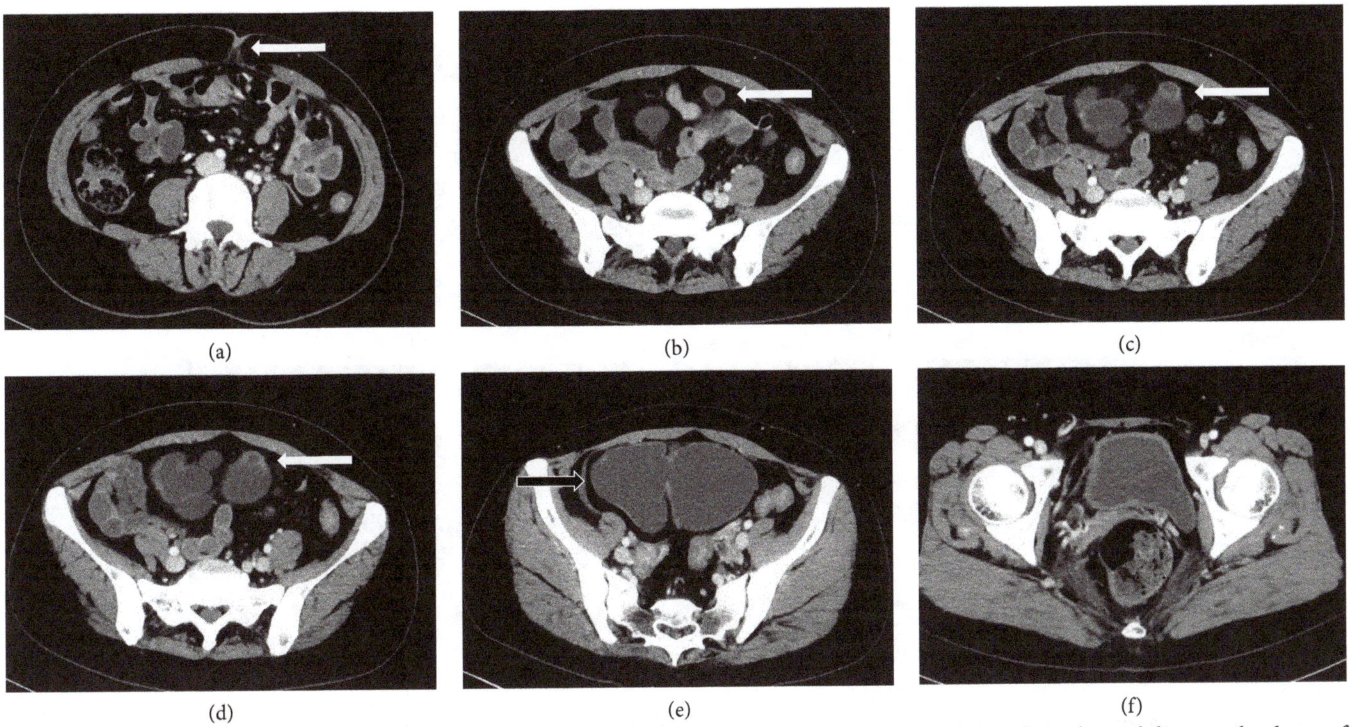

FIGURE 1: Abdominal CT shows urachal remnant and bladder diverticulum. (a–d) The fibrous cord runs from the umbilicus to the dome of the bladder (arrow). (e) A large bladder diverticulum locates in the right lateral wall (arrow). (f) CT findings nine months after the operation revealing no recurrence of the diverticula.

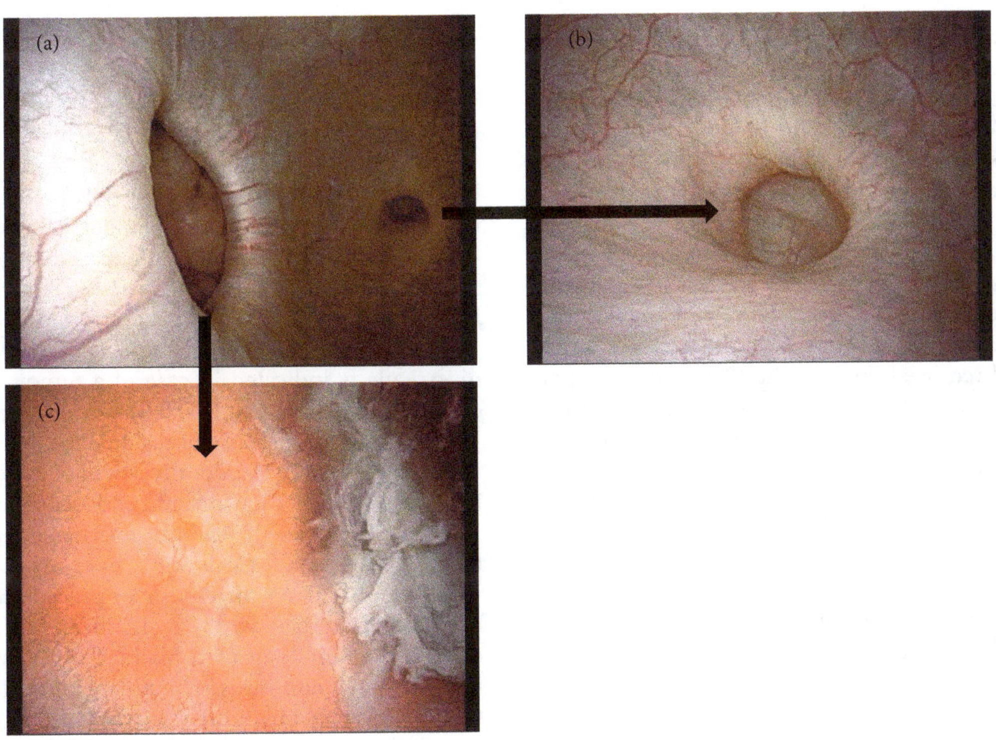

FIGURE 2: Cystoscopic examination showed a diverticulum neck at the right wall and urachal diverticulum at the dome of bladder. (a, b) The diverticular mucosa was redness, and (c) erosion.

dropped into the abdominal cavity. The 12-mm camera port was placed in the umbilical hole. We prepared the five working ports (Figure 3(a)). Two were inserted at the height of the umbilicus on the bilateral middle clavicular line, and the other three were inserted at the inside of the right upper abdomen and outside of the bilateral lower abdomen. First, we inserted a camera into the right side working port of the umbilicus height and dissected the urachal ligament and adjacent tissues

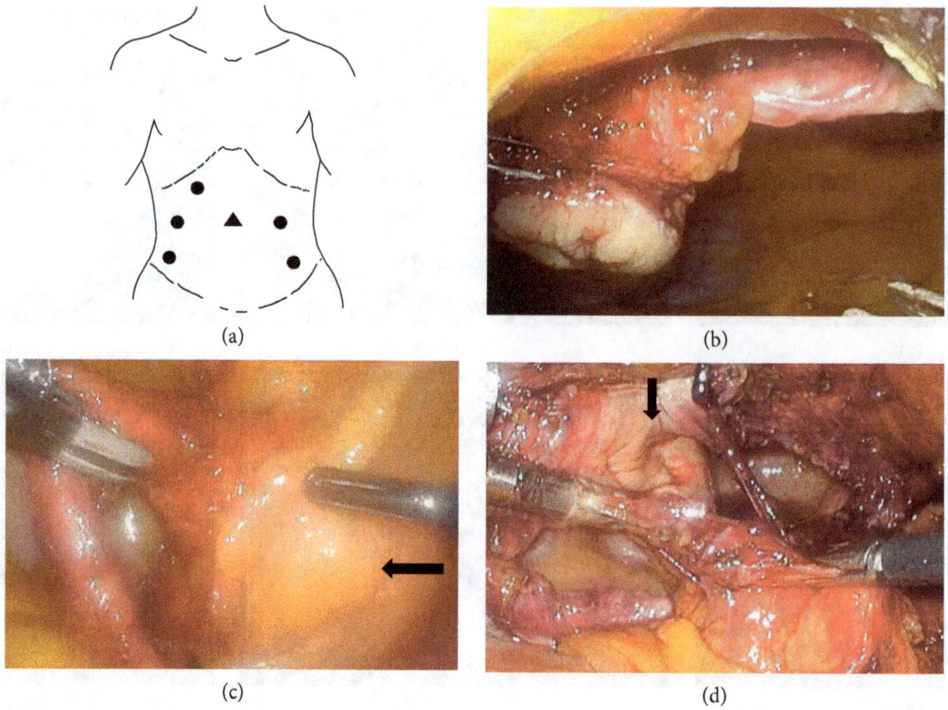

FIGURE 3: (a) The placements of the trocar port. ●: operator's and assistant's port; ▲: camera port. (b) The umbilicus and umbilical ligament viewed from the right working port. (c) Excision of the umbilical ligament just above the bladder dome. The bulging of the bladder diverticulum is identified just to the right side of the bladder dome (arrow). (d) After resection of the bladder diverticulum. The urachal diverticulum is identified just to the left of the resection site (arrow).

toward the bladder using the remaining right working port (Figure 3(b)). We transferred the camera to the central camera port and dissected the umbilical ligament until just above the bladder dome. We could confirm the bulging of the bladder diverticulum just to the right side of the bladder dome (Figure 3(c)). We used the cystoscopy to visualize the diverticular neck. The cystoscopic light could be observed from the abdominal cavity, and the bladder diverticulum was circumferentially resected at its neck. The resection line was extended to the bladder dome, and the urachal diverticulum was also resected (Figure 3(d)). The specimens were placed in an organ retrieval bag and removed through the 12-mm camera port site. The bladder defect was closed in 2 layers with a running 3-0 V-loc suture. The total operative time was 216 min with minimal blood loss.

The Foley catheter was removed on the seventh postoperative day, and she was discharged home on the same day. For 18 months after the operation, she was able to void without residual urine, urinary tract infection ceased to develop, and had no recurrence of the diverticula (Figure 1(f)). Microscopic hematuria also disappeared.

3. Discussion

Urachal remnants; that is a rare congenital anomaly, represent a failure in the obliteration of the allantois at birth that connects the bladder to the umbilicus. The most common symptoms and signs at diagnosis is umbilical discharge, while an incidental diagnosis is increasing as diagnostic imaging improves [1]. Spontaneous resolution without further intervention has been reported; however, it has also been suggested that chronic exposure to urinary stasis, infection, and inflammation in the remnant may predispose to urachal carcinoma. Therefore, there is no consensus on the management of Urachal remnants.

Bladder diverticula represent herniation of the urothelial lining that project through a congenital or acquired weakness in the muscular wall of the bladder [2]. Acquired bladder diverticula are associated with increased intravesical pressure secondary to bladder outlet obstruction but are often clinically insignificant and most of the bladder diverticula do not require intervention. On the other hand, surgical treatment of bladder diverticula is indicated in case of a tumor or stones in the diverticulum, persistent LUTS despite medications, recurrent UTIs, and a large amount of residual urine [2]. Several treatment strategies for bladder diverticula have been advocated, including surgical excision, and endoscopic management.

The patients with bladder diverticula were reported to have a higher risk for development of urothelial carcinoma, which can occur synchronously or precede carcinoma of the nondiverticular bladder [3]. A significantly higher percentage of diverticulum-associated bladder carcinomas are said to be high-grade and invasive compared with their non-diverticulum-associated counterparts because attenuation of the muscle layer associated with diverticulum formation may facilitate tumor invasion into peridiverticular soft tissues. Follow-up must be taken for the patients such as the present case.

Laparoscopic diverticulectomy is said to be technically feasible and safe and thought of as representing an alternative to the standard open procedure [4]. In the present case, the patient complained of intractable bladder diverticulitis and underwent laparoscopic bladder diverticulectomy and excision of urachal remnant simultaneously. Endoscopic fulguration of bladder diverticula was not recommended for this young patient because of the possibility of the remaining diverticulum and the risk of development urothelial carcinoma. The previous report suggested a laparoscopic approach for each of these diseases can be used safely, effectively, and minimally invasive.

4. Conclusion

We reported a patient who underwent laparoscopic bladder diverticulectomy and excision of urachal remnant simultaneously. Laparoscopic surgery was performed without any complications. Moreover, postoperative urination was good. Follow-up must be taken for the patients such as the present case because of a higher risk for the development of urothelial carcinoma.

Abbreviations

LUTS: Lower urinary tract symptoms
UTIs: Urinary tract infections
CT: Computed tomography.

Acknowledgments

This research project received no specific grant from funding agencies in the public or commercial sectors.

References

[1] J. A. Naiditch, J. Radhakrishnan, and A. C. Chin, "Current diagnosis and management of urachal remnants," *Journal of Pediatric Surgery*, vol. 48, no. 10, pp. 2148–2152, 2013.

[2] M. X. Kong, X. Zhao, E. Kheterpal et al., "Histopathologic and clinical features of vesical diverticula," *Urology*, vol. 82, no. 1, pp. 142–147, 2013.

[3] M. T. Idrees, R. E. Alexander, J. B. Kum, and L. Cheng, "The spectrum of histopathologic findings in vesical diverticulum: implications for pathogenesis and staging," *Human Pathology*, vol. 44, no. 7, pp. 1223–1232, 2013.

[4] A. M. Abdel-Hakim, A. El-Feel, H. Abouel-Fettouh, and I. Saad, "Laparoscopic vesical diverticulectomy," *Journal of Endourology*, vol. 21, no. 1, pp. 85–89, 2007.

Penile Glans Amputation following Circumcision: A Case Report of a Rare Complication

Salman Soltani,[1] Mahdi Mottaghi,[2] Amir Jafarpisheh,[3] and Mahmoud Tavakkoli[4]

[1]*Kidney Transplantation Complications Research Center, Mashhad University of Medical Sciences, Mashhad, Iran*
[2]*Students Research Committee, Faculty of Medicine, Mashhad University of Medical Sciences, Mashhad, Iran*
[3]*Department of Urology, Faculty of Medicine, Mashhad University of Medical Sciences, Mashhad, Iran*
[4]*Kidney Transplantation Complications Research Center, Mashhad University of Medical Sciences, Mashhad, Iran*

Correspondence should be addressed to Mahmoud Tavakkoli; tavakkolim@mums.ac.ir

Academic Editor: Nicola Zampieri

Circumcision is the most prevalent surgery among men. Like any other surgical intervention, it is associated with several complications. A rare shocking complication is glans amputation which is a urologic emergency. Herein, we present a 4-year-old boy with penile glans amputation following circumcision. The reimplantation was performed in less than two hours. We approximated the ends over a size 4 : 0 catheter. The urethral anastomosis was performed via 6 : 0 Vicryl sutures. Then, we sutured amputated glans in place via Vicryl 4 : 0. We immobilized the penis for a week via bandages used in penile reconstruction surgeries. We also used pentoxifylline to treat glans ischemia after surgery. The patient and his parents did not mention any difficulties or abnormalities while voiding, and the cosmetic result was favorable after three months of follow-up.

1. Introduction

Circumcision is an ancient surgical procedure and remains the most frequent surgery until today. About 25 to 35% of the male population around the world are circumcised [1–3]. Muslims, Jews, Christians (especially in North America), and native Australians are accounted for the majority of this fraction [4].

2. Case Presentation

A 4-year-old boy was brought to the emergency department due to the glans amputation during the circumcision procedure. The procedure performed by a general practitioner in an outpatient office, using the Mogen clamp. The responsible physician had covered the amputated part in sterile moist gauze and a plastic bag, then put it in an ice pack and urgently sent him to our tertiary referral hospital where he was prepared for surgery in less than an hour (Figure 1).

In the operating room, both amputated surfaces were irrigated via 0.9% saline and 10% povidone-iodine. The amputated part appeared completely white. After the preparation for replantation, a 6 Fr transurethral catheter inserted through the amputated part of the glans and then inserted further to the urethra and bladder. Urethra anastomosed via interrupted sutures (6 : 0 Vicryl suture). Then, the amputated part of the glans reattached to the penis via Vicryl sutures 4 : 0 and finally, circumcision completed. After an hour in the postoperation room, the first signs of reperfusion started to appear like bright pink appearance, but poor capillary reperfusion (about 2-3 seconds) (Figure 2). The patient's vital signs were stable and he was transferred to the ward. The penis immobilized via a splint. The next morning, parents complained about minor discoloration of the tip of the glans. After consultation with a vascular surgeon, we started him on pentoxifylline (200 mg twice a day, orally). We also managed the wound by keep soaking the bandages and the gauzes. We carefully watched the glans penis appearance, and after two days, the discoloration faded. The patient was discharged home one week after the surgery with a Foley catheter and antibiotics. After 21 days, the Foley catheter was removed while the appearance of the penis was normal.

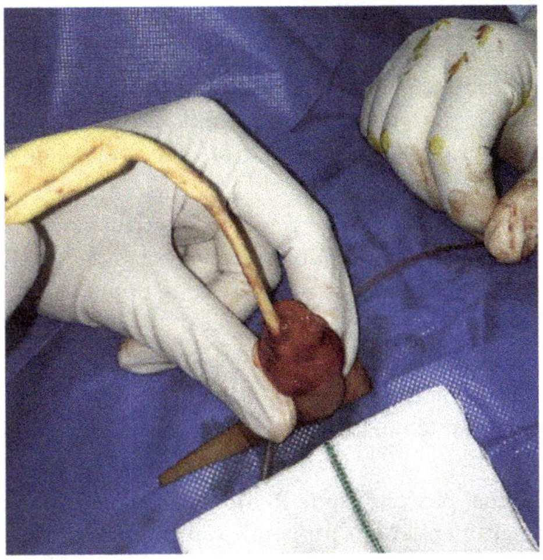

Figure 1: Amputated glans and complete injury of the urethra.

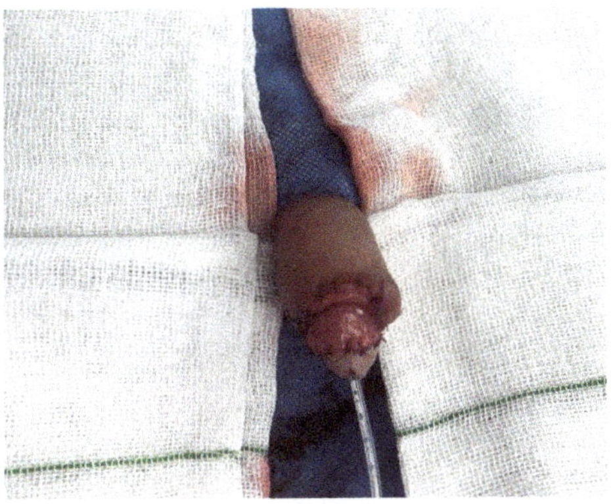

Figure 2: Penis pink appearance in the postoperation room.

Ultrasound showed normal urinary residue. We also performed a urinary flowmetry which was normal. After three months, his parents reported normal voiding stream and examination revealed no stenosis with satisfactory cosmetic results. Parents look agitated during all visits and did not consent for taking a follow-up image and said that it makes their son uncomfortable. Finally, they agreed to take a picture themselves (Figure 3).

3. Discussion

Although several medical benefits are proposed for circumcision, it is mainly done due to religious beliefs or as a routine cultural behavior [4]. Medically, it decreases urinary tract infection (especially in the first year of life), penile cancer, cervical cancer in one's partner, and sexually transmitted infections (HSV, HPV, HIV, trichomoniasis, syphilis, and chancroid) [5]. The Joint United Nations Programme on HIV and AIDS (UNAIDS) advises performing circumcision to prevent HIV. It provides lifetime partial protection against HIV transmission from female to male. It is advised to be performed in the first month of life because of its less complication rate during this period [5]. Circumcision's complication rate was about 0.19% to 3.1% which reported in a systematic review in 2010 [6]. Interventions of the health care system on training the circumcisers probably affect the complication rate. In Israel where traditional circumcisers (Mohels) are trained by the ministry of health and ministry of religion, the complication rate is about 0.34%, while in Nigeria, this rate is about 20% and this high complication rate is probably due to inadequate training of circumcisers [2, 4]. Circumcision's complications might present early or delayed. Bleeding and infection are the most frequent early complications which are generally easy to control [2, 4]. Delayed complications include excessive foreskin, shortage of penile skin, skin bridges, fistula, buried penis, meatal stenosis, and glans injures [2, 4]. Penile glans amputation is rare but it is a urologic emergency and needs prompt replantation. The surgeon should focus on restoring the function of the glans and urethra while preserving the cosmetic appearance of the glans to avoid the future psychological burden. The amputated part should be dressed via a sterile moist gauze in a plastic bag and kept in the ice and water. Direct contact of the amputated part with the ice can cause tissue damage and replantation failure [1, 7]. The replantation should be performed under eight hours from injury to achieve the best functional and cosmetic results [1, 8]. A urinary catheter should be placed for at least a week to decrease the tension on the urethra and subsequently decrease the chance of fistula development [7].

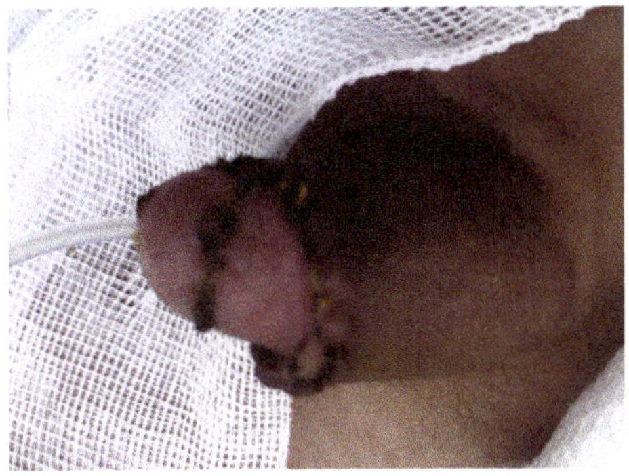

Figure 3: Follow-up image after 3 weeks of operation.

The etiology of glans amputation during circumcision is not well understood but Salle et al. found a similar pattern of penis injury (the ventrolateral aspect of the glans is cut accompanying urethral injury) and remnant adhesions in one amputated glans [1]. They hypothesized that remaining adhesions between prepuce and glans, especially on the ventral aspect of the penis, can cause clamping the glans partially or completely. They also declare that poor releasing of adhesions on the ventral side might be due to the location of the frenular artery. Injury to this artery can cause profuse bleeding; therefore, inexperienced circumcisers might avoid this area to reduce the probability of bleeding; thus, more adhesions remain [1]. Another risk factor for glans amputation is the technique in which the circumcision performed. There are three basic patterns for circumcision: Guillotine-like clamps (like Mogen clamp), glans protective clamps (like Plastibell and Gomco clamps), and free-hand approach (usually used in the operating room) with no device. Each type is associated with advantages and disadvantages. Mogen clamp is commonly used because it is time-saving and provides good cosmetic outcome. But its major disadvantage is that glans is hidden during clamping and cutting the prepuce [1]. The experience of the circumciser is another determining factor for the complication rate. Circumcision is usually performed by traditional circumcisers, nurses, general practitioners, and rarely surgeons and urologists [2]. The study of Okeke et al. showed that traditional circumcisers had lower complication rate but it is probably due to underestimation. Traditional circumcisers probably report only major complications [2].

For treatment, it is advised to perform penile shaft replantation in a microvascular fashion, but glans vessels are low-gauge and macroscopic replantation seems to be the best choice [8, 9]. Urethral injury almost always a company glans amputation. Reanastomosis of the urethra decreases the chance of fistula and meatal stenosis but increases the chances of urethral shortage and subsequent ventral chordee [9]. Faydaci et al. performed replantation without urethral reanastomosis to gain better cosmetic outcomes [9].

Glans discoloration and edema were seen in the same studies on the second postoperative day [7, 9]. Different strategies were used in different settings. Faydaci et al. used a hyperbaric oxygen chamber; Roche et al. used leech medicinal therapy; and we used pentoxifylline after consultation with vascular surgeons, and all methods provide satisfactory outcomes [7, 9]. As expected, patients' parents act agitatedly during the treatment course and a lack of a psychologist to control the situation caused several difficulties for the patient, his parents, and physicians. Glans amputation can cause psychological complications (short and long term) in the patient and his family, so we suggest referring the patients to get further consultation and support from a psychologist.

4. Conclusion

Penile glans amputation is a rare complication of circumcision. It can be prevented by educating circumcisers. Guillotine-like procedures increase the risk and proper removal of adhesions, especially on the ventral aspect of the penis might decrease the risk. Treatment is replantation of amputated part within eight hours of the accident. Hyperbaric oxygen chamber, medicinal leech therapy, and pentoxifylline can be used to provide reperfusion to the amputated part after the replantation.

References

[1] J. L. Pippi Salle, L. E. Jesus, A. J. Lorenzo et al., "Glans amputation during routine neonatal circumcision: mechanism of injury and strategy for prevention," *Journal of Pediatric Urology*, vol. 9, no. 6, pp. 763–768, 2013.

[2] L. I. Okeke, A. A. Asinobi, and O. S. Ikuerowo, "Epidemiology of complications of male circumcision in Ibadan, Nigeria," *BMC Neurology*, vol. 6, no. 1, p. 21, 2006.

[3] I. Sasmaz, B. Antmen, G. Leblebisatan, B. Şahin Karagün, Y. Kilinç, and R. Tuncer, "*Circumcision and complications in patients with haemophilia in southern part of Turkey: Çukurova experience*," *Haemophilia*, vol. 18, no. 3, pp. 426–430, 2012.

[4] J. B. Chaim, P. M. Livne, J. Binyamini, B. Hardak, D. Ben-Meir, and Y. Mor, "*Complications of circumcision in Israel: a one year multicenter survey*," *Israel Medical Association Journal*, vol. 7, no. 6, pp. 368–370, 2005.

[5] B. J. Morris, J. N. Krieger, and J. D. Klausner, "*CDC's male circumcision recommendations represent a key public health measure.*," *Global Health: Science and Practice*, vol. 5, no. 1, pp. 15–27, 2017.

[6] H. A. Weiss, N. Larke, D. Halperin, and I. J. B. Schenker, "Complications of circumcision in male neonates, infants and children: a systematic review," *BMC Urology*, vol. 10, no. 1, 2010.

[7] N. A. Roche, B. Vermeulen, P. Blondeel, and F. Stillaert, "Technical recommendations for penile replantation based on lessons learned from penile reconstruction," *Journal of Reconstructive Microsurgery*, vol. 28, no. 4, pp. 247–250, 2012.

[8] J. H. Kim, J. Y. Park, and Y. S. Song, "Traumatic penile Injury: from circumcision injury to penile amputation," *BioMed Research International*, vol. 2014, Article ID 375285, 6 pages, 2014.

[9] G. Faydaci, K. Uğur, C. Osman, Ş. Şermin, and E. Bilal, "Amputation of glans penis: a rare circumcision complication and successful management with primary anastomosis and hyperbaric *oxygen therapy.*," *Korean Journal of Urology*, vol. 52, no. 2, pp. 147–149, 2011.

42

An Unusual Location for a Nonurachal Bladder Adenocarcinoma

George Khludenev, Akshay Reddy, Sinan Akosman, and Michael J. Whalen

George Washington University School of Medicine, 2300 I St NW, Washington, DC 20052, USA

Correspondence should be addressed to Akshay Reddy; reddyak@gwu.edu and Michael J. Whalen; mwhalen@mfa.gwu.edu

Academic Editor: Tun-Chieh Chen

Malignant bladder neoplasms represent a significant disease burden not only for urologists but also the broader medical community. While the majority of bladder tumors are urothelial in origin, up to two percent are found to be adenocarcinomas. Among bladder adenocarcinomas, roughly one-tenth are urachal and are frequently located at the dome of the bladder where urachal remnants can often be found. We describe a case of bladder adenocarcinoma that presented at the dome of the bladder but ultimately exhibited a nonurachal histology. A 65-year-old male with a history of myocardial infarction and cerebrovascular accident with residual right-sided hemiparesis and aphasia was referred to our clinic for evaluation of a bladder mass discovered in the setting of painless gross hematuria. Diagnostic cystoscopy demonstrated a large mass at the dome of the bladder, and subsequent transurethral resection revealed stage T1 mucinous adenocarcinoma arising in a villous adenomatous lesion without the presence of muscle in the specimen. The patient underwent a robotic-assisted laparoscopic partial cystectomy with extended bilateral pelvic lymph node dissection. Postoperatively, the patient experienced short-lived paralytic ileus and was discharged on postoperative day 5. Follow-up surveillance imaging at 6 months with CT chest, abdomen, and pelvis, repeat office cystoscopy, and negative tumor markers postoperatively indicated no evidence of disease recurrence. Characterization of bladder adenocarcinomas into urachal and nonurachal subtypes is critical in differentiating the operative management and oncologic outcomes of the respective neoplasms. However, given the paucity of literature describing treatment approaches to bladder adenocarcinoma in general, existing methods have largely mirrored genetically similar neoplasms, including ovarian and colon adenocarcinomas. Although there is still much to be understood regarding the potential mechanisms of carcinogenesis of nonurachal adenocarcinomas, further investigation may pave the way for a more standardized treatment paradigm and provide insight into the potential utility of modern immunotherapies.

1. Introduction

With an overall lifetime risk of approximately 2.2% in the general population, bladder cancer represents the sixth most common cancer in the United States and is expected to affect one out of every 27 men and one out of every 89 women during their lifetime [1, 2]. While most bladder tumors demonstrate urothelial histology, adenocarcinoma accounts for only 0.5-2% of cases and typically exhibits invasive behavior. Adenocarcinomas of the bladder are further classified based on their developmental origin from the urachus, an embryological remnant of the fibrous allantois that connects the developing bladder to the umbilicus [3]. Since the allantois connects the umbilicus to the dome of the bladder, urachal adenocarcinomas are often found in this location. They are actually far less common than their nonurachal counterparts, only accounting for an estimated 10% of bladder adenocarcinomas [2]. Nonetheless, given the rarity of adenocarcinoma of the bladder (0.5-2% in the United States) compared to other, more prevalent histological subtypes such as urothelial or squamous cell, there is a paucity of data and literature discussing either urachal or nonurachal bladder malignancies [3]. Here, we describe the presentation and management of a patient with nonurachal, primary bladder adenocarcinoma at the dome of the bladder.

2. Case Presentation

A 65-year-old male was referred to our clinic for evaluation of a bladder mass discovered in the setting of painless gross hematuria. The patient's past medical history was notable for a myocardial infarction 4 years prior, and a cerebrovascular accident 3 years prior with residual right-sided hemiparesis and aphasia, rendering him wheelchair bound.

Cross-sectional imaging via CT abdomen and pelvis revealed an exophytic mass at the bladder dome measuring 7.8 × 5.9 cm with central necrosis and a thick, enhancing wall as well as probable communication with the lumen of the urinary bladder (Figures 1 and 2). There was no hydronephrosis or pelvic lymphadenopathy. Metastatic survey was negative. Diagnostic cystoscopy demonstrated a large mass at the dome of the bladder, and subsequent transurethral resection revealed stage T1 mucinous adenocarcinoma arising in a villous adenomatous lesion without the presence of muscle in the specimen. Serum tumor markers revealed elevated CEA at 131 ng/mL (ULN 4.7 ng/mL).

After thorough counseling and informed consent about the potential role of perioperative chemotherapy the patient elected for surgical management and underwent a robotic-assisted laparoscopic partial cystectomy with extended bilateral pelvic lymph node dissection. Although no muscle-invasion had been seen on TURBT pathology, the advanced radiographic appearance of the tumor, with concern for extravesical extension, justified the surgical approach. Intraoperatively, no gross metastatic lesions in the abdomen were seen and the tumor was resected with 1.5 cm margins. All twenty-four dissected lymph nodes were negative for carcinoma. Final pathology revealed pT2b with tumor involvement of the surface urothelium and invasion of the deep muscularis propria. Pathologic evaluation further revealed that, although the location of this tumor at the dome of the bladder suggested urachal adenocarcinoma as the final diagnosis, no urachal glandular remnants were identified and so the features were most strongly suggestive of a primary nonurachal bladder adenocarcinoma (Figures 3 and 4).

Postoperatively, the patient experienced paralytic ileus but otherwise did well and was discharged on postoperative day 5. He was counseled about the role of adjuvant chemotherapy but elected to defer given the lack of robust evidence. Follow-up surveillance imaging at 6 months with CT chest, abdomen, and pelvis revealed no evidence of disease recurrence. He also underwent a normal office cystoscopy and had negative tumor markers, indicating no evidence of disease. The patient remained disease free at 24-month follow-up.

Molecular profiling of the tumor using the Foundation One CDx test reported microsatellite stability and a tumor mutational burden of 4 mutations per megabase. The test also described four genomic alterations: G12D on the KRAS gene, R201C on the GNAS gene, Q604 on the RMB10 gene, and R248W on TP53 gene. Targeted therapeutic options for this tumor type are limited; however, treatments targeting similar tumor subtypes have shown promise.

3. Discussion

Beyond the origin of disease, urachal and nonurachal adenocarcinoma can also be differentiated by their presentation, management, and oncologic outcomes (Table 1). The nonurachal subtype is more common in younger patients (median 69 yo vs. 56 yo) and, historically, has been noted to present later in the disease course with metastatic or lymph node spread [2, 4]. Although bladder dome involvement was noted in the pathology of our patient with nonurachal adenocarcinoma, it is important to note that the anterior wall and dome are most often associated with urachal tumors [2, 4]. The etiology of bladder adenocarcinomas is not entirely well established but is hypothesized to be a result of a metaplastic transformation of the cells within von Brunn's nests to cystitis glandularis/cystica and later to adenocarcinoma, a sequence triggered by chronic inflammation [5]. Histologically, urachal tumors are classified broadly into two categories: mucinous cystic and noncystic adenocarcinomas. Primary adenocarcinomas are similar in nature to noncystic adenocarcinomas and are classified enteric-type, mucinous (with or without signet ring cells) and not otherwise specified [4]. Specific variants may resemble salient features similar to colon or ovarian adenocarcinoma such as signet ring carcinoma or those originating from villous adenomas, as seen in our patient [5]. From a purely histological standpoint, these bladder neoplasms do differ from colonic and ovarian adenocarcinoma in staining patterns of B-catenin (membranous in bladder, nuclear in colonic), positivity of keratin 7 (more common in bladder), and keratin 20 (more common in colonic) and usually negative for OC125 (typically positive in ovarian/cervical glandular tumors) [5]. Genetically, however, both urachal and nonurachal subtypes tend to express molecular markers more similar to colorectal or ovarian adenocarcinomas, rather than urothelial bladder tumors. Both glandular neoplasms of the bladder and colon are more likely to express mutations in the TP53, APC (Wnt pathway), and KRAS [6, 7]. The genetic profiling data from our patient's tumor is consistent with what has been described in the existing literature. Broadly characterized for bladder neoplasms in general, TP53 mutations have been far more thoroughly described (up to 50%) as potential drivers of carcinogenesis [8]. More specifically, though limited by patient sample sizes, the current genetic profiling data of mucinous type primary bladder adenocarcinomas highlight KRAS (MAPK pathway) mutations in up to 67% of tumors [7]. Likewise, the specific G12D mutation in our patient is also a characteristic of glandular neoplasms in gastrointestinal sites, including the pancreas and colon. Though no viable immunotherapies have been determined to specifically target this KRAS mutation, several novel contenders do exist from other primary sites and have potential to be extrapolated to benefit a wider range of solid malignancies, including the bladder. Though preliminary, the use of primed cytotoxic T cell therapies to target KRAS mutations in colorectal carcinoma have shown some oncologic success in targeting neoantigens produced by the mutant G12D tumor cells and presented on HLA class I molecules [9].

As with any rare disease, it is difficult to make conclusive outcome-based statements with a high degree of power. However, when exclusively evaluating survival differences, Luzzago et al. have retrospectively provided the most comprehensive and recent data comparing the survival outcomes

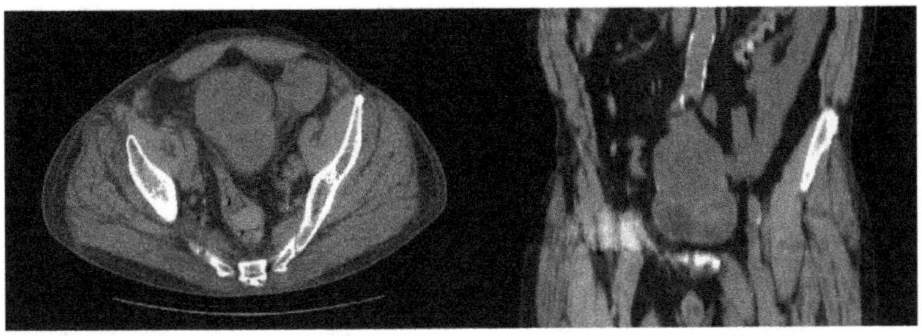

FIGURE 1: Axial and coronal cross-sectional imaging via CT abdomen and pelvis revealing an exophytic mass arising at dome of bladder.

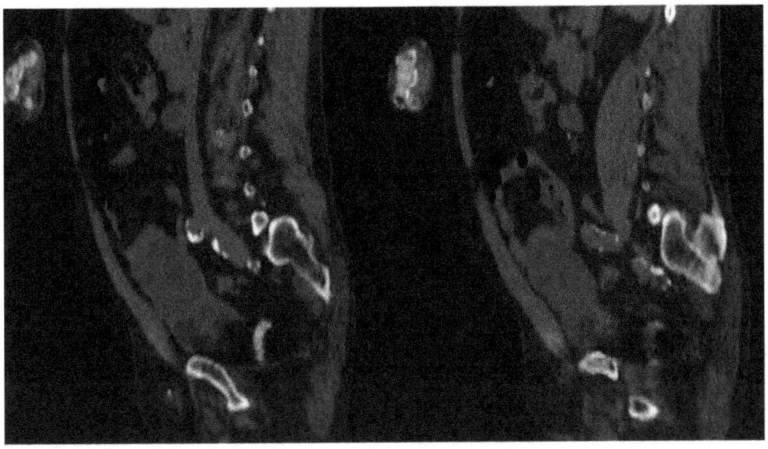

FIGURE 2: Sagittal cross-sectional imaging via CT abdomen and pelvis revealing an exophytic mass arising at the dome of the bladder.

of urachal vs. nonurachal subtypes using the Surveillance, Epidemiology and End Results (SEER) database [10]. Despite the fact that it is less common, five-year cancer-specific survival in the nonmetastatic setting was shown to favor urachal versus nonurachal (68 vs. 49%, respectively, HR 0.6; $p = 0.01$) [10]. Though these comparisons were adjusted for potential confounding variables, discrepancies in treatment approach and unmeasured clinicopathologic features may have influenced these findings.

From a treatment perspective, urachal tumors are more likely to be managed with partial cystectomy (73.9 vs. 14.8%), with some older studies indicating up to 83% of patients with urachal tumors treated with partial cystectomy (PC) [10, 11]. There is greater variation in the management of nonurachal tumors, and recently, there has been an increasing interest in the utility of adjuvant chemotherapy and even external beam radiation therapy (EBRT) in the setting of locally advanced disease and/or positive surgical margin. In our patient, partial cystectomy was an appropriate option due to the concern for urachal pathology due to location at the dome, exophytic nature of the tumor, and ability to maintain adequate postoperative functional bladder capacity. In assessing the outcomes of PC vs. RC (radial cystectomy), a recent retrospective study evaluating the SEER database has shown no significant difference in the five-year overall survival in nonmetastatic, T1-2 adenocarcinoma treated with PC vs. RC (PC = 27% and RC = 21%, $P = 0.9$). Of note, such retrospective analysis is subject to treatment selection bias, since more PC patients were stage T1 as opposed to T2 [12].

While the role of adjuvant chemotherapy in bladder urothelial carcinoma has been explored in the literature, there is less robust evidence for the role in adenocarcinomas. A meta-analysis by Leow et al. demonstrated a 23% reduction in relative risk of death (HR 0.77) for patients with muscle-invasive bladder cancer undergoing cisplatin-based adjuvant chemotherapy after radical cystectomy [13]. For primary bladder adenocarcinoma, the situation is more complicated given the lack of standardized chemotherapy regimens. Most of the approach is extrapolated from the colorectal cancer literature for which locally advanced (stage 3 disease) treatment regimens generally consist of FOLFOX (5-FU, leucovorin, and oxaliplatin) or CapeOx (capcitabine and oxaliplatin) and may not be directly applicable [14]. Berg et al. have recently reported no improvement in median survival in patients with nonmetastatic, muscle-invasive adenocarcinoma/urothelial cancer with glandular dedifferentiation (pT2N+M0 or ≥pT3N0/N+M0) who underwent RC with adjuvant chemotherapy compared to those who received RC alone (21.79 months vs. 22.60 months) [15]. Davaro et al. described similar findings while evaluating the benefit of EBRT in patients with nonmetastatic cT2-4 nonurachal adenocarcinoma. Five-year survival significantly ($P < 0.001$) favored those who received cystectomy alone (39.6%) compared to cystectomy and EBRT (26.9%), although this finding was likely a consequence of

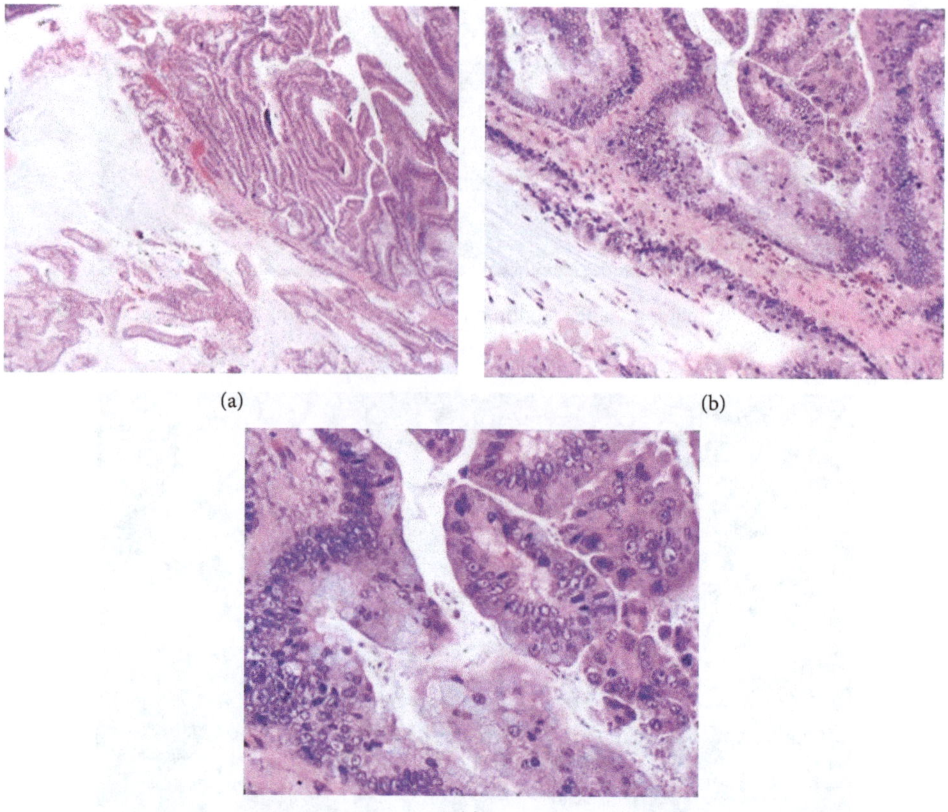

FIGURE 3: Representative pathology at (a) 4x and (b) 20x demonstrating villous architecture arising from mucinous adenocarcinoma and (c) 40x with presence of mucin producing goblet cells.

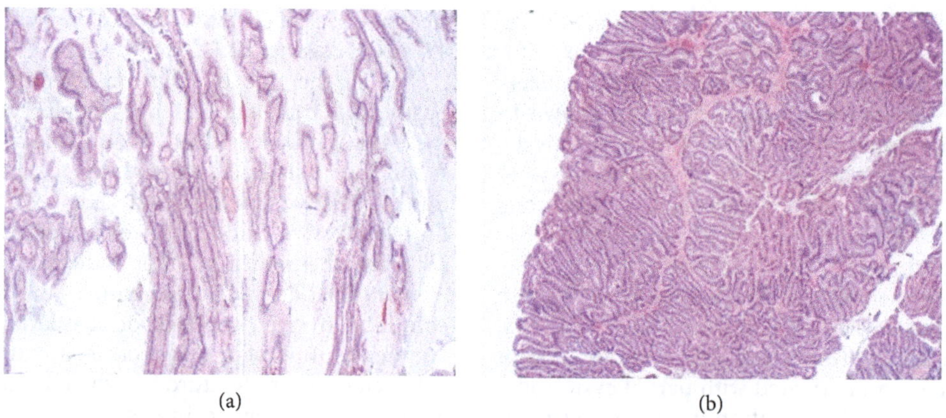

FIGURE 4: (a) Villous architecture 4x. (b) Glandular architecture of nonurachal adenocarcinoma 4x.

TABLE 1: Comparison of urachal vs. nonurachal bladder adenocarcinoma presentation.

	Urachal [3]	Non-urachal [3, 5]
Origin of disease	Urachal remnant	Bladder urothelium
Age	5-6th decade of life	6-7th decade of life
Location of disease	Bladder dome, anterior wall	Trigone, posterior wall, but can arise throughout
Immunohistochemical staining	CK20, CDX2 (+/- CK7, B-catenin, HM cytokeratin)	Variable based on histological phenotype
Possible symptoms	Umbilical discharge/bleeding, hematuria, lower urinary tract symptoms	Hematuria, lower urinary tract symptoms

the higher stage and positive margin status of the cystectomy +EBRT group [16]. Data regarding the role of neoadjuvant chemotherapy is also limited, with one small study consisting of 6 patients (3 with urachal and 3 with nonurachal locally advanced disease) showing modest benefit in downstaging of the primary tumor and preventing micrometastasis with a gemcitabine/cisplatin and S-1 (5-FU alternative) regimen [17]. The role of more modern adjuvant immunotherapies in nonurothelial bladder cancers has also not yet been well established. As mentioned previously, recent genetic and molecular evidence suggests greater similarities between bladder to colon adenocarcinomas rather than urothelial tumors. These findings may be indicative of the utility of more novel immunotherapeutics, similar to those used in adenocarcinoma of the colon, though yet to be extensively studied [7]. For example, current ongoing clinical trials of immunotherapeutic agents nivolumab and ipilimumab in addition to targeted molecular therapy (cabozantinib) for rare genitourinary cancers that have metastasized promise to add valuable information [18].

In summary, adenocarcinoma of the bladder is a relatively uncommon and aggressive urologic malignancy that can be subclassified based on the origin of the disease. Neoplasms of the urachus are far more rare than primary adenocarcinoma. In addition, there is much greater variation in the management of nonurachal tumors, especially regarding the role of perioperative chemotherapy and radiation as adjuvant modalities in treating nonurachal adenocarcinoma. Continued research on this specific subclassification of bladder cancer is needed to further characterize and understand its behavior and the associated clinical outcomes.

Abbreviations

CT: Computed tomography
SEER: Surveillance, Epidemiology and End Results (database)
PC: Partial cystectomy
RC: Radical cystectomy
ERBT: External beam radiation therapy
FOLFOX: 5-FU, leucovorin, and oxaliplatin
CapeOx: Capecitabine and oxaliplatin.

Consent

Written consent was obtained for the surgery and for the use of patient's case and associated images for research purposes.

Authors' Contributions

GK obtained the radiographic images and was a major contributor in writing the manuscript. AR obtained the pathologic images and was a major contributor in writing the manuscript. SA performed a review of the relevant literature and contributed to the planning of the manuscript. MW performed all surgical intervention and patient care, determined the scope and focus of the manuscript, was a major contributor in writing the manuscript, and was responsible for the global and critical review of the manuscript. All authors have read and approved of this manuscript.

Acknowledgments

We thank Dr. Masoumeh K. Rezaei and Dr. William Gesztes for providing the pathologic images presented in the manuscript.

References

[1] American Cancer Society, *Cancer Facts and Figures 2020*, National Cancer Institute, Atlanta, 2020.

[2] J. L. Wright, M. P. Porter, C. I. Li, P. H. Lange, and D. W. Lin, "Differences in survival among patients with urachal and nonurachal adenocarcinomas of the bladder," *Cancer*, vol. 107, no. 4, pp. 721–728, 2006.

[3] V. Dadhania, B. Czerniak, and C. C. Guo, "Adenocarcinoma of the urinary bladder," *American Journal of Clinical and Experimental Urology*, vol. 3, no. 2, pp. 51–63, 2015.

[4] A. S. Taylor, R. Mehra, and A. M. Udager, "Glandular tumors of the urachus and urinary bladder: a practical overview of a broad differential diagnosis," *Archives of Pathology and Laboratory Medicine*, College of American Pathologists, Northfield, Illinois, 2018.

[5] J. R. Goldblum, L. W. Lamps, J. K. McKenney, and J. L. Myers, *Rosai and Ackerman's Surgical Pathology*, E-Book. Elsevier Health Sciences. Chapter: 25, 11th edition, 2017.

[6] S. Roy, D. Pradhan, W. L. Ernst et al., "Next-generation sequencing-based molecular characterization of primary urinary bladder adenocarcinoma," *Modern Pathology*, vol. 30, no. 8, pp. 1133–1143, 2017.

[7] A. S. Pires-Luis, P. Martinek, R. Alaghehbandan et al., "Molecular genetic features of primary nonurachal enteric-type adenocarcinoma, urachal adenocarcinoma, mucinous adenocarcinoma, and intestinal metaplasia/adenoma: review of the literature and next-generation sequencing study," *Advances in Anatomic Pathology*, vol. 27, no. 5, pp. 303–310, 2020.

[8] G. Wu, F. Wang, K. Li et al., "Significance of TP53 mutation in bladder cancer disease progression and drug selection," *PeerJ*, vol. 7, no. 12, article e8261, 2019.

[9] E. Tran, P. F. Robbins, Y. C. Lu et al., "T-cell transfer therapy targeting mutant KRAS in cancer," *The New England Journal of Medicine*, vol. 375, no. 23, pp. 2255–2262, 2016.

[10] S. Luzzago, C. Palumbo, G. Rosiello et al., "Survival of contemporary patients with non-metastatic urachal vs. non-urachal adenocarcinoma of the urinary bladder," *World Journal of Urology*, vol. 38, no. 11, pp. 2819–2826, 2020.

[11] J. R. Molina, J. F. Quevedo, A. F. Furth, R. L. Richardson, H. Zincke, and P. A. Burch, "Predictors of survival from urachal cancer: a mayo clinic study of 49 cases," *Cancer*, vol. 110, no. 11, pp. 2434–2440, 2007.

[12] S. Luzzago, C. Palumbo, G. Rosiello et al., "Survival after partial cystectomy for variant histology bladder cancer compared with urothelial carcinoma: a population-based study," *Clinical Genitourinary Cancer*, vol. 18, no. 2, pp. 117–128.e5, 2020.

[13] J. J. Leow, W. Martin-Doyle, P. S. Rajagopal et al., "Adjuvant Chemotherapy for Invasive Bladder Cancer: A 2013 Updated Systematic Review and Meta-Analysis of Randomized Trials," *European Urology*, vol. 66, no. 1, pp. 42–54, 2014.

[14] J. M. Loree, A. Sha, M. Soleimani et al., "Survival impact of CAPOX versus FOLFOX in the adjuvant treatment of stage III colon cancer," *Clinical Colorectal Cancer*, vol. 17, no. 2, pp. 156–163, 2018.

[15] S. Berg, D. D'Andrea, M. W. Vetterlein et al., "Impact of adjuvant chemotherapy in patients with adverse features and variant histology at radical cystectomy for muscle-invasive carcinoma of the bladder: does histologic subtype matter?," *Cancer*, vol. 125, no. 9, pp. 1449–1458, 2019.

[16] F. Davaro, J. Schaefer, A. May, J. Raza, S. Siddiqui, and Z. Hamilton, "Invasive non-urachal adenocarcinoma of the bladder: analysis of the National Cancer Database," *World Journal of Urology*, vol. 37, no. 3, pp. 497–505, 2019.

[17] B. Yu, J. Zhou, H. Cai et al., "Neoadjuvant chemotherapy for primary adenocarcinomas of the urinary bladder: a single-site experience," *BMC Urology*, vol. 15, no. 1, 2015.

[18] 2019, Testing the effectiveness of two immunotherapy drugs (nivolumab and pilimumab) with one anti-cancer targeted drug (cabozantinib) for rare genitourinary tumors. Clin Identifier NCT03866382.

43

Use of Cadaveric Pericardial Tissue in the Surgical Treatment of Neurogenic Bladder

Madison Caja,[1,2] **Michaela Lamonde,**[1,2] **John Barnard,**[1,3] **Stanley Zaslau,**[1,2,3] **and Robert E. Shapiro**[1,2,3]

[1] *West Virginia University School of Medicine, Morgantown, WV 26506, USA*
[2] *Department of Obstetrics & Gynecology, West Virginia University School of Medicine, Morgantown, WV 26506, USA*
[3] *Department of Urology, West Virginia University School of Medicine, Morgantown, WV 26506, USA*

Correspondence should be addressed to Robert E. Shapiro; rshapiro@hsc.wvu.edu

Academic Editor: Sigurdur Gudjonsson

The surgical treatments for neurogenic bladder are extremely variable. The lack of specific treatment guidelines makes this disease process even more challenging to treat. We present a case of a 55-year-old female with neurogenic bladder secondary to spinal cord injury (SCI). Her incontinence was conservatively managed with indwelling Foley drainage. Despite continued upsizing of the Foley catheters, the patient continued to have urinary leakage. The patient subsequently underwent a transvaginal bladder neck closure (BNC) with suprapubic bladder neck diversion (SPC). The urethra was successfully closed and uniquely supported with the use of cadaveric pericardial tissue (CPT). This surgical approach of neurogenic bladder provides durable continence with short operative times, minimal patient morbidity, decreased hospital length, and low risk of progressive renal dysfunction. BNC with SPC can provide an excellent management solution for neurogenic bladder from spinal cord injury refractory to conservative management.

1. Introduction

Spinal cord injuries (SCI) arising from trauma or surgical complications are an unfortunate common occurrence with approximately 54 per million per year in the United States [1]. The sequalae that occur after SCI can often be severe. One of the most common complications from SCI is voiding dysfunction [2]. SCI causes loss of both motor and sphincter control of the bladder. As a result, patients often require intermittent catheterization or placement of indwelling catheters. These treatments, however, are not always curative. Patients with even the most intensive bladder regimens will often suffer from urinary incontinence.

For patients with intractable incontinence despite indwelling catheters, bladder neck closure (BNC) with suprapubic catheter placement (SPC) is a treatment option. Limited published data exist on this treatment option and the data that exists primarily involves an abdominal surgical approach. Moreover, this data also suggests that complications such as bladder outlet fistulae can occur in 20–30 % of patients [3].

We present a case of a patient with neurogenic bladder that underwent a transvaginal BNC with SPC diversion. The urethra was successfully closed and uniquely supported with the use of cadaveric pericardial tissue (CPT) to prevent fistula formation.

2. Case Report

A 55-year-old female suffered a spinal cord injury (SCI) following a spinal surgery in 2015 and consequently became wheel chair bound. Her health history was significant for morbid obesity, type 2 diabetes, hypertension, chronic obstructive pulmonary disease (COPD), history of deep venous thrombosis (DVT), recurrent urinary tract infections (UTIs), and sacral decubitus ulcers. The patient was treated by the urology department for kidney stones prior to her SCI. Her past surgical history was significant for pelvic laparoscopy, tubal ligation, exploratory laparotomy, and colostomy placement.

The patient's urinary incontinence was initially managed conservatively with Foley catheters and anticholinergic

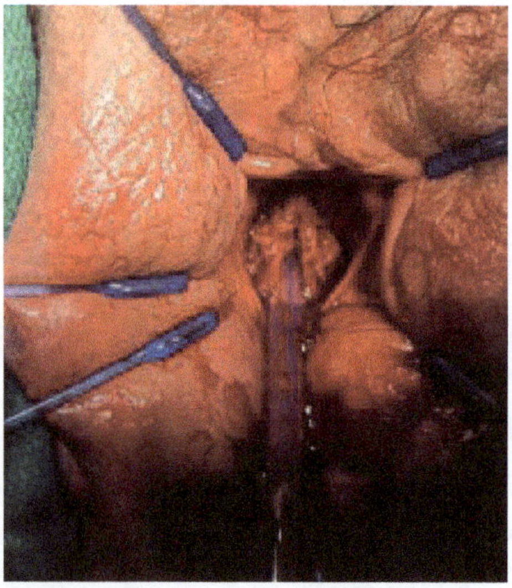

FIGURE 1: Patulous urethra is clearly observed circumferentially surrounding the Foley catheter.

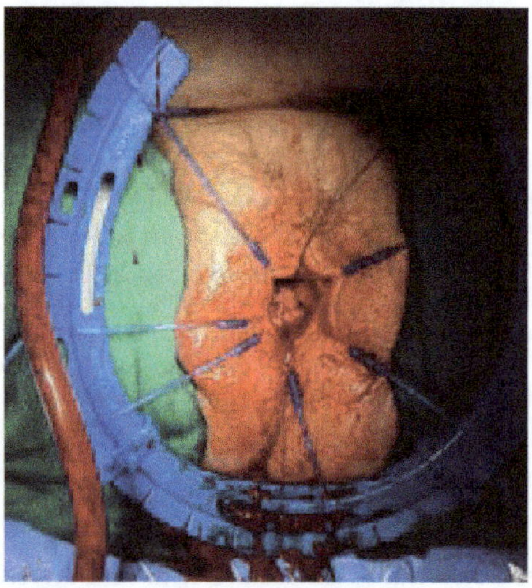

FIGURE 2: The bladder neck closure is seen with both the interrupted and imbricating layer of 2-0 vicryl closed.

medications. She required multiple upsizing of catheters due to continued urinary leakage. The persistent urinary incontinence was significantly affecting the patient's quality of life and was further complicating her sacral decubitus ulcers. The patient elected to proceed with BNC with SPC diversion. Secondary to medical comorbidities and history of prior abdominal surgery, the decision was made to use a transvaginal approach. This case was a combined surgical approach with urology and urogynecology.

Once in the operating room, the full defect of the urethra was appreciated (Figure 1). The urethra was patulous with significant erosions on the dorsal side. The urethra was dissected and mobilized to the level of the bladder neck. The bladder neck was then closed in four layers. An interrupted layer followed by imbricating layers of 2-0 vicryl was used (Figure 2). A layer of cadaveric pericardial tissue (CPT)

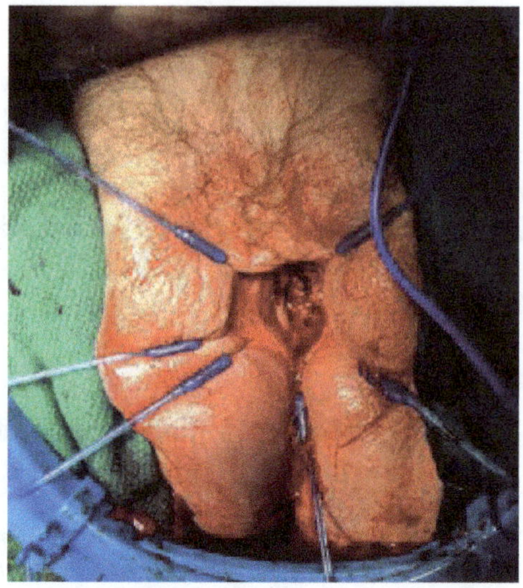

FIGURE 3: The third layer of the bladder neck closure can be appreciated. The cadaveric pericardial tissue in place to prevent vesicovaginal fistula formation.

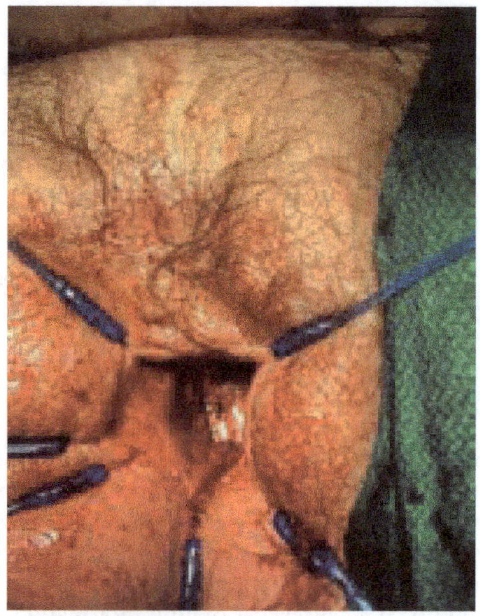

FIGURE 4: Final layer of bladder neck closure with the cadaveric pericardial tissue in place.

was incorporated in the bladder neck closure for enhanced support and to prevent the occurrence of fistula (Figures 3 and 4). Finally, the vaginal mucosa was closed with running 3-0 vicryl. A SPC was then placed. The patient tolerated the procedure well and was discharged to home the same day.

The patient has been seen for SPC exchange at 3 and 6 months postoperatively. She is doing well and has no further incontinence. Her decubitus ulcers have greatly improved.

3. Discussion

Since 1985, there have been only a handful of published studies that describe transvaginal bladder neck closure (BNC) and suprapubic catheter (SPC) placement in the treatment of neurogenic bladder [4]. Most of these studies cite bladder outlet fistulae as a significant complication [3]. Our case is unique with the usage of cadaveric pericardial tissue (CPT) to augment the closure and thereby reduce the risk of fistula formation. One study successfully combated the risk of fistula formation by using a posterior urethral flap to secure the suture line [5]. In our case, the decision was made to use CPT to help augment the native tissue repair secondary to the concern over the patient's medical comorbidities interfering with wound healing. Due to the low cost, ease of handling, and less immunogenicity, we feel that CPT is a good option to augment native tissue repairs [6]. A paucity of studies exist on biologic grafts used to prevent fistula formation. However, literature from colon and rectal surgery reports good success with utilizing porcine submucosa to close fistula tracts of the anus [7].

The traditional abdominal approach of a BNC and SPC has a reported 15% complication rate and average length of stay of 4 days [3]. Our approach offers an excellent alternative for patients who are poor candidates for abdominal surgery. We were able to safely send our patient home on postoperative day 0 and without the risk of a significant abdominal wound infection or further abdominal surgery. It has been shown that transvaginal BNC, compared to abdominal approach, is associated with decreased short-term complications and additionally both a shorter operative time and hospital stay [8].

The chronic use of an indwelling catheter, irrespective of whether it travels via the urethra or via the suprapubic route, has been associated with a number of undesired and cumbersome problems such as irritation, leakage, infections, stone formation, catheter dislocation, cuff rupture, and metaplastic malformation [9]. Another option for these patients could instead be a catheterizable vesicostoma in combination with a bladder neck closure. Unfortunately, the most common reported complication of catheterizable vesicostomas is incontinence. According to the most recent literature, this can be as high as 30 percent [10]. In addition, approximately 20 percent of these patients require reoperation for stomal stenosis [10]. As this patient already suffered from intractable incontinence and had significant medical comorbidities that prohibited major surgery, we elected to proceed with SPC.

Another consideration in this case would have been to perform a Martius modified labial fat pad flap (MMLFPF), commonly known as the Martius flap. The Martius flap has been described in the literature most commonly for vaginal fistula repair [11]. This technique has been noted to be successful in cases where vaginal tissue integrity is a concern [12]. We chose cadaveric pericardial tissue over a MMLFPF to diminish risk of potential long term patient sequelae such as labial pain, numbness, and distortion, all of which have been described in the literature [13].

We hope this case report adds to a body of evidence in support of CPT in tissue closure and negates the risk of fistulas. This case also highlights the importance of a multidisciplinary team and the benefit of combined surgical cases when appropriate. By combining skills of gynecologic and urologic surgeons, we were able to safely and efficiently treat a major problem for our patient.

4. Conclusion

Bladder neck closure with suprapubic catheter should be considered in patients with neurogenic bladder refractory to conservative treatment. The transvaginal approach, with the adjunct use of cadaveric pericardial tissue (CPT), offers comparable outcomes to the abdominal approach with considerably less morbidity. The use of CPT for tissue interposition potentially decreases the risk of failure and vesicovaginal fistula formation, although more research is needed on this subject. Using a multidisciplinary surgical approach, both urologists and urogynecologists should be made aware of this option.

Disclosure

This case report was presented as a poster at the Van Liere Research Symposium at West Virginia University on 3/21/2019.

Authors' Contributions

Madison Caja, Michaela Lamonde, John Barnard, Stanley Zaslau, and Robert Shapiro carried out conception and design, acquisition, analysis, an interpretation of data, and drafting. They reviewed the paper and gave final approval.

References

[1] National Spinal Cord Injury Statistical Center, *Annual Report for the Model Spinal Cord Injury Care Systems*, Birmingham, AL, USA, 2017.

[2] D. D. Cardenas, J. M. Hoffman, S. Kirshblum, and W. McKinley, "Etiology and incidence of rehospitalization after traumatic spinal cord injury: a multicenter analysis," *Archives of Physical Medicine and Rehabilitation*, vol. 85, no. 11, pp. 1757–1763, 2004.

[3] J. Colli and L. K. Lloyd, "Bladder neck closure and suprapubic catheter placement as definitive management of neurogenic bladder," *The Journal of Spinal Cord Medicine*, vol. 34, no. 3, pp. 273–277, 2011.

[4] P. E. Zimmern, H. R. Hadley, G. E. Leach, and S. Raz, "Transvaginal closure of the bladder neck and placement of a suprapubic catheter for destroyed urethra after long-term indwelling catheterization," *The Journal of Urology*, vol. 134, no. 3, pp. 554–556, 1985.

[5] E. S. Rovner, C. M. Goudelocke, A. Gilchrist, and B. Lebed, "Transvaginal bladder neck closure with posterior urethral flap for devastated urethra," *Urology*, vol. 78, no. 1, pp. 208–212, 2011.

[6] J. Hosseini, S. Hosseini, M. A. Hosseini, and Y. Rezaei, "Pericardium in reconstructive urologic surgeries: a systematic review and meta-analysis," *Urologia Internationalis*, pp. 1–14, 2018.

[7] E. Bubbers and K. Cologne, "Management of complex anal fistulas," *Clinics in Colon and Rectal Surgery*, vol. 29, no. 01, pp. 043–049, 2016.

[8] H. Willis, N. A. Safiano, and L. K. Lloyd, "Comparison of transvaginal and retropubic bladder neck closure with suprapubic catheter in women," *The Journal of Urology*, vol. 193, no. 1, pp. 196–202, 2015.

[9] J. M. Hollingsworth, M. A. Rogers, S. L. Krein et al., "Determining the noninfectious complications of indwelling urethral catheters," *Annals of Internal Medicine*, vol. 159, no. 6, p. 401, 2013.

[10] D. G. Holmes, J. Thrasher, G. Y. Park, D. C. Kueker, and J. W. Weigel, "Long-term complications related to the modified Indiana pouch," *Urology*, vol. 60, no. 4, pp. 603–606, 2002.

[11] T. E. Elkins, J. O. DeLancey, and E. J. McGuire, "The use of modified Martius graft as an adjunctive technique in vesicovaginal and rectovaginal fistula repair," *Obstetrics & Gynecology*, vol. 75, no. 4, pp. 727–733, 1990.

[12] A. Wilson, S. Pillay, and T. Greenwell, "How and why to take a Martius labial interposition flap in female urology," *Translational Andrology and Urology*, vol. 6, no. S2, pp. S81–S87, 2017.

[13] D. Lee, B. E. Dillon, and P. E. Zimmern, "Long-term morbidity of martius labial fat pad graft in vaginal reconstruction surgery," *Urology*, vol. 82, no. 6, pp. 1261–1266, 2013.

Rare Case of Multiple Perirenal, Extra-Adrenal Myelolipoma: Case Report, Current Management Options and Literature Review

Goran Benko,[1] **Andrina Kopjar**,[2] **Marin Plantak**,[1] **Danijel Cvetko**,[3] **Vicko Glunčić**,[4] **and Anita Lukić**[5]

[1]*Department of Urology, Varaždin General Hospital, I. Meštrovića 1, Varaždin, Croatia*
[2]*Department of Pathology, Varaždin General Hospital, I. Meštrovića 1, Varaždin, Croatia*
[3]*Department of Radiology, Dubrava Clinical Hospital, Av. Gojka Šuška 6, Zagreb, Croatia*
[4]*Department of Anesthesia, Advocate Illinois Masonic Medical Center, 836 W Wellington Ave, Chicago, IL 60657, USA*
[5]*Department of Anaesthesiology, Reanimatology, and Intensive Care, Varaždin General Hospital, I. Meštrovića 1, Varaždin, Croatia*

Correspondence should be addressed to Goran Benko; goran.benko@gmail.com

Academic Editor: Claudio Simeone

Extra-adrenal myelolipomas are rare, asymptomatic entities, although large tumors may cause local symptoms or hemorrhage. When these lesions occur outside the adrenals in the retroperitoneum, they are radiographically easily confused with both primary and secondary retroperitoneal tumors, which tend to be aggressive. Although myelolipomas are benign and can be managed conservatively, if malignancy is suspected, a surgical procedure is an option. We report a case of a 68-year-old patient with multiple perirenal extra-adrenal myelolipomas. Initial abdominal ultrasound reviled an inhomogeneous mass surrounding the left kidney. Subsequent CT examination of the abdomen showed four separate, extrarenal, well-circumscribed, round-shaped, fat-containing retroperitoneal tumors. Given the significant size of the masses, that compressed major abdominal vessels and the suspicion of liposarcoma, a surgical excision of the lesions was performed. The tumors were easily separated, all surrounding structures were spared, and they were removed completely. Histologically, all masses consisted of hematopoietic and mature fat tissue and the final diagnosis was extra-adrenal myelolipoma. The patient was released from the hospital 7th day after surgery in good condition and at his baseline. Since myelolipomas are, by definition, nonfunctional benign tumors, there was no need for further follow-up. The radiological evaluation and fine needle biopsy are usually sufficient to establish the diagnosis, but in some cases of well-differentiated liposarcoma, the differentiation between myelolipoma and liposarcoma can be challenging. Therefore, considering that myelolipomas and liposarcomas have opposite prognoses, which affects the surgeon's decision on the extent of surgical procedure and further treatment, we also emphasize the importance of intraoperative assessment of the tumor, both by the surgeon and by intraoperative pathology consultation.

1. Introduction

Myelolipomas are rare tumorous mixtures of adipose and relatively normal trilineage hematopoietic tissue. They usually occur as adrenal tumors (incidence is estimated at lower than 0.1%.), but extra-adrenal myelolipomas have also been described, occurring as head and neck, chest, intra-abdominal, or pelvic masses in up to 15% of all cases (Table 1) [1–4]. Perirenal extra-adrenal myelolipomas are especially rare and occur as single retroperitoneal perirenal masses [5].

Both adrenal and extra-adrenal myelolipomas are typically asymptomatic, although large tumors may cause local symptoms or hemorrhage [6]. Tumors could vary in size and often exceed 10 cm in diameter.

Although adrenal myelolipomas can be managed conservatively, when myelolipomas occur as large multiple retroperitoneal masses, they are radiographically easily confused with both, primary or secondary retroperitoneal tumors. Those could be aggressive neoplasms, such as liposarcoma, requiring different treatment [6].

Table 1: Extra-adrenal location of myelolipoma [2].

Location*	
Head	Retroorbital
	Nasal cavity
	Mandible
Thorax	Endobronchial
	Pulmonary
	Pleural
	Mediastinal (posterior, anterior, middle)
	Chest wall
	Costal
Abdomen	Renal (hilum, sinus, extramedullary)
	Perirenal
	Periureteric
	Retroperitoneal
	Mesenterical (omental)
	Gastric
	Hepatic
	Splenic
	Perisplenic
Pelvis	Presacral
	Ovarian
	Lower pelvis
	Perivesical
Spinal	
Paravertebral	
Lymphonodal	

*Myelolipomas can occur at location site or at multiple locations simultaneously.

In this report, we pinpoint the possibility that, although extremely rare, myelolipomas can occur as large, multiple, retroperitoneal, perirenal masses that could be initially mistaken for aggressive neoplasms.

2. Case Report

A 68-year-old man with lower urinary tract symptoms (LUTS) and well-controlled hypertension was referred to the department of urology. Initial abdominal ultrasound detected an inhomogeneous mass surrounding the left kidney. Complete laboratory exams were normal.

Subsequent CT examination of the abdomen reviled four separate, extrarenal, well-circumscribed, round-shaped, and fat-containing retroperitoneal masses (12.0 × 12.0 cm, 12.0 × 8.0 cm, 6.0 × 3.5 cm, and 5.0 × 4.5 cm). Due to the volume of the masses, the aorta and inferior vena cava were compressed, as well as branches of the superior mesenteric artery. There was no hydronephrosis, and suprarenal glands and other organs appeared normal (Figures 1(a) and 1(b)). Based on the radiological findings, the initial differential diagnosis was liposarcoma.

Given the significant size of the masses that compressed the major abdominal vessels and the suspicion of liposarcoma, a decision was made to surgically excise the lesions. The surgical procedure was performed using an open transabdominal approach, under general anesthesia. Tumors were soft and well encased by a thin capsule, intimately attached to the renal adipose capsule, ureter, and abdominal aorta. They were easily separated, all surrounding structures were spared, and the tumors were completely removed (Figure 2). Both surgical procedures and anesthesia were uneventful, with no significant blood loss.

Gross pathology revealed encapsulated, well-defined, soft masses measuring 11.5 × 8.5 × 6.0 cm, 15.0 × 10.0 × 6.5 cm, 6.0 × 5.5 × 3.5 cm, and 2.0 × 2.0 × 2.0 cm. Histologically, all the masses consisted of hematopoietic and mature fat tissue (Figure 3). The dominant tissue component was granulopoietic cells in various developmental stages, with the normal morphology of the megakaryocyte lines. There was no suprarenal gland tissue in the tumor, so the definitive diagnosis was extra-adrenal myelolipoma.

The patient was released from the hospital 7th day after the surgery, in good condition and at his baseline. Since myelolipomas are, by definition, nonfunctional benign tumors, there was no need for any further follow-up.

3. Discussion

The vast majority of myelolipoma cases have been presented as a single mass. They are asymptomatic, incidentally found on imaging studies, and can be managed conservatively [7, 8]. On ultrasonography, they present as a hyperechoic mass if the tumor is predominantly fatty, or as a hypoechoic mass, if the tumor is composed of myeloid cells. Small areas of hemorrhage within the mass can eventually calcify [9]. Most tumors are unilateral and vary in size from 2 to 26 cm at the time of diagnosis, but bilateral and even multifocal tumors have been described [5]. Spontaneous rupture of myelolipomas has been reported, usually when the tumor exceeded 10 cm.

Usually, extra-adrenal myelolipoma can be diagnosed by CT or MRI scans with great certainty [5, 7], and additional confirmation can be obtained by fine needle biopsy under ultrasound and/or CT guidance. Even so, the differentiation between (extra)adrenal myelolipoma and other fat-containing retroperitoneal tumors could be difficult. Indeed, the majority of fat-containing tumors are well-differentiated liposarcomas [10], which can be misleading and can represent a challenge for radiologists, since many myelolipomas are actually often misdiagnosed as liposarcomas [8].

Open surgery is a gold standard for the treatment of large myelolipomas. On the other hand, a transperitoneal or retroperitoneal approach with minimally invasive surgery is possible, as shown by Arezzo et al. [11]. Furthermore, Cochetti et al. showed that even large suprarenal myelolipomas can be treated by minimally invasive robotic surgery for the treatment of large adrenal myelolipoma [12]. Despite that, our decision for transabdominal open surgery was undertaken regarding the size of the tumor and easier approach to large vessels surrounding the tumor itself.

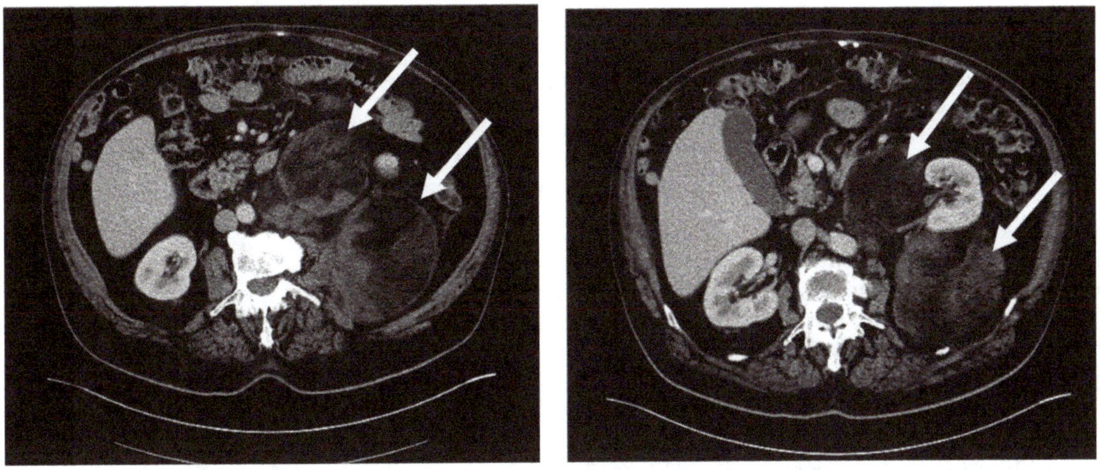

(a) (b)

Figure 1: CT scan with multiple retroperitoneal myelolipomas (arrows).

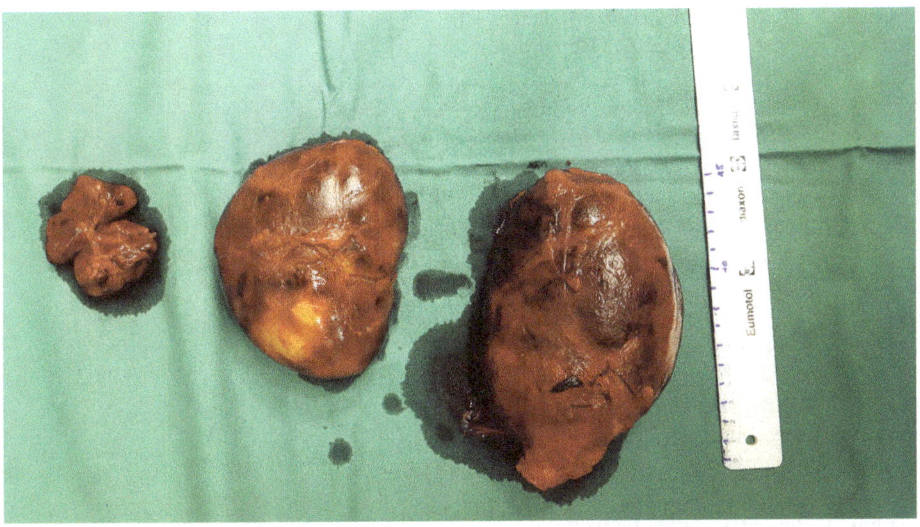

Figure 2: Gross appearance of surgically removed myelolipomas.

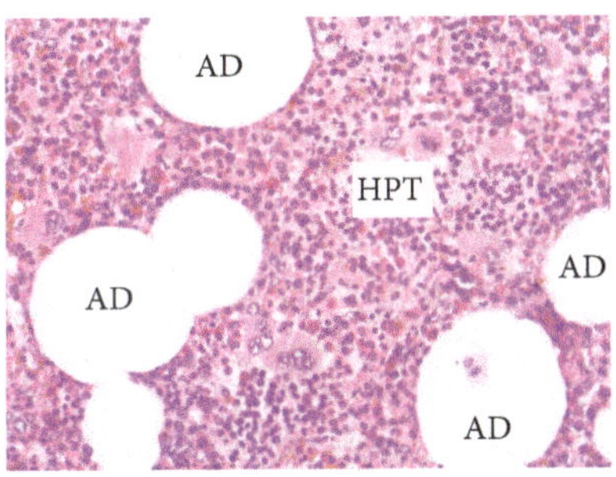

Figure 3: Microscopic appearance of myelolipoma with normal adipocytes (AD) and normal trilineage hematopoietic tissue (HPT) (hematoxylin-eosin staining, original magnification 40x).

Currently, there are no consensus recommendations for postoperative surveillance of myelolipoma [9]. Classically, asymptomatic or small (<4 cm) myelolipomas are treated conservatively with routine cross-sectional surveillance imaging, while surgical resection is usually reserved for symptomatic or large (>7 cm) lesions [7]. On the other hand, low-grade liposarcomas, which myelolipoma could be mistaken for, are treated aggressively (extensive surgery is required) and have a worse prognosis.

Although myelolipomas are rare, and especially multiple extra-adrenal retroperitoneal types, we would like to remind the surgeons, radiologists, and pathologists to be aware of these tumors. The radiological evaluation supported by histological examination upon the fine needle biopsy is usually sufficient to establish the diagnosis, but in some cases of well-differentiated liposarcoma, telling the difference between myelolipoma and liposarcoma can be challenging. Therefore, considering that myelolipomas and liposarcomas have a diametrically opposite prognosis, which then drives the surgeon's decision on the treatment, we also emphasize the importance of intraoperative assessment of the tumor, both by the surgeon as well as by intraoperative pathological evaluation.

References

[1] A. Hakim and C. Rozeik, "Adrenal and extra-adrenal myelolipomas – a comparative case report," *Journal of Radiology Case Reports*, vol. 8, no. 1, pp. 1–12, 2014.

[2] 2020, https://pubmed.ncbi.nlm.nih.gov/?term=extraadrenal+myelolipoma&sort=date.

[3] J. A. Nitz, J. Huckleby, E. H. Hwang, M. G. Medina, S. J. Pera, and S. T. Orcutt, "Symptomatic extra-adrenal myelolipoma in the spleen," *Case Reports in Surgery*, vol. 2020, Article ID 8839178, 3 pages, 2020.

[4] A. Conley, E. Klein, E. Edhayan, and R. Berri, "Extra-adrenal myelolipoma presenting as efferent limb obstruction," *Case Reports in Surgery*, vol. 2012, Article ID 718383, 4 pages, 2012.

[5] A. Hajiran, C. Morley, R. Jansen et al., "Perirenal extra-adrenal myelolipoma," *World Journal of Clinical Cases*, vol. 2, no. 7, pp. 279–283, 2014.

[6] J. R. Wagner, D. E. Kleiner, M. C. M. Walther, and W. M. Linehan, "Perirenal myelolipoma," *Urology*, vol. 49, no. 1, pp. 128–130, 1997.

[7] A. J. Wein, L. R. Kavoussi, A. W. Partin, and C. A. Peters, *Campbell-Walsh Urology*, Elsevier, Philadelphia, 11th edition, 2016.

[8] M. Itani, A. P. Wasnik, and J. F. Platt, "Radiologic-pathologic correlation in extra-adrenal myelolipoma," *Abdominal Imaging*, vol. 39, no. 2, pp. 394–397, 2014.

[9] K. S. Baker, D. Lee, M. Huang, and E. S. Gould, "Presacral myelolipoma: a case report and review of imaging findings," *J Radiol Case Rep.*, vol. 6, no. 6, pp. 1–9, 2012.

[10] D. Zieker, I. Königsrainer, S. Miller et al., "Simultaneous adrenal and extra-adrenal myelolipoma – an uncommon incident: case report and review of the literature," *World Journal of Surgical Oncology*, vol. 6, no. 1, p. 72, 2008.

[11] A. Arezzo, A. Bullano, G. Cochetti et al., "Transperitoneal versus retroperitoneal laparoscopic adrenalectomy for adrenal tumours in adults," *Cochrane Database of Systematic Reviews*, vol. 12, 2018.

[12] G. Cochetti, A. Paladini, A. Boni et al., "Robotic treatment of giant adrenal myelolipoma: a case report and review of the literature," *Mol Clin Oncol.*, vol. 10, no. 5, pp. 492–496, 2019.

45

Use of the T-1470 LiteTouch™ Laser in the En Bloc Resection of an Upper Tract Urothelial Cancer

Ezra Shoen, Benjamin Zollinger, Tripp Gresham, Katayoon M. Rezaei, and Michael Whalen

School of Medicine and Health Sciences, The George Washington University, Washington, D.C., 20037, USA

Correspondence should be addressed to Ezra Shoen; eshoen@gwmail.gwu.edu

Academic Editor: Fumitaka Koga

Background. Endoscopic laser-ablative therapy of upper tract urothelial carcinoma offers kidney-sparing treatment for well-selected low-risk tumors. The traditional technique consists of tumor biopsy with flexible forceps or nitinol basket for pathologic assessment of stage and grade, followed by laser ablation of the tumor. In this case, we present the use of the new T-1470 LiteTouch™ laser for intraoperative tumor en bloc resection, affording both tissue acquisition and tumor ablation. *Case Presentation.* An 81-year-old female with a past medical history significant for stage 4 chronic kidney disease, peripheral artery disease, coronary artery disease, type 2 diabetes mellitus, and gout was diagnosed with a 2 cm left upper tract high-grade papillary urothelial carcinoma confirmed by cytology with cell block preparation. Using a novel approach, the tumor was resected, en bloc, using the T-1470 LiteTouch™ laser which allowed for sufficient tissue resection for pathologic examination and strong hemostasis. This new technique is the first recorded example of tumor en bloc resection using the T-1470 LiteTouch™ laser of an upper tract urothelial carcinoma. *Conclusion.* The use of the T-1470 LiteTouch™ laser offers promise for its use as a novel laser for the endoscopic treatment of upper tract urothelial carcinoma. It shows potential for advantages over current techniques through its ability to achieve en bloc resection and superior hemostasis.

1. Introduction

Endoscopic management of an upper tract urothelial carcinoma (UTUC) allows for kidney preservation compared to the historical standard of care of a radical nephroureterectomy (RNU), and is therefore an attractive treatment option for patients with underlying chronic kidney disease. The standard technique for endoscopic UTUC surgery includes tumor biopsy by forceps or nitinol basket, and then tumor ablation by holmium:yttrium-aluminum-garnet (Ho:YAG) and/or neodymium:yttrium-aluminum-garnet (Nd:YAG) lasers [1, 2]. In this study, we present the use of a novel laser, the T-1470 LiteTouch™ diode laser, produced by Convergent Laser Technologies, for the en bloc resection of a UTUC.

2. Case Presentation

An 81-year-old female with stage 4 chronic kidney disease, peripheral artery disease, coronary artery disease, type 2 diabetes mellitus, and gout was referred for management of suspected left upper tract malignancy in the setting of gross hematuria. Noncontrast CT abdomen and pelvis demonstrated mild left hydronephrosis and high-attenuation tissue density material in the left upper pole calyx, concerning for blood products and/or malignancy.

After informed consent, the patient was taken to the operating room for cystoscopy, ureteroscopy, and biopsy. Intraoperatively, at least 2 cm left upper pole/renal pelvis tumor nodule was observed with surrounding blood clot, obscuring the true extent of the disease burden. Tissue was obtained with the Piranha forceps and brush biopsy. An attempt was made with the Ho:YAG laser to fulgurate the lesion, but total ablation was not performed given the obscuring clot burden. A ureteral stent was placed. Postoperatively, she did well. Cytologic examination with cell block preparation demonstrated high-grade urothelial carcinoma among nonviable papillary fragments (Figures 1(a) and 1(b)). Results from cytology/biopsy found no evidence of invasion

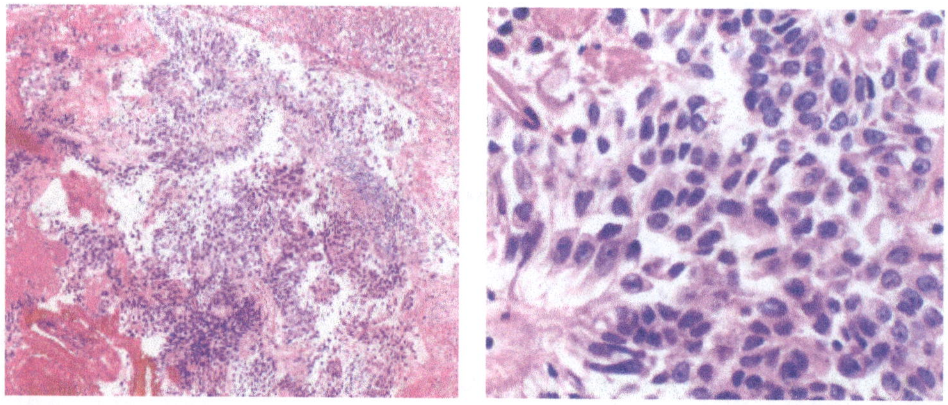

(a) (b)

FIGURE 1: (a) Papillary urothelial carcinoma fragments; cell block (H&E, medium power 10x). (b) High-grade cytologic atypia with enlarged hyperchromatic nuclei and high N/C ratio; cell block (H&E, high power 40x).

(a) (b)

FIGURE 2: (a) Uteroscopic view of UTUC prior to en bloc resection. (b) Uteroscopic view of UTUC after en bloc resection. Hemostasis was achieved with no evidence of bleeding postresection.

and had a preliminary stage of pTa. This staging, however, may not have been fully representative of the tumor. A subsequent nuclear medicine renal scan revealed equal split renal function, increasing the risk of hemodialysis after standard of care nephroureterectomy. She therefore refused this treatment option, along with percutaneous resection and endocavitary therapy. After being lost to follow-up for several months, restaging cross-sectional imaging showed no retroperitoneal lymphadenopathy or metastatic disease. Again refusing percutaneous antegrade resection, she consented to ureteroscopy with laser ablation. The T-1470 LiteTouch™ laser was selected for performance characteristics, including superior efficacy of hemostasis compared to the Ho:YAG laser.

The patient returned to the operating room for left ureteroscopy and biopsy with placement of an 11/13 ureteral access sheath and intended tumor laser ablation and ureteral stent placement. However, upon commencing the ablation, it was discovered that the laser was adept at creating a controlled and even tissue plane deep to the urothelium that enabled enucleation of the tumor largely en bloc (Figures 2(a) and 2(b)).

At the conclusion of the procedure, the enucleation bed was inspected and found to be hemostatic without concern of perforation (Figure 2(b)). Three large fragments of the tumor were evacuated with a nitinol basket via the ureteral access sheath and sent for pathological analysis. A ureteral stent was placed, and the case was concluded. Cytologic examination with cell block preparation again demonstrated high-grade papillary urothelial carcinoma (Figures 1(a) and 1(b)). Although sufficient tissue had been acquired for a thorough assessment of grade, pathologic staging was confounded by cautery artifacts caused by the laser (see Discussion Literature Review below for lessons learned). The patient is currently awaiting adjuvant endocavitary chemotherapy.

3. Discussion and Literature Review

To our knowledge, this case represents the first use of the T-1470 LiteTouch™ laser for UTUC treatment. While traditionally lasers have been used solely for endoscopic tumor ablation, the T-1470 LiteTouch™ laser's unique advantages make it an ideal candidate for both en bloc resection and hemostasis. Some limitations of endoscopic management include limited tissue yield afforded by traditional biopsy instruments, as well as tumor understaging due to inadequate assessment of the depth of penetration.

The T-1470 LiteTouch™ Laser system is a diode laser with a wavelength of 1470 nm, allowing for deep soft tissue penetration into fat, as well as absorption by water. Additionally, the wavelengths are well absorbed by oxyhemoglobin which allows for effective coagulation. These characteristics therefore offer superior soft tissue penetration for tissue acquisition without significant bleeding that would otherwise obscure the ablation zone. Such real-time hemostasis affords accurate assessment and adjustment of the resection plane, which are integral features to afford successful tumor en bloc resection. Furthermore, en bloc resection increases the pathologic yield and minimizes tissue loss during pathologic processing. The combined use of the 11/13 ureteral access sheath allows for rapid, real-time extraction of the resulting large tissue fragments.

The ability to obtain accurate grade-diagnostic biopsies prior to tumor ablation is a documented limitation to endoscopic UTUC treatment [3]. Because endoscopic management is typically only appropriate for low-risk UTUC, an accurate stage and grade are vital for informing the clinical decision on whether RNU is necessary [4]. The use of the T-1470 LiteTouch™ laser for en bloc resection allows for the pathological staging and grading of the fully excised tissue instead of a pre-op biopsy by forceps or basket. While Ho:YAG or Nd:YAG lasers have ablative capabilities, given the very limited depth of tissue penetration as well as limited hemostatic potential, tumor en bloc resection is not reliably performed with these technologies. At 5 W, the power settings for this case, the T-1470 LiteTouch™ achieves a depth of penetration of roughly 0.4 mm. Given the limited anatomical working space during ureteroscopy, tumor en bloc resection has been challenging and relatively inaccessible in the past. Additionally, achieving hemostasis is always a concern for endoscopic UTUC surgery, and failure to do so can pose serious risks to patient safety. The presence of intraoperative bleeding could reduce or eliminate the visualization of the surgical field during the procedure. Moreover, it may be challenging to identify and coagulate the source of the bleed. While the Ho:YAG laser's hemostatic ability is appropriate in the enucleation of the prostate [5], the upper tract offers a smaller working space, making a laser with improved hemostasis a more ideal option. The T-1470 LiteTouch™ Laser's size, precision, tissue absorptive capacity, and strong hemostatic potential offer ideal characteristics to perform this surgery. We believe this technique can be reproduced using the T-1470 LiteTouch™ Laser in future patients.

Other fields that have employed a 1470 nm laser include otolaryngology, colorectal surgery, and vascular surgery [6–8]. In each of these fields, the laser was similarly selected for its strong hemostatic and ablative capacity. As the laser is relatively new, the nascent experience is growing, and literature regarding the use of this technology is limited.

While the aforementioned case illustrates a successful example of this procedure, there were several limitations encountered that should be noted to improve future procedures. Due to excess thermal injury, cautery artifact partially obstructed pathologic evaluation (Figure 3). This was likely a consequence of the frequency of the laser being set too high during this pilot experience. In the aforementioned case, the laser was set at 5 Watts and 30 Hz. The T-1470 LiteTouch™ Laser offers a 30 Hz, 20 Hz, and 10 Hz setting for frequency options. Reducing the frequency decreases the temperature during tissue en bloc resection and thereby reduces cautery artifact. One limitation of this approach is reduced tissue energy absorption at this frequency could potentially prolong procedural time. Nonetheless, for future procedures, we recommend decreasing the frequency to the 20 Hz or 10 Hz setting which will maintain the depth of penetration and hemostasis, as the wavelength is held constant, but minimize cautery artifact. In fact, the lower frequency increases the latency time between pulses and allows oxyhemoglobin more time to absorb the laser energy which theoretically may improve hemostasis.

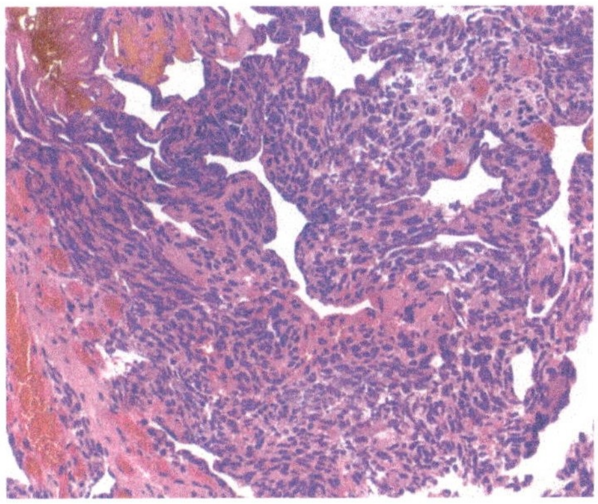

Figure 3: Marked thermal artifact; cell block (H&E, high power 40x).

Another limitation, to this novel approach, is identifying the appropriate margin of resection. Given en bloc resection of an upper tract urothelial carcinoma has not, to our knowledge, been performed previously, no literature exists to indicate an optimal margin. This limitation is further complicated by the grade, stage, architecture, use of neoadjuvant chemotherapy, and location of the tumor, all of which may affect the desired margin. One approach could be to resect a wide margin similar to that ablated during a laser ablation for low-risk disease. More data is needed to identify an appropriate margin.

4. Conclusion

Endoscopic management of UTUC offers a less invasive, kidney-sparing treatment for properly selected patients. The traditional endoscopic approach with Ho:YAG/Nd:YAG lasers is limited to just tumor ablation, given the limitations in tissue penetration depth and most importantly hemostasis. In this case, we illustrated the successful management of UTUC by tumor en bloc resection using the T-1470 LiteTouch™ Laser. Historically 1470 nm diode lasers have been used for tumor resection in other medical specialties such as otolaryngology [9]. Tumor en bloc resection using the T-1470 LiteTouch™ Laser is a novel technique and technology for the management of UTUC. The laser provided strong hemostasis and offered a potential advantage over current methods by yielding abundant tissue for accurate pathologic examination. As experience with this technology mounts, a more reliable assessment of the tumor grade and stage has the potential to expand the indication for endoscopic management to patients with higher risk features.

Consent

Consent to publish this information was obtained from the study participant.

References

[1] F. G. Petros, R. Li, and S. F. Matin, "Endoscopic approaches to upper tract urothelial carcinoma," *The Urologic Clinics of North America*, vol. 45, no. 2, pp. 267–286, 2018.

[2] D. P. Verges, C. D. Lallas, S. G. Hubosky, and D. H. Bagley Jr., "Endoscopic treatment of upper tract urothelial carcinoma," *Current Urology Reports*, vol. 18, no. 4, pp. 1–12, 2017.

[3] A. Breda, A. Territo, F. Sanguedolce et al., "Comparison of biopsy devices in upper tract urothelial carcinoma," *World Journal of Urology*, vol. 37, no. 9, pp. 1899–1905, 2019.

[4] M. Rouprêt, M. Babjuk, E. Compérat et al., "European Association of urology guidelines on upper urinary tract urothelial carcinoma: 2017 update," *European Urology*, vol. 73, no. 1, pp. 111–122, 2018.

[5] F. Shigemura, "Current status of holmium laser enucleation of the prostate," *International Journal of Urology*, vol. 25, no. 3, pp. 206–211, 2018.

[6] S. Havel, "Intraindividual comparison of 1,470 nm diode laser versus carbon dioxide laser for tonsillotomy: a prospective, randomized, double blind, controlled feasibility trial," *Lasers in Surgery and Medicine*, vol. 44, no. 7, pp. 558–563, 2012.

[7] G. Giamundo, "Closure of fistula-in-ano with laser - FiLaC™: an effective novel sphincter-saving procedure for complex disease," *Colorectal Disease*, vol. 16, no. 2, pp. 110–115, 2014.

[8] S. Doganci and U. Demirkilic, "Comparison of 980 nm laser and bare-tip fibre with 1470 nm laser and radial fibre in the treatment of great saphenous vein varicosities: a prospective randomised clinical trial," *European Journal of Vascular and Endovascular Surgery*, vol. 40, no. 2, pp. 254–259, 2010.

[9] F. Liang, Z. Xiao, R. Chen et al., "Transoral 980-nm/1470-nm dual-wavelength fiber laser microsurgery for early-stage glottic carcinoma," *Oral Oncology*, vol. 96, pp. 66–70, 2019.

46

Rare Associations with Posterior Urethral Valves

Ahmed Osama Mohamed, Bala Eradi, Anthony Owen, and Ashok Rajimwale

Department of Paediatric Surgery, Leicester Royal Infirmary, Infirmary Square, leicester, LE1 5WW, UK

Correspondence should be addressed to Ahmed Osama Mohamed; dr.ahmed.osama.salama@gmail.com

Academic Editor: Claudio Simeone

Posterior urethral valves are a common cause of congenital bladder outlet obstruction. Known associations include cardiac malformations and gastrointestinal abnormalities. In this case series, we report on two cases of PUV associated with anorectal malformations along with a case of PUV in monochorionic diamniotic twins. We explore the difficulty in achieving a diagnosis and the final management. The association of posterior urethral valves in a patient with anorectal malformation should be suspected in case of associated oligohydramnios or oliguria postnatally. There should be a high index of suspicion in twin pregnancy even if only one of the twins is suspected of bladder outlet obstruction.

1. Introduction

Posterior urethral valves (PUV) are the most common congenital cause of bladder outlet obstruction in children and a leading cause of end-stage renal failure. The estimated incidence of PUV is 1 in 3800 live births in the UK, of which 40% of patients are diagnosed antenatally [1]. Nonurological common anomalies associated with PUV include cardiac malformations, gastrointestinal abnormalities, and aneuploidy in about 40% of cases [2]. We describe 3 cases of PUV with rare associations and their management.

2. Case 1: PUV Associated with Imperforate Anus

A baby boy born at 34 + 6 weeks by emergency C-section weighing 2.735 kg with antenatal scans suggestive of oligohydramnios and dilated bowel loops however with a normal renal tract. At birth, he was found to have an imperforate anus; hence, a sigmoid colostomy was performed.

Postoperatively, he was noticed to have oliguria and worsening renal functions. Interestingly at the same time, the colostomy bag was filling with faeces and watery effluent. Close inspection revealed watery discharge from defunctioning limb of colostomy explaining rising blood urea and creatinine levels and acidosis. We suspected bladder outflow obstruction and regurgitation of urine through the recto urethral fistula. Renal ultrasound scan (USS) showed bilateral hydronephrosis and hydroureters. Perineal USS showed dilated posterior urethra. Attempted urethral catheterisation proved difficult, so a suprapubic catheter was inserted.

Micturating cystourethrogram (MCUG) through suprapubic catheter revealed a dilated posterior urethra and a rectobulbar fistula (Figure 1). On day 13 of life and after stabilisation of general condition, the patient was taken to theatre for cystoscopic ablation of the valves. The suprapubic catheter was removed, and a urinary catheter was left for one week.

Subsequently, he suffered from persistent nonbilious vomiting along with metabolic alkalosis. Abdominal USS revealed coexisting pyloric stenosis. Laparoscopic pyloromyotomy was performed and made good postoperative recovery. At the age of 4 months, posterior sagittal anorectoplasty (PSARP) with dissection and ligation of the rectobulbar fistula was done. Under the same anaesthetic, repeat cystoscopy was done to confirm the absence of any residual valves. After regular dilatation and achieving a good size neo-anus, stoma closure was performed at the age of 7 months. On follow-up at 3 years, he is thriving well with improvement of the bilateral hydronephrosis and hydroureter on serial ultrasound scans

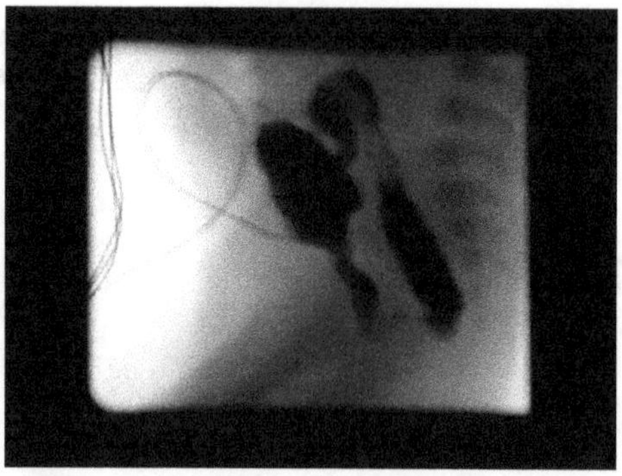

Figure 1: MCUG showing evidence of PUV and rectobulbar fistula.

and no history of urinary tract infections (UTI). He has achieved bladder control and has been progressing well with bowel continence.

3. Case 2: PUV Associated with Rectoperineal Fistula

This full-term baby boy was born after an uneventful pregnancy and normal antenatal scans. At birth, he was found to have a rectoperineal fistula, accessory nipples, and preauricular skin tags. He underwent primary PSARP on day two of life for the rectoperineal fistula. Echocardiography revealed a patent foramen ovale and tricuspid valve thickening. The rest of his VACTERYL screening—including a renal ultrasound—were normal. Unfortunately, this child later presented with two confirmed episodes of E-coli urinary tract infections in the first 4 months of life. Although a repeat USS did not reveal any anomalies, we proceeded for a MCUG, which showed a dilated posterior urethra suggestive of PUV (Figure 2). Cystoscopic valve ablation was then performed with good postoperative recovery. At the age of 8 years, this child has done well with normal renal function and has achieved both urinary and faecal continence with the aid of regular laxatives.

4. Cases 3 and 4: PUV in Monochorionic Twins

We report a case of PUV in monochorionic diamniotic twins born at 36 weeks by Emergency C-section due to breech presentation. Antenatal scans in twin 1 showed bilateral hydroureter and hydronephrosis and oligohydramnios. Postnatal renal USS showed bilateral hydronephrosis with loss of corticomedullary differentiation and a dilated left ureter.

Antenatal scan in twin 2 showed left hydronephrosis. Postnatal renal USS showed thick wall bladder and bilateral hydronephrosis and hydroureters. MCUG in twin 2 revealed a dilated posterior urethra and grade V left ureteric reflux (Figure 3) While in twin 1 revealed a grossly dilated posterior urethra and a trabeculated urinary bladder (Figure 4). Bladder drainage was achieved using urethral catheters in both twins. Due to the low birth weights of twins and circumstances related to the COVID-19 Pandemic, ablation was performed at 8 weeks of age. Currently, twins are doing well and awaiting check cystoscopy (accepted unit policy in our hospital) and circumcision.

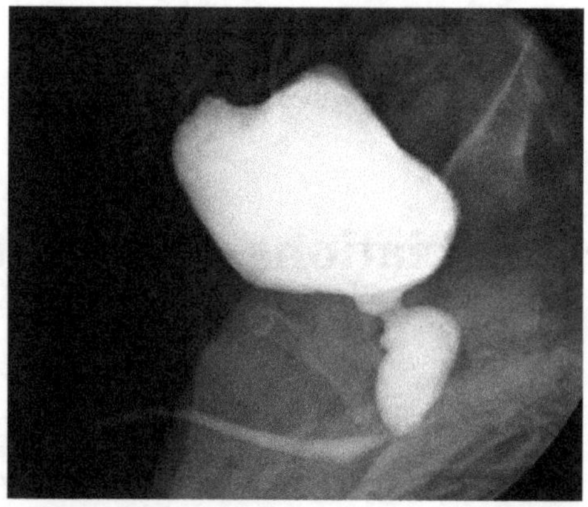

Figure 2: Dilated posterior urethra on MCUG.

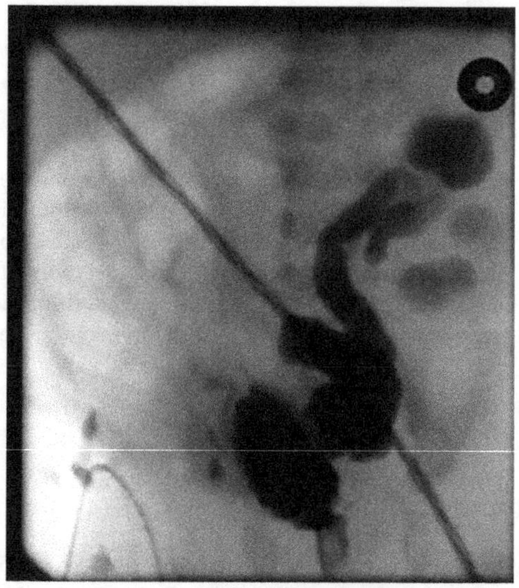

Figure 3: Dilated posterior urethra and left grade V reflux.

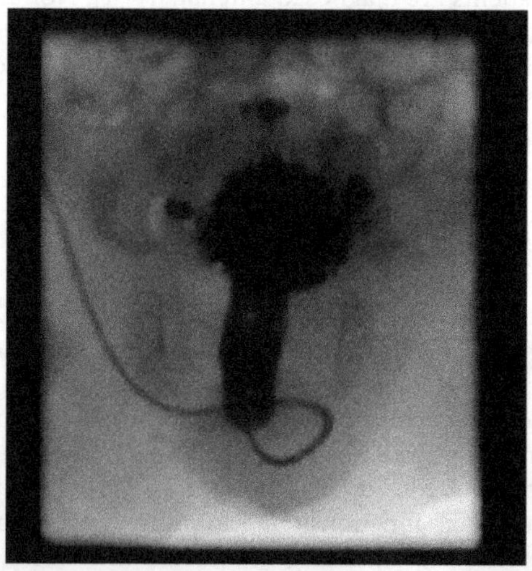

Figure 4: Dilated posterior urethra and a trabeculated urinary bladder.

5. Discussion

Posterior urethral valves (PUV) are thought to result from an anomalous insertion of the mesonephric duct into the urogenital sinus, preventing normal migration of these ducts and their anterior fusion forming the abnormal ridges in the membranous urethra [3]. Young's [4] classification of 3 types of PUV has recently been challenged, and a newer concept was proposed by Dewan and Goh that in bladder outlet obstruction, the uninstrumented urethra looks more like a circumferential obstructing membrane with a small central or eccentric opening named congenital obstructing posterior urethral membrane (COPUM) [5]. Various associations (up to 40%) with PUV have been reported including cardiovascular abnormalities, absent external auditory meatus, bilateral adrenal agenesis, hypospadias, micro/macrophallus, and anterior urethral valves [6–8].

The association of PUV with anorectal malformations is exceedingly rare and can pose a diagnostic and therapeutic challenge. Few reports [6, 9, 10] exist of this association; however, only one report had a presentation similar to our first case explaining the dilemma and difficulty identifying or suspecting PUV with anorectal malformations. Case 2 highlights the false-negative diagnosis of PUV on antenatal scans and normal postnatal scans (as a normal VACTREL screening tool in our institution); however, a diagnosis was made following investigation for recurrent UTI.

Comparing both cases, the presence of a rectourethral fistula in the first case could have served as a "pop-off" mechanism and protected the upper urinary tracts. This is evident when comparing the degree of posterior urethral dilatation in both cases.

Familial occurrence of PUV has been reported, particularly in dizygotic twins; however, P. Burttet in an extensive review of literature found 12 cases of familial nontwin sibling with PUV [11]. Interestingly, he also found that diagnosis in the second sibling was delayed in most cases if not suspected antenatally. It has been a known fact that the prevalence of structural defects is 1.2–2 times higher twin pregnancies compared to singletons, with increased rates in monochorionic twins [12]. This is also the case with PUV whose association with twins has been previously reported [13–15]. In one report, antenatal presentation in the identical twins was different in both including one twin showing urinary ascites and bilateral dysplastic kidneys while the other twin presenting a less severe form of the disease [15]. However, our twins had shown almost identical antenatal image of bilateral hydroureter and hydronephrosis though oligohydramnios was present in twin 1. Postnatal MCUG revealed the presence of reflux in one of the twins only. Although there is no established genetic link to this anomaly, the association of PUV in twins and nontwin siblings has led to the speculation of a possibility of an autosomal recessive pattern of inheritance or some form of genetic predisposition [14, 16]. This has led to the general recommendation of urologic evaluation of the male sibling and family member of a male child with PUV [13, 17].

6. Conclusion

Although exceedingly rare, the association of posterior urethral valves in a patient with anorectal malformation (ARM) should be suspected in case of associated oligohydramnios, postnatal oliguria, or watery effluents in colostomy bag with rising renal function and acidosis. There should also be a high index of suspicion in twin pregnancy even if only one of the twins is suspected of bladder outlet obstruction.

References

[1] E. Brownlee, R. Wragg, A. Robb, H. Chandran, M. Knight, and L. McCarthy, "Current epidemiology and antenatal presentation of posterior urethral valves: outcome of BAPS CASS National Audit," *Journal of Pediatric Surgery*, vol. 54, no. 2, pp. 318–321, 2019.

[2] T. T. Chao and J. S. Dashe, *Posterior Urethral Valves*, Elsevier Inc., Second edition, 2017.

[3] A. Krishnan, A. De Souza, R. Konijeti, and L. S. Baskin, "The anatomy and embryology of posterior urethral valves," *The Journal of Urology*, vol. 175, no. 4, pp. 1214–1220, 2006.

[4] H. H. Young, W. A. Frontz, and J. C. Baldwin, "Congenital obstruction of the posterior urethra," *The Journal of urology*, vol. 3, no. 5, pp. 289–366, 1919.

[5] P. A. Dewan and D. G. Goh, "Variable expression of the congenital obstructive posterior urethral membrane," *Urology*, vol. 45, no. 3, pp. 507–509, 1995.

[6] S. A. Hayden, P. D. Russ, D. H. Pretorius, M. L. Manco-Johnson, and W. H. Clewell, "Posterior urethral obstruction. Prenatal sonographic findings and clinical outcome in fourteen cases," *Journal of Ultrasound in Medicine*, vol. 7, no. 7, pp. 371–375, 1988.

[7] J. Carvell and R. Mulik, "A case of hypospadias, anterior and posterior urethral valves," *Journal of surgical case reports*, vol. 2013, no. 2, 2013.

[8] K. L. Rao, B. Eradi, and P. Menon, "Anterior and posterior urethral valves: a rare association," *Journal of Pediatric Surgery*, vol. 38, no. 7, pp. 1-2, 2003.

[9] C. E. Carlton, F. J. Harberg, and F. M. Fry, "Urologic complications of imperforate anus," *The Journal of Urology*, vol. 109, no. 4, pp. 737–739, 1973.

[10] M. P. Singh, A. Haddadin, R. B. Zachary, and D. W. Pilling, "Renal tract disease in imperforate anus," *Journal of Pediatric Surgery*, vol. 9, no. 2, pp. 197–202, 1974.

[11] L. M. Burttet, "Posterior urethral valves disorder in non-twin siblings: case report and literature review," *Medical and Surgical Urology*, vol. 3, no. 2, 2014.

[12] V. J. Baldwin and V. J. Baldwin, *Anomalous development of twins*, Pathology of Multiple Pregnancy, 1994.

[13] J. V. Thomalla, M. E. Mitchell, and R. A. Garett, "Posterior urethral valves in siblings," *Urology*, vol. 33, no. 4, pp. 291–294, 1989.

[14] P. M. Livne, J. Delaune, and E. T. Gonzales, "Genetic etiology of posterior urethral valves," *The Journal of Urology*, vol. 130, no. 4, pp. 781–784, 1983.

[15] G. M. Maruotti, A. Agangi, P. Martinelli, and D. Paladini, "Early prenatal diagnosis of concordant posterior urethral valves in male monochorionic twins," *Prenatal Diagnosis*, vol. 26, no. 1, pp. 67–70, 2006.

[16] F. Morini, M. Ilari, A. Casati, A. Piserà, L. Oriolo, and D. A. Cozzi, "Posterior urethral valves and mirror image anomalies in monozygotic twins," *American Journal of Medical Genetics*, vol. 111, no. 2, pp. 210–212, 2002.

[17] A. O. Talabi, O. A. Sowande, O. Adejuyigbe, J. A. Owa, and A. O. Igwe, "Posterior urethral valves in fraternal twins," *Annals of Pediatric Surgery*, vol. 14, no. 3, pp. 190-191, 2018.

A Giant Solitary Adrenal Plasmacytoma in a Patient with HIV: A Rare Case Report and Review of the Literature

Mehdi Chennoufi,[1] **Ibrahim Boukhannous**,[1] **Mohamed Mokhtari**,[1] **Anouar El Moudane**,[1] **Mohamed Irzi**,[1] **Abdelghani Ouraghi**,[1] **Issam Jandou**,[1] **Achraf Miry**,[2] **and Ali Barki**[1]

[1]*Department of Urology, Mohamed VI University Hospital Center, Mohamed I University, Oujda, Morocco*
[2]*Department of Pathology, Mohamed VI University Hospital Center, Mohamed I University, Oujda, Morocco*

Correspondence should be addressed to Mehdi Chennoufi; dr.mehdi.chennoufi@gmail.com

Academic Editor: Claudio Simeone

Solitary extramedullary plasmacytoma (EMP) involving the adrenal gland is an extremely rare malignancy. We report a case of a solitary adrenal plasmacytoma in an HIV-positive 50-year-old woman on antiretroviral therapy who presented with a rapidly progressing lumbar left masse. A CT scan objectified a locally advanced left adrenal mass measuring 135mm long axis. A biopsy was taken, and the histopathology with the immunohistochemical study objectified an adrenal gland plasmacytoma. The skeletal survey and the sternal suction biopsy did not show any abnormalities. The diagnosis of a solitary EMP of the adrenal gland was made. There are only 10 cases of solitary adrenal plasmacytoma with only one case associated with an HIV-positive patient reported in the literature. Therefore, this paper is aimed at presenting the second case of an HIV-positive patient diagnosed with solitary adrenal plasmacytoma.

1. Introduction

Extramedullary plasmacytoma (EMP) is a proliferation of monoclonal plasmatic soft tissue, without bone marrow involvement in patients with no clinical evidence of multiple myeloma (MM) [1]. It represents less than 4% of all plasma cell malignancies, of which 15% progress to MM and 80% are developing in the upper respiratory system and the head [2]. Any extraosseous organ can also be affected. Solitary adrenal gland plasmacytoma is extremely rare in an HIV-positive patient [3], unlike plasmablastic lymphomas [4]. It has been proven that the solitary EMP is touching this category of patients with younger age, atypical clinical course, and higher aggressivity. The diagnosis is a histopathological dilemma, while its management is still controversial. In the literature, there is no evidence of the superiority of laparoscopic retroperitoneal adrenalectomy compared with laparoscopic transperitoneal adrenalectomy in regard to the duration of surgery, operative blood loss, and conversion to open surgery, while late morbidity might be reduced following the retroperitoneal approach for small lesions (less than 6 cm to 7 cm) [5]. This case is proof that the plasma cell malignancies associated with a human immunodeficiency virus (HIV) could have an unusual localization, an unpredictable evolution, and a poor prognosis.

2. Case Report

A 50-year-old female patient who had been diagnosed with HIV 6 months previously under highly active antiretroviral therapy (HAART) was admitted for abdominal pain and mass syndrome of the left flank evolving for a month with a weight loss of 12 kg, in whom the clinical examination found a conscious patient, normotensive, with tenderness in the left flank, absence of clinical Cushing syndrome, or hyperandrogenism; the rest of the clinical examination is unremarkable.

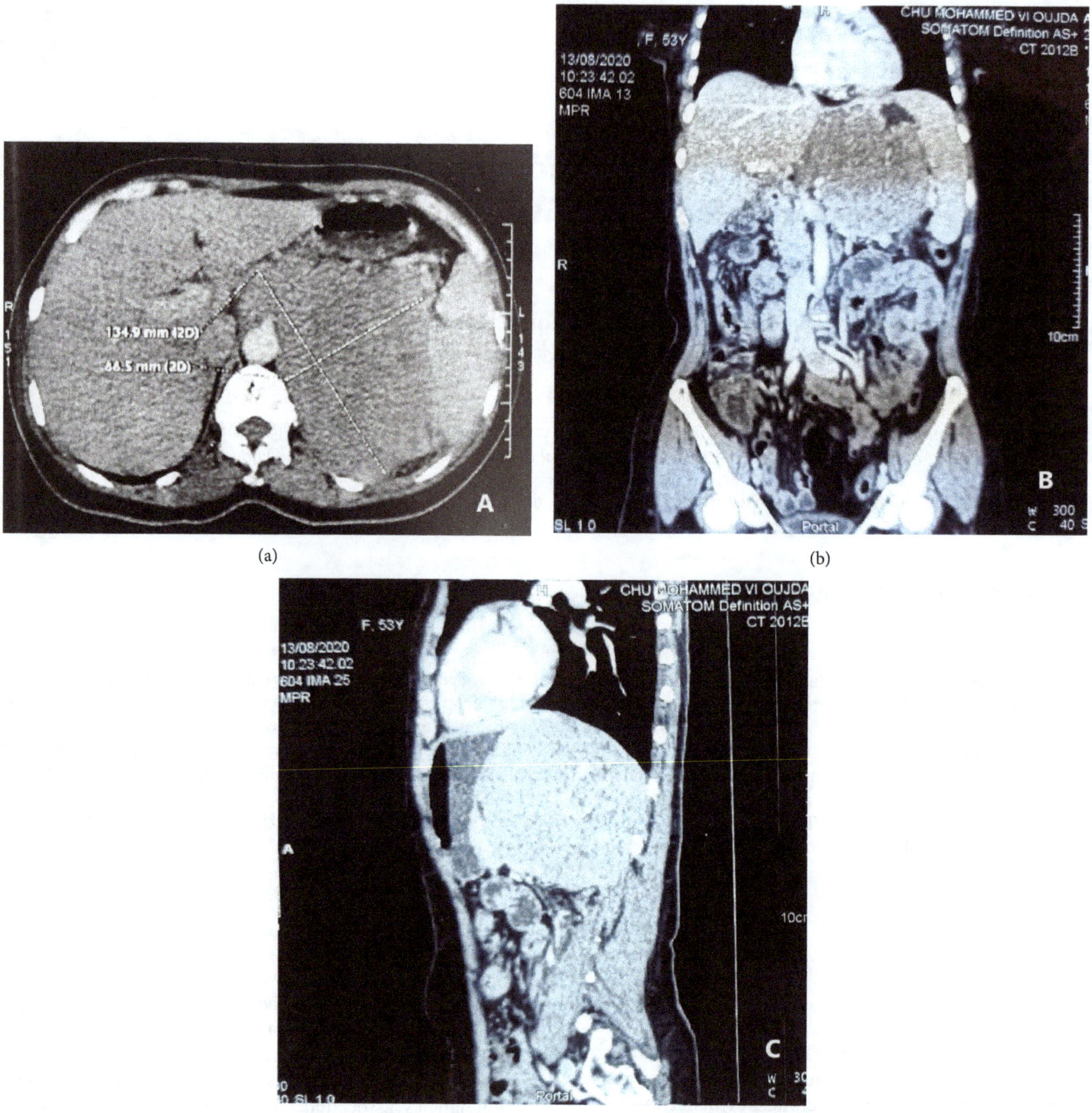

Figure 1: Abdominal CT scan: (a) axial, (b) frontal, and (c) sagittal images show the reports of the locally advanced left adrenal mass of 13.5 cm long axis.

The thoracic abdominopelvic scan (Figure 1) objectified a voluminous retroperitoneal tumor process centered on the left adrenal compartment badly limited irregular, containing zones of necrosis, measuring135 × 110 × 129 mm 10 HU of density, which infiltrates the great gastric curvature, the body and the tail of the pancreas without a dividing line, and the splenic vein which is laminated. Outside comes at intimate contact with a spleen includes the upper pole of the left kidney. Posteriorly, it arrives at the contact of the vertebral bodies D10, 11, and 12 and invades the left diaphragmatic pillar, the psoas muscle, and the square of the left lumbar region. Thus, it encompasses the celiac trunk and the renal artery over their entire circumference and the abdominal aorta over a circumference > 180° comes into contact with the superior mesenteric artery, and the common hepatic artery without a sign of invasion comes into contact with the inferior vena cava with a border of separation in places, associated with perilesional lymphadenopathy the largest 19 mm, left inferior lobar parenchymal nodule of 7 mm, and left supraclavicular lymphadenopathy the largest 13 mm.

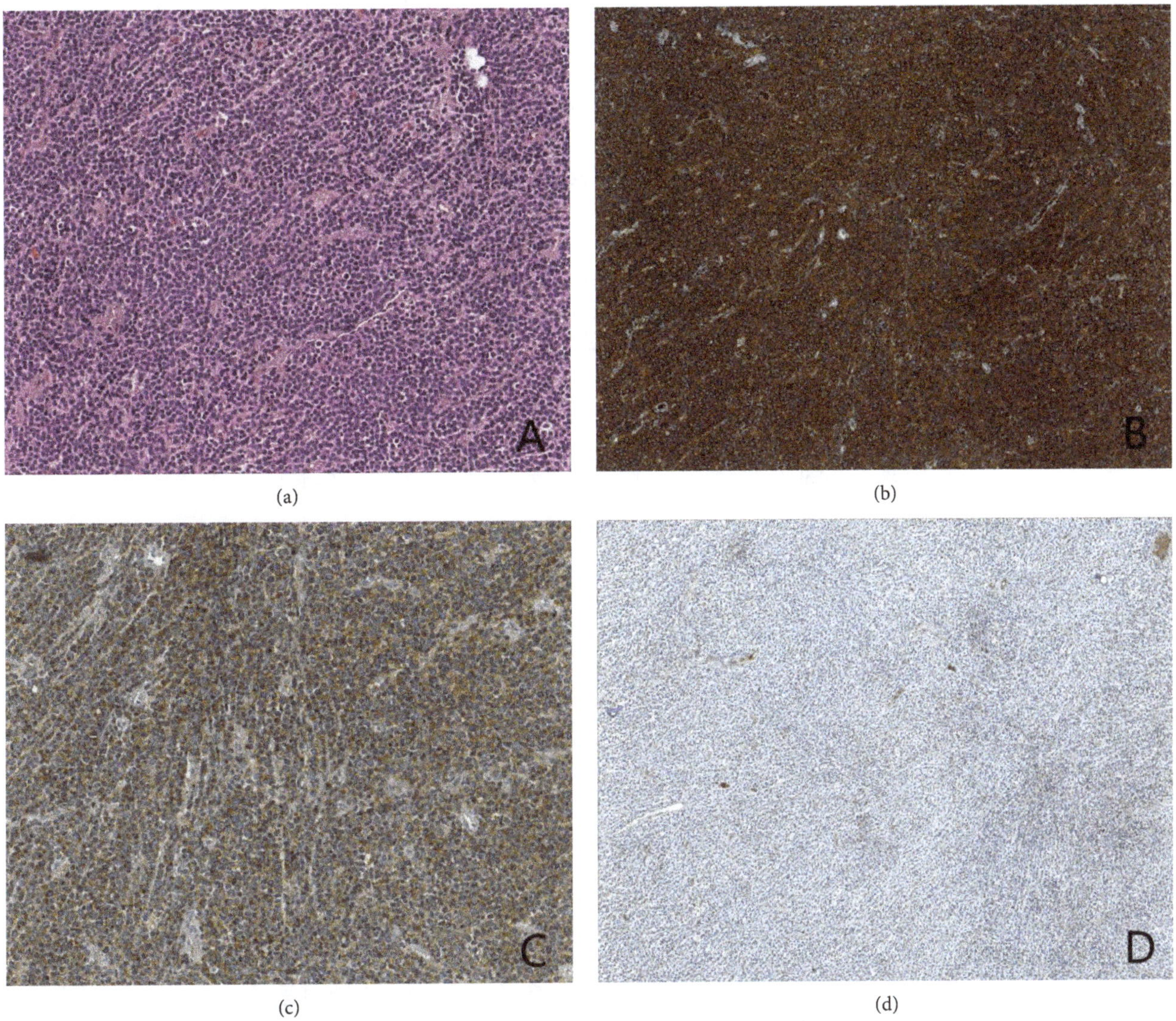

FIGURE 2: Microphotography showing sheets of atypical plasma cells (a). (HE, 100x). Immunohistochemical staining shows that the tumor cells were positive for CD138 (b), positive for lambda (c), and negative for kappa (d).

Biological exploration revealed a negative endogenous hypersecretion of cortisol, negative urinary methoxylated metabolites, and no hypersecretion of androgens.

Creatinine was 5.56 mg/L, urea 0.27 g/L, natremia 139 mEq/L, kalmia 3.6 mEq/L, calcemia 100 mg/L, hemoglobin 12.3 g/dL, white blood cells 3110/mm^3, and platelets 198,000/mm^3, and the liver function test was unremarkable.

The patient was placed on level 2 analgesic treatment. A percutaneous biopsy of the mass was taken, showing a proliferation of atypical plasma cells. No intact tissue of the adrenal gland was found. Immunohistochemistry study revealed a negative expression of CD3 and CD20 excluding a plasmablastic lymphoma and a positive expression of CD138 and lambda light chains confirming the diagnosis of adrenal plasmacytoma (Figure 2).

Further serum investigation by immunoelectrophoresis of Bence-Jones proteins was made showing a high level of lambda light chains at 45.8 mg/L (normal level between 4 and 25.1 mg/L) with the normal level of kappa light chains at 6.2 mg/L (normal level between 5.2 and 22.17 mg/L). X-rays of the skeleton did not show lesions. A sternal suction biopsy did not show any plasmacytic infiltration. The diagnosis of a solitary adrenal plasmacytoma was established.

The patient was transferred to the oncology for chemotherapy and radiotherapy. But unfortunately, she died after 3 months of following up.

3. Discussion

Four categories of plasma cell malignancies exist: MM, plasma cell leukemia, solitary plasmacytoma of the bone, and EMP [4]. This latter is a rare malignant monoclonal plasma cell proliferation in patients with no clinical signs of MM. It represents less than 4% of all plasma cell malignancies [6] with 15% usually developing to MM [4]. 80% arise in the head, the oral cavity, and the upper respiratory tract, while 20% occur in the thyroid, breast, gastrointestinal tract, spleen, retroperitoneum, kidney, bladder, and testes. EMP is very rarely involving the adrenal gland [7].

Table 1: Solitary extramedullary adrenal gland plasmacytoma reported in the literature.

Study	Years	Country	Age	Gender	Side	Tumor size (cm)	Function	Treatment	HIV +	Serum protein electrophoresis	Kappa	Lambda	Follow-up (month)
Kahara [15]	2001	Japan	52	Male	Right	4	No	LCA	No	+	No	Specimen	12
Asahi [16]	2001	Japan	52	Male	Right	4	No	LCA+C +R	No	+	No	Specimen	
Fujikata [12]	2002	Japan	77	Male	Right	10	Yes	OA+nephrectomy+R		+	Specimen	Blood	12
Rogers [17]	2004	USA	75	Female	Right	3.5	No	LCA+R	No	—	No	Specimen	NP
Li [18]	2007	China	64	Female	Bilateral	6 right/4left	No	OA	No	—	No	Specimen	NP
Ahmed [13]	2009	Saudi Arabia	47	Male	Bilateral	8 right/8 left	No	C+autologous hematopoietic stem cell transplantation	No	+	Specimen + urine	No	47
Blanco [19]	2011	Spain	76	Female	Left	6	No	Adrenalectomy+R	No	NP	NP	NP	40
Cao [20]	2014	China	26	Male	Right	4.5	No	LCA	No	+	Specimen	No	72
Cao [14]	2016	China	35	Male	Right	3.5	No	LCA	Yes	+	No	Specimen	24
Townend/Graus [21]	2016	Australia	57	Male	Bilateral	5.5 right/9.5 left	No	Bilateral OA	No	+	Specimen +serum+urine	No	NP
Chennoufi	2020	Morocco	50	Female	Left	13.5	No	C+R	Yes	+	No	Specimen +blood	3

LCA: laparoscopic adrenalectomy; C: chemotherapy; R: radiotherapy; OA: open adrenalectomy; NP: no report.

Several retrospective studies revealed that the incidence of monoclonal gammopathy was from 3.8% to 26% in HIV-positive patients [8, 9] vs. 3.2% in the general population older than 50 years old [10]. The mechanisms of the high risk of plasma cell disorders in HIV patients are still poorly elaborated. However, two mechanisms were proposed to explain this situation: antigen stimulation and immunodeficiency. HIV viral antigens could stimulate the proliferation of B cells and the secretion of an immunoglobulin without the interference of T cells, most often due to chronic antigenic stimulation. Also, HIV can cause T cell dysfunction thus activating B cells without viral antigen stimulation [11].

The diagnosis is established on the findings of a plasma cell tumor in the exerted specimen or biopsy, the immunohistochemistry study, the immunological analysis of serum and urine, the absence of multiple myeloma on bone marrow suction biopsy, and the absence of skeletal lesions [3].

There are only 10 cases reported in the literature (Table 1). Most cases were reported in the Asian population. The age ranges from 26 to 77 years with a medium at 61 years. Sex ratio was 2.3 male/1 female. Our patient was a 50-year-old female. The right adrenal gland was more affected with three cases of bilateral tumors, and only one case of left adrenal plasmacytoma. The mean maximum dimension was 5.8 cm (range, 3.5 cm to 10 cm). Our case was the largest adrenal gland plasmacytoma reported to date with 13.5 cm in the long axis. Fujikata et al. [12] reported high levels of noradrenaline in the endocrinologic function with an elevation of monoclonal IgG-lambda at serum immunoelectrophoresis, contrasted with a monoclonality of IgG-kappa at immunohistochemical study, from where the diagnosis of extramedullary plasmacytoma independent of simultaneous benign M proteinemia was established. Ahmed et al. [13] reported bilateral regression of the adrenal tumors with calcification and fibrosis after two consecutive autologous hematopoietic stem cell transplantation. Cao et al. [14] reported the first case of extramedullary plasmacytoma involving the adrenal gland in an HIV-positive 35-year-old male patient. Of the six cases that have reported follow-up data on adrenal EMP, the follow-up ranging was from 12 to 72 months, with no recurrences.

Most HIV-positive patients are excluded from clinical trials. There are no guidelines for managing these specific patients. HAART is essential in the treatment of plasma cell disorders in HIV-positive patients. Yet, it is unclear how long the patients need to be on it before and during the course of chemotherapy. The role of RT is not clear unless there is a suspicion of residual disease [11]. The autologous hematopoietic stem cell transplantation is a possible alternative that needs more long-term studies.

4. Conclusion

Solitary EMP involving the adrenal gland in patients with HIV is extremely uncommon. The diagnosis is established on clinical, radiological, immunohistochemical, and histological data. The management is still controversial. More case reports and long-term-studies are needed to establish well-supported guidelines for these specific patients.

References

[1] World Health Organization, *Pathology and Genetics of Tumours of Soft Tissue and Bone*, IARC Press, Lyon, France, 2002.

[2] P. Galieni, M. Cavo, A. Pulsoni et al., "Clinical outcome of extramedullary plasmacytoma," *Haematologica*, vol. 85, no. 1, pp. 47–51, 2000.

[3] P. de Camargo Moraes, L. A. Thomaz, V. A. Montalli, J. L. C. Junqueira, C. M. B. Ribeiro, and L. B. Oliveira, "Extramedullary Plasmacytoma Diagnosed in an HIV-Positive Patient by an Unusual Clinical Presentation," *Case Reports in Dentistry*, vol. 2016, Article ID 6305173, 5 pages, 2016.

[4] A. A. Joseph, S. Pulimood, M. T. Manipadam, A. Viswabandya, and E. Sigamani, "Extramedullary plasmacytoma: an unusual neoplasm in a HIV-positive patient," *International Journal of STD & AIDS*, vol. 27, no. 10, pp. 909–911, 2016.

[5] A. Arezzo, A. Bullano, G. Cochetti et al., "Transperitoneal versus retroperitoneal laparoscopic adrenalectomy for adrenal tumours in adults," *Cochrane Database of Systematic Reviews*, vol. 12, no. 12, article CD011668, 2018.

[6] World Health Organization, *Patology & Genetics—Head and Neck Tumors*, IARC Press, Lyon, France, 2005.

[7] S. Herranz, M. Sala, M. Cervantes, M. Sasal, A. Soler, and F. Segura, "Neoplasia of plasma cells with atypical presentation and infection by the human immunodeficiency virus. A presentation of two cases," *American journal of hematology*, vol. 65, no. 3, pp. 239–242, 2000.

[8] B. J. Dezube, D. M. Aboulafia, and L. Pantanowitz, "Plasma cell disorders in HIVinfected patients: from benign gammopathy to multiple myeloma," *The AIDS reader*, vol. 14, no. 7, pp. 372–374, 2004.

[9] A. S. Fiorino and B. Atac, "Paraproteinemia, plasmacytoma, myeloma and HIV infection," *Leukemia*, vol. 11, no. 12, pp. 2150–2156, 1997.

[10] R. A. Kyle, T. M. Therneau, S. V. Rajkumar et al., "Prevalence of monoclonal gammopathy of undetermined significance," *The New England Journal of Medicine*, vol. 354, no. 13, pp. 1362–1369, 2006.

[11] W. J. Coker, A. Jeter, H. Schade, and Y. Kang, "Plasma cell disorders in HIV-infected patients: epidemiology and molecular mechanisms," *Biomarker Research*, vol. 1, no. 1, 2013.

[12] S. Fujikata, N. Tanji, K. Aoki, H. Ohoka, N. Hojo, and M. Yokoyama, "Extramedullary plasmacytoma arising from an adrenal gland," *Urology*, vol. 60, no. 3, 2002.

[13] M. Ahmed, A. Al-ghamdi, M. Al-omari, M. Aljurf, and Y. Al-kadhi, "Autologous bone marrow transplanation for extramedullary plasmacytoma presenting as adrenal incidentaloma," *Annals of Saudi Medicine*, vol. 29, no. 3, pp. 219–222, 2009.

[14] D. Cao, Y. Hu, L. Li, W. Xiao, and Q. Wei, "Retroperitoneal laparoscopic management of a solitary extramedullary plasmacytoma associated with human immunodeficiency virus infection: a case report," *Oncology Letters*, vol. 11, no. 1, pp. 767–769, 2016.

[15] T. Kahara, Y. Nagai, H. Yamashita, E. Nohara, K. Kobayashi, and T. Takamura, "Extramedullary plasmacytoma in the adrenal incidentaloma," *Clinical Endocrinology*, vol. 55, no. 2, pp. 267–270, 2001.

[16] H. Asahi, Y. Iwasa, K. Komatsu, A. Hirata, K. Koshida, and M. Namiki, "A case of plasmacytoma involving adrenal gland," *Acta urologica Japonica*, vol. 47, no. 9, pp. 629–631, 2001.

[17] C. G. Rogers, P. A. Pinto, and E. G. Weir, "Extraosseous (extramedullary) plasmacytoma of the adrenal gland," *Archives of Pathology & Laboratory Medicine*, vol. 128, no. 7, pp. e86–e88, 2004.

[18] Y. Li, Y. K. Guo, Z. G. Yang, E. S. Ma, and P. Q. Min, "Extramedullary plasmacytoma involving the bilateral adrenal glands on MR imaging," *Korean Journal of Radiology*, vol. 8, no. 3, pp. 246–248, 2007.

[19] F. Blanco Antona, S. Bahamonde Cabria, L. Blanco Antona, and A. Marín Pérez-Tabernero, "Adrenal extramedullary plasmacytoma," *Cirugía Española*, vol. 89, no. 10, pp. 690-691, 2011.

[20] D. Cao, L. Li, L. Liu et al., "Solitary extramedullary plasmacytoma of the adrenal gland: a rare case report with review of the literature," *International journal of clinical and experimental pathology*, vol. 7, no. 12, pp. 9072–9075, 2014.

[21] P. J. Townend, G. Kraus, L. Coyle, D. Nevell, A. Engelsman, and S. B. Sidhu, "Bilateral extramedullary adrenal plasmacytoma: case report and review of the literature," *International Journal of Endocrine Oncology*, vol. 4, no. 2, pp. 67–73, 2017.

Abdominoscrotal Hydrocele: An Uncommon Cause of Abdominoscrotal Cystic Swelling

Manish Swarnkar[1] **and Pathan Tanveer Khan**[2]

[1]*Department of Surgery, LN Medical College, Madhya Pradesh, 462042, Bhopal, India*
[2]*Department of General Surgery, JNMC, Maharashtra, 442001, Wardha, India*

Correspondence should be addressed to Manish Swarnkar; mswarnkar1971@gmail.com

Academic Editor: Claudio Simeone

Abdominoscrotal hydrocele (ASH) consists of fluid-filled intercommunicating inguinoscrotal and abdominal sac with a characteristic hourglass-like picture on CECT, which usually affects single testis and a rare cause of abdominoscrotal cystic swelling. The precise etiology of ASH is not known. Ultrasonography is the initial diagnostic modality of choice as it demonstrates the intercommunication between the two sacs and also identifies any abnormality of the testis and genitourinary tract. We are reporting a case of a 27-year-old patient presented in the General Surgery OPD of Acharya Vinoba Bhave Hospital in 2019 with bilateral scrotal and abdominal swelling. On examination, cross fluctuation was positive between left hydrocele and abdominal swelling, raising suspicion of ASH, which was confirmed on CECT. The patient underwent excision of sac through left inguinoscrotal approach and an uneventful postoperative course.

1. Introduction

Abdominoscrotal hydrocele is a rare clinical entity seen only in 0.18%-3.1% of hydrocele cases [1, 2]. ASH is a dumbbell or hourglass-shaped hydrocele that extends from the scrotum to the abdominal cavity extraperitonealy through the inguinal canal. ASH is usually unilateral, but few bilateral cases have been described in literature. Here, we present a case of left-sided ASH with review of literature.

2. Case Report

A 27-year-old male patient presented in the General Surgery OPD of Acharya Vinoba Bhave Hospital in 2019 with bilateral scrotal and lower abdominal swelling (Figure 1(a)), which was insidious in onset with dull aching dragging pain. There was no previous history of trauma or fever. On physical examination, bilateral hydrocele was present, and both swellings were nonreducible, transluminant, and fluctuant. Abdominal swelling was extending up to the umbilicus, and cross fluctuation was present with left side hydrocele, raising the possibility of left-sided ASH. The CECT abdomen revealed a large intercommunicating homogeneous hourglass-shaped fluid collection involving the lower abdomen and left scrotum (Figure 2), confirming the diagnosis. The patient underwent uneventful, complete excision of the sac through the left inguinoscrotal approach (Figure 1(b)).

3. Discussion

Since the first description by Dupuytren in 1834 when it was called hydrocele en bisac, many titles have been used until Bickle in 1919 suggested the abdominoscrotal hydrocele as a proper descriptive term [1, 3]. ASH is most commonly seen in the pediatric age group of less than five years and second and third decade in adults. It is a congenital anomaly of processus vaginalis which starts as an inguinoscrotal hydrocele and gradually extends into the abdomen forming a two-compartment intercommunicating hydrocele [1]. Free intercommunication is a cardinal feature giving rise to characteristic clinical and radiological features [1]. The concepts of ASH etiopathogenesis are basically based on intraoperative findings. The three most commonly proposed theories

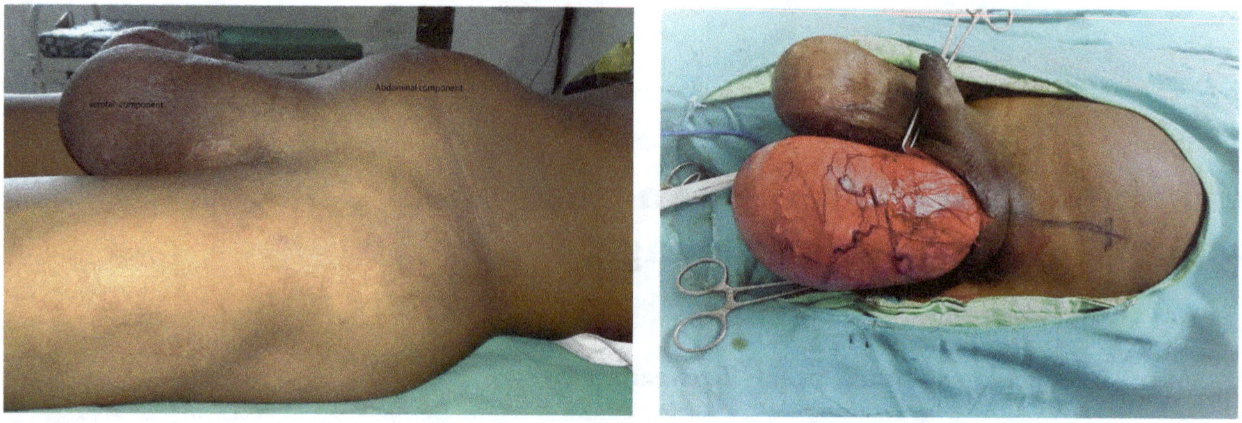

(a) (b)

Figure 1: (a) Photograph showing abdominal and scrotal components of abdominoscrotal hydrocele. (b) Excision of sac through inguinoscrotal incision.

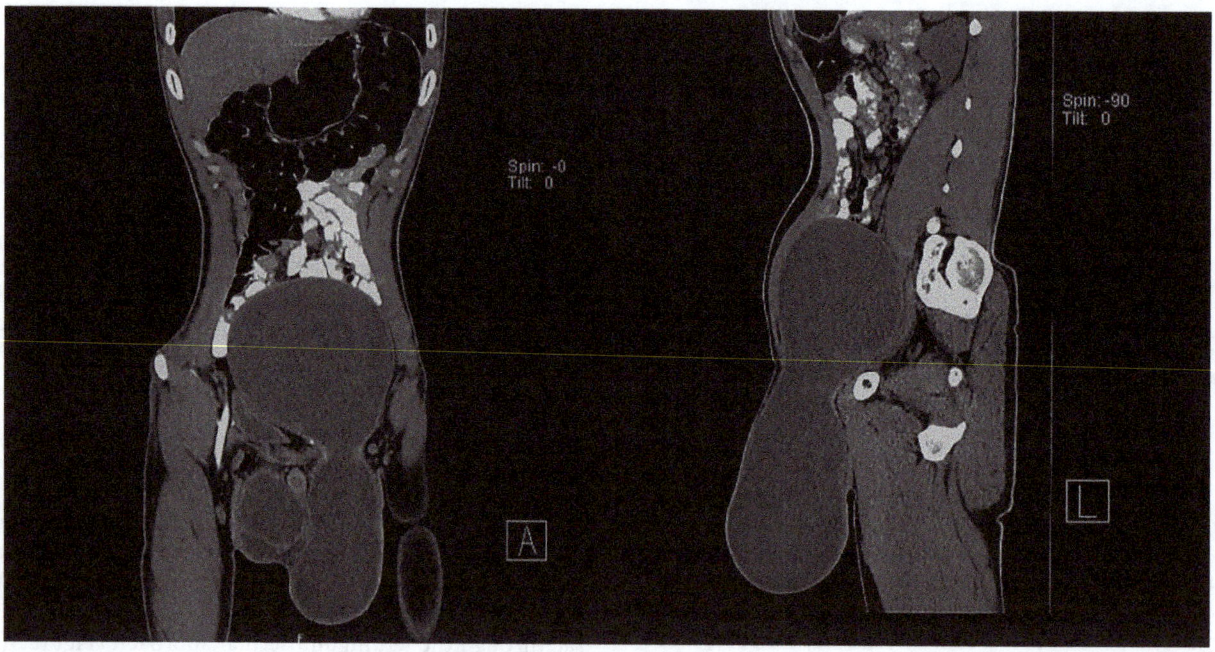

Figure 2: CECT showing hourglass appearance of ASH with intercommunicating scrotal and abdominal sac.

are "(1) cephalad extension of a simple hydrocele, (2) high obliteration of processus vaginalis (PPV), and (3) PPV acting as a one-way valve with cephalad extension of hydrocele sac." However, the most widely accepted theory is Dupuytren's original theory of high intracystic pressure in the scrotal component that leads to cephalad extension through the musculofascial inguinal canal and formation of the abdominal sac [4]. The natural history of ASH varies in pediatrics and adults; in children, it is a rapidly evolving observable lesion with the possibility of spontaneous resolution, but in adults, it is a long-standing, nonresolving progressive cystic lesion [1]. "Springing back ball sign" firstly suggested by Wlochynski et al. in which compression of the scrotum makes the abdominal component more prominent and once pressure is released scrotum regains its size is more characteristic than the cross fluctuation test [1, 5]. Testicular ectopia or cryptorchidism is the most common congenital anomalies associated with ASH [1].

USG is the initial modality of investigation in which ASH appears as an anechoic homogeneous lesion and intercommunication can be delineated on graded compression during USG [1, 6]. The CECT abdomen is required to prove definitive intercommunication and in complex cases. Magnetic resonance imaging is required to detect vascular complication like deep vein thrombosis and for suspicion of malignant transformation [1, 6].

ASH should be differentiated from hernia, chord lymphangioma, spermatocele, cystic abdominal mass, and ascites. Long-standing ASH leads to pressure-related complication like hydroureteronephrosis, deep vein thrombosis, leg edema, testicular dysraphism, and impaired spermatogenesis and rarely malignant transformation [4, 7, 8].

Malignancy with ASH seen only in 0.86% of cases, because of low incidence and serial pathological examination of specimens to rule out malignancy, could not provide any evidence that ASH is responsible for malignant transformation [1].

Surgical excision of the sac is the cornerstone of treatment in adult patients because of the unlikelihood of spontaneous resolution, to avoid pressure-related complications [4]. Different surgical techniques like scrotal, inguinal, inguinoscrotal, and laparoscopic-assisted scrotal approaches have been described in literature. The inguinoscrotal approach provides excellent exposure, and further dissection can be facilitated by decompression of sac or cutting of deep inguinal ring which helps in identification and mobilization of vas deferens and spermatic vessels for orchidopexy. In difficult cases, paramedian laparotomy may be required to dissect the sac away from the urinary bladder and other retroperitoneal structure [4]. Conservative management has been described in asymptomatic, uncomplicated pediatric ASH where spontaneous resolution is possible, or the patient is a poor candidate for surgery [1, 9].

4. Conclusion

ASH is a rare cause of abdominoscrotal swelling, which has different etiological hypotheses and multiple clinicopathological variants. Clinical examination and USG are initial modalities sufficient to make diagnoses, but CECT is required to prove intercommunication and other associated complexities. Despite available minimal invasive techniques for treatment, complete excision of the sac via inguinoscrotal incision remains the standard approach.

References

[1] R. A. Gadelkareem, "Abdominoscrotal hydrocele: a systematic review and proposed clinical grading," *African Journal of Urology*, vol. 24, no. 2, pp. 83–92, 2018.

[2] F. Luks, S. Yazbeck, Y. Homsy, and P. Collin, "The abdominoscrotal hydrocele," *European journal of pediatric surgery*, vol. 3, no. 3, pp. 176–178, 1993.

[3] G. C. Prather, "Abdominoscrotal hydrocele," *New England Journal of Medicine*, vol. 226, no. 7, pp. 255–260, 1942.

[4] A. D. Doudt, J. E. Kehoe, R. C. Ignacio, and M. S. Christman, "Abdominoscrotal hydrocele: a systematic review," *Journal of pediatric surgery*, vol. 51, no. 9, pp. 1561–1564, 2016.

[5] T. Wlochynski, J. Wassermann, and Z. Generowicz, "Abdominoscrotal hydrocele in childhood," *Journal of pediatric surgery*, vol. 28, no. 2, pp. 248–250, 1993.

[6] P. M. Kamble, A. A. Deshpande, V. B. Thapar, and K. Das, "Large abdominoscrotal hydrocele: uncommon surgical entity," *International journal of surgery case reports*, vol. 15, pp. 140–142, 2015.

[7] B. Klin, Y. Efrati, A. Mor, and I. Vinograd, "Unilateral hydroureteronephrosis caused by abdominoscrotal hydrocele," *The Journal of urology*, vol. 148, 2 Part 1, pp. 384–386, 1992.

[8] I. H. Krasna, M. Solomon, and R. Mezrich, "Unilateral leg edema caused by abdominoscrotal hydrocele: elegant diagnosis by MRI," *Journal of pediatric surgery*, vol. 27, no. 10, pp. 1349–1351, 1992.

[9] V. Upadhyay, M. Abubacker, and R. Teele, "Abdominoscrotal hydrocele-is there a place for conservative management?," *European journal of pediatric surgery*, vol. 16, no. 4, pp. 282–284, 2006.

A Conservative Approach to Inflammatory Myofibroblastic Tumor of the Bladder: A Case Report and Review of Literature

Rawad Abou Zahr,[1] **Elie Ghabi**,[2] **Mehdi Idrissi-Kaitouni**,[1] **and Thierry Roumeguere**[1]

[1]*Urology Department, Erasme Hospital, Université Libre de Bruxelles, Brussels, Belgium*
[2]*Urology Department, Saint George Hospital University Medical Center, University of Balamand, Beirut, Lebanon*

Correspondence should be addressed to Rawad Abou Zahr; rawad.abouzahr@gmail.com
and Thierry Roumeguere; thierry.roumeguere@erasme.ulb.ac.be

Academic Editor: Fumitaka Koga

Inflammatory myofibroblastic tumors (IMTs) are particularly rare tumors that have been described in various anatomic locations, of which the urinary bladder is the most common. These benign tumors are amendable to conservative therapy but are notoriously difficult to diagnose given their mimicry of malignant sarcomas and sarcomatoid carcinomas, making an accurate diagnosis paramount to spare a patient radical and unnecessary treatment. We hereby present the case of a 37-year-old female patient who was diagnosed with an IMT of the urinary bladder during workup for painless gross hematuria. Patient was successfully managed with a laparoscopic partial cystectomy and is free of recurrence 5 years after surgery. IMTs are rare benign tumors that share the same clinical presentation as malignant bladder tumors. Deep biopsy and experienced pathologist are crucial in establishing diagnosis and avoiding patient radical treatment. This case is a classical demonstration of a remarkably rare tumor that was adequately managed with conservative therapy, achieving excellent clinical outcomes.

1. Introduction

Inflammatory myofibroblastic tumors (IMTs) are particularly rare tumors that have been described in various anatomic locations such as the lungs, pancreas, bladder, and prostate [1–5]. First described by Roth in 1980, this rare entity came to be commonly reported in urinary bladders and the lungs as the most common sites [1, 4]. These tumors are characterized by a spindle cell proliferation loosely distributed in a congested myxoid stroma with variable populations of inflammatory cells [1, 3, 4]. IMTs share similar features with sarcomas and sarcomatoid carcinomas which makes the diagnosis of IMTs challenging, as these tumors tend to present with similar clinical presentation as urothelial bladder tumors. Hence, an accurate diagnosis is critical as IMTs have a benign course, are unlikely to recur or metastasize, and are amendable to conservative therapy [1, 3]. Our case is that of a 37-year-old female patient who was diagnosed with an IMT during workup for painless gross hematuria. She was successfully managed with a laparoscopic partial cystectomy and is free of recurrence 5 years postoperatively.

2. Case Presentation

A 37-year-old female, nonsmoker, presented to our institution for painless gross hematuria. She had no previous history of abdominopelvic surgery, urinary or gynecologic instrumentation, nor any history of recurrent or chronic urinary infections. Physical examination and serum biochemical investigations were unremarkable. Urine analysis and microscopy revealed numerous morphologically normal red blood cells with the presence of inflammatory cells. Significant wall thickening of the right lateral wall of the urinary bladder centered around a 2×2 cm exophytic mass was seen on computed tomography (CT) scan, as seen in Figure 1. Further assessment was done using magnetic resonance imaging (MRI) that revealed tumoral extension into the detrusor muscle. No pelvic or retroperitoneal lymphadenopathy was noted. A transurethral deep biopsy of the tumor was performed.

Histologic analysis of the resection fragments revealed evidence of ulcerations in the urothelium with submucosal proliferation of fusiform spindle cells with mild cytonuclear

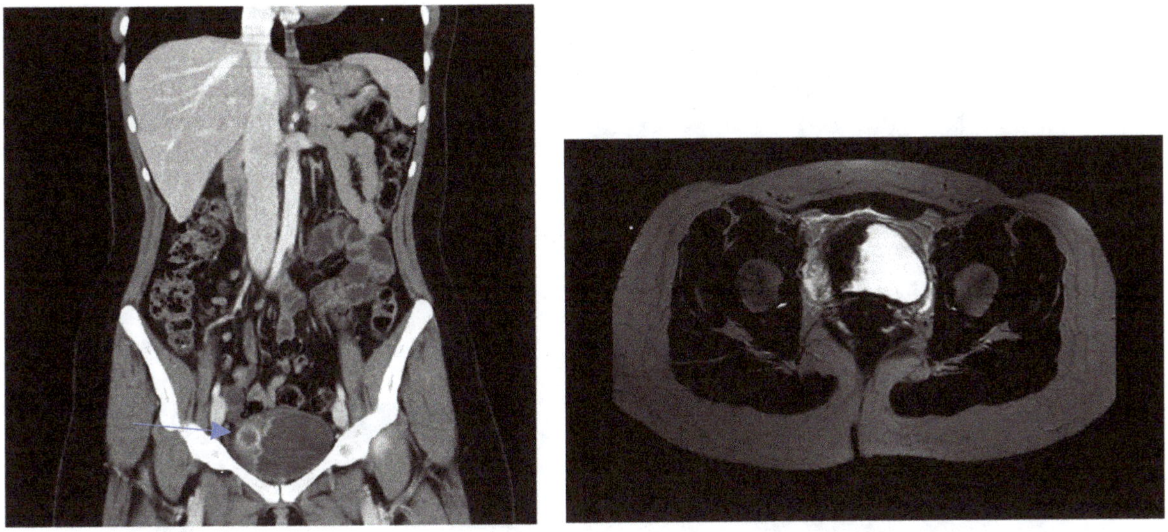

(a) (b)

FIGURE 1: Coronal CT scan (a) and axial MRI (b) demonstrating 2×2 cm exophytic polyp (arrow) associated with significant bladder wall thickening of the urinary bladder with invasion of detrusor muscle.

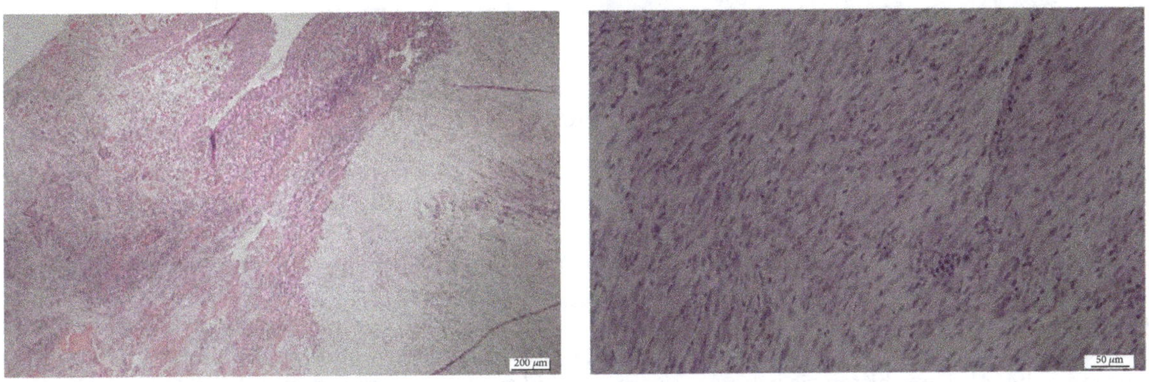

(a) (b)

FIGURE 2: Wright and Giemsa stain demonstrating fusiform spindle cells with cellular atypia and an edematous myxoid stroma under low (a) and high power (b) magnification.

atypia and minimal mitotic activity in a richly vascularized and edematous myxoid stroma. Certain foci of necrosis were noted. A dense inflammatory infiltrate composed of lymphocytes, polynuclear neutrophils, and polynuclear eosinophils was present in the tumoral tissue (Figure 2). Immunohistochemistry was positive for AE1/AE3 along the entire urothelium and less so in the spindle cell foci and positive for SMA in the spindle cell foci.

Given the histologic features and the immunohistochemical profile, diagnosis of a pseudosarcomatous myofibroblastic tumor of the urinary bladder was made. The patient successfully underwent a laparoscopic partial cystectomy to resect the remaining tumor mass (Figure 3). Histologic evaluation revealed similar findings with negative resection margins. No adjuvant treatment was offered. Close follow-up by yearly CT scan imaging and biannual cystoscopy revealed no evidence of disease recurrence 5 years postoperatively.

3. Discussion

Nonepithelial tumors of the urinary bladder make up 2% to 5% of primary neoplasms of the bladder [6]. Inflammatory myofibroblastic tumors belong to this class of neoplasms, and though numerous cases have been described yet the incidence of these rare tumors is largely unknown. They are observed across all ages but generally occur in children and young adults, with most reported cases belonging to the pediatric population, and with a slight female predominance [1, 3, 6]. IMTs are associated with smoking, prior abdominopelvic surgery, and bladder instrumentation, yet cases with no discernable risk factors have also been described [6, 7].

Pathologically, IMTs are described as gray-white or tan-yellow firm well-circumscribed lesions with sizes ranging from 1 to 20 cm and a variable degree of focal necrosis, hemorrhage or cystic changes, or calcification [8]. A cross-section of the tumor seen in our case is similar to the classical

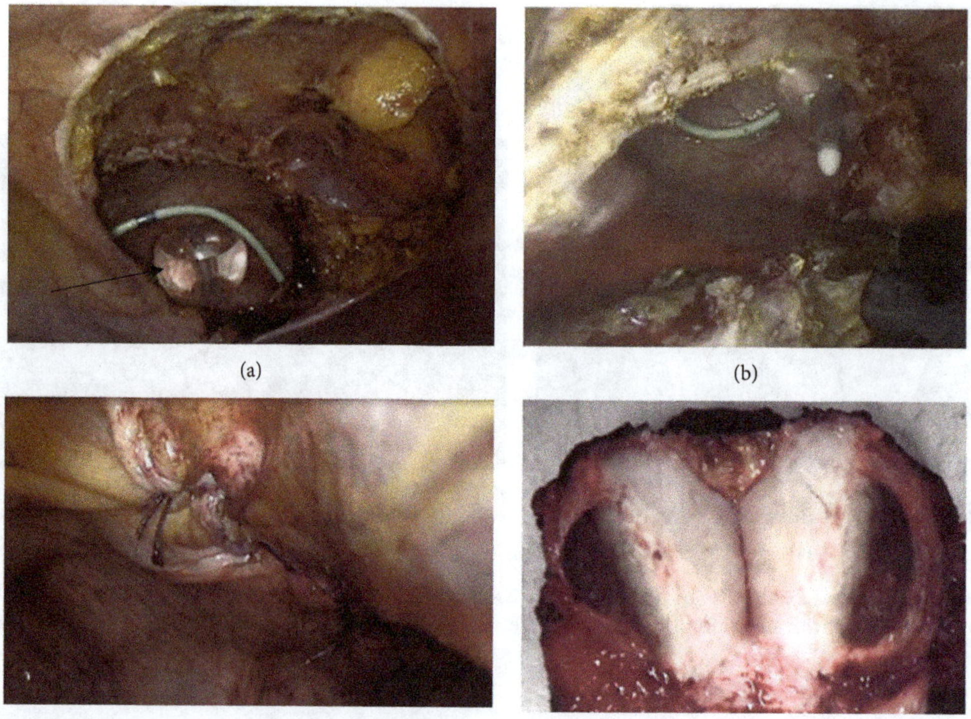

FIGURE 3: Intraoperative view of the bladder defect post partial cystectomy, arrow on foley catheter (a and b), view of the bladder post defect repair (c), and a cross-section of the tumor revealing a white soft myxoid mass (d).

appearance recognized in the literature. Histologically, the tumor is characterized by a dense proliferation of myofibroblast and fibroblast spindle cells in an edematous myxoid stroma with a large infiltrate of inflammatory cells predominantly composed of lymphocytes, neutrophils, and eosinophils [8]. The histologic features may however vary between tumors at the same site [4]. Three histologic patterns are generally recognized, the first has the appearance of granulation tissue and nodular fasciitis characterized by spindle cells in a myxoid pattern with an abundant eosinophilic cytoplasm [4, 8]. The second pattern involves densely packed spindle cells with a more prominent inflammatory component and the third is relatively hypocellular with an abundance of collagen, plasma cells, lymphocytes, and eosinophils [4, 8]. These patterns, however, are similar to those seen in malignant sarcomas and spindled carcinomas such as leiomyosarcoma, sarcomatoid carcinoma, and rhabdomyosarcoma [8]. Importantly, low degrees of cellular and nuclear atypia and a low number of mitotic figures are important distinguishing factors that may help in diagnosing an IMT [6].

The immunohistochemical profile of IMTs often overlaps with other malignancies, which makes the diagnosis of an IMT more difficult. In general, IMTs stain positive for vimentin, desmin, smooth muscle actin, muscle-specific actin, and keratin [1]. ALK positivity is recognized as a particularly useful and specific immunological marker for IMTs [1]. IMTs also characteristically stain negative for myogenin (Myf4) and MyoD1 which are generally positive in embryonal rhamdomyosarcomas, a malignant soft tissue tumor that shares similar histologic features with IMTs [1].

Clinically, IMTs are slow-growing benign tumors that are amendable to conservative treatment [1, 3]. Generally, management is surgical with complete resection with negative margins being critical. Hence, conservative management can consist of a partial cystectomy preserving the quality of life of the patient and avoiding the complications and morbidity of radical cystectomy. A limited role for chemotherapy exists; they are almost exclusively used in the management of unresectable tumors, incomplete resections, or if resections would lead to significant morbidity [1, 2]. IMTs generally do not recur following complete resection; however, recurrence in genitourinary cases has been observed in up to 2.7% of patients [1]. Timely follow-up is therefore crucial with imaging or endoscopy as appropriate, to identify recurrent disease or possible metastasis.

4. Conclusion

In conclusion, inflammatory myofibroblastic tumors are remarkably rare nonepithelial benign neoplasms of unknown pathogenesis that presents similarly to malignant diseases. These tumors present a diagnostic challenge due to the overlap of histologic and immunohistochemical features seen in malignant neoplasms such as leiomyosarcoma, embryonal rhabdomyosarcoma, carcinoid sarcoma, and other malignant soft tissue neoplasms. Certain histologic and immunohistochemical findings are somewhat specific to IMTs which aids in differentiating them. A deep transurethral resection biopsy and an experienced pathologist are paramount in establishing the diagnosis and avoiding the patient radical treatments.

The standard of care is surgical resection with negative margins with chemotherapy and radiotherapy reserved for unresectable or incompletely resected tumors. These tumors generally do not recur or metastasize; however, cases of recurrence or metastasis have been reported. Our case is a classical demonstration of an IMT discovered in a 37-year-old female managed with a laparoscopic partial cystectomy and remains recurrence free after 5 years.

Acknowledgments

The authors have no acknowledgments to declare.

References

[1] J. C. V. Laylo, N. L. Lim, and J. J. V. Remo, "Inflammatory myofibroblastic tumor of the urinary bladder: a prognostically favorable spindle cell neoplasm," *Urology Case Reports*, vol. 34, article 101474, 2021.

[2] Z. Chen, Y. Lin, M. Li et al., "Pancreatic inflammatory myofibroblastic of the pancreatic neck: a case report and literature review," 2020, https://www.researchsquare.com/article/rs-131102/v2.

[3] A. Higazy and M. Kandel, "Prolapsing inflammatory myofibroblastic tumor of the urinary bladder: a case report and a review of literature," *Urology Case Reports*, vol. 31, article 101191, 2020.

[4] S. Kovach, A. Fischer, P. Katzman et al., "Inflammatory myofibroblastic tumors," *Journal of Surgical Oncology*, vol. 94, no. 5, pp. 385–391, 2006.

[5] M. S. Kim and S. C. Lim, "A rare case of inflammatory myofibroblastic tumor of the prostate and review of the literature," *In Vivo*, vol. 34, no. 4, pp. 2043–2048, 2020.

[6] A. Lekas, A. Parasi, T. Papathomas et al., "Pseudosarcomatous myofibroblastic lesion of the urinary bladder: a rare entity posing a diagnostic challenge and therapeutic dilemma," *Diagnostic Pathology*, vol. 3, no. 1, p. 11, 2008.

[7] T. Vasilakaki, K. Koulia, A. Tsavari et al., "Pseudosarcomatous myofibroblastic proliferation of the urinary bladder: a rare entity," *Urology*, vol. 83, no. 6, pp. 1409–1411, 2014.

[8] L. Cheng, S. Foster, G. Mac Lennan, A. Lopez-Beltran, S. Zhang, and R. Montironi, "Inflammatory myofibroblastic tumors of the genitourinary tract—single entity or continuum?," *Journal of Urology*, vol. 180, no. 4, pp. 1235–1240, 2008.

50

Penile Glans Necrosis following Prostatic Artery Embolization for the Treatment of Benign Prostatic Hyperplasia: A Rare but Serious Complication

Eric Chung[1,2,3]

[1]AndroUrology Centre, Brisbane QLD, Australia
[2]University of Queensland, Princess Alexandra Hospital, Brisbane, QLD, Australia
[3]Macquarie University Hospital, Sydney, NSW, Australia

Correspondence should be addressed to Eric Chung; ericchg@hotmail.com

Academic Editor: Mohamed A. Ghoneim

Background. Prostate artery embolization (PAE) is a novel endovascular procedure to treat men with benign prostatic hyperplasia (BPH) symptoms who wish to maintain sexual potency postoperatively. However, serious treatment-related adverse events (TRAEs) of PAE such as penile glans necrosis (PGN) can be devastating and require urgent attention. *Case presentation.* Mr GM is a 65-year-old sexually active Anglo-Saxon man who have long-standing BPH symptoms unresponsive to medical therapy. While he had an uneventful bilateral superselective PAE using gel foam, there were signs to suggest of PGN, and this was treated conservatively. The patient presented to the emergency department 5 days later with a painful, dark penile glans and accompanying urinary dysuria and hematuria. Clinical examination confirmed evolving PGN. He received 10 courses of hyperbaric oxygen therapy (HBOT) with complete resolution of his PGN. *Conclusion.* While superselective embolization is usually always performed, nontarget embolization may occur, as intravascular particles may reflux into adjacent vessels. In this unique and extremely rare case report of PGN following PAE, complete resolution was achieved with HBOT. Proposed benefits of HBOT include anti-inflammation, promotion of neovascularization, and induced rate of collagen deposition, resulting in a faster and more effective resolution of PGN.

1. Introduction

Prostatic artery embolization (PAE) is a relatively safe and effective treatment for men with lower urinary tract symptoms secondary to benign prostatic hyperplasia (BPH) [1, 2]. The mechanism of action for PAE to achieve targeted prostate tissue apoptosis occurs through catheter-directed particulate microembolic agents injected directly into the prostatic artery under fluoroscopic guidance [3, 4]. Given its unique and minimally invasive approach, PAE has gained considerable interest as an alternative to other contemporary minimally invasive BPH surgery that offers preservation of the sexual function postoperatively.

Common treatment-related adverse events (TRAE) include urinary tract infection, acute urinary retention, dysuria, and persistent urinary symptoms [1, 2]. However, serious TRAE can occur when nontarget embolization of intravascular particles refluxes into adjacent penile, vesical, or rectal arteries causing bladder wall ischemia, ischemic glans of the peni,s and ischemic rectitis [1, 5, 6]. We present a rare case of penile glans necrosis (PGN) secondary to nontarget embolization during PAE and the role of hyperbaric oxygen therapy (HBOT).

2. Case Report

This case report has received institutional ethics review board approval and patient informed consent. Mr GM is a 65-year-old sexually active man who has long-standing BPH symptoms. He has tried oral Tamsulosin therapy with minimal clinical efficacy and is bothered by the retrograde ejaculation. He has a normal erectile function and is sexually active. His other medical history includes hypertension, hyperlipidemia, and gout.

Following discussion regarding various minimally invasive BPH surgeries, he has elected to undergo PAE to improve his urinary flow while at the same time preserve his sexual function. Preoperative planning was undertaken using computer tomography angiography (CTA) pelvis which showed a prostatic volume of 138 cc (68 × 60 × 65 mm).

A single operator, who had 15 years of experience in endovascular procedures and 5 years of experience in PAE, performed bilateral superselective PAE under local anesthesia with mild sedation. The total time taken for PAE was 118 minutes. Under ultrasound-guided left brachial artery puncture, a 4 French CXI guide catheter placed into the anterior division of the internal iliac arteries on both sides. Headway duo microcatheter was used for selective right prostate artery catheterization. This was uneventful with good uptake of embolic into the prostate with no observed collateral circulation. On the left access to the prostate artery was difficult. It came off the anterior division of the internal iliac artery with two other vessels, both of which went to the bladder. It was very difficult to select the prostate artery despite it being quite large. This was eventually catheterized using a synchrosoft guidewire with a very marked hook shape on the end. Flat-panel CT showed a satisfactory appearance to the pre-embolization picture with the only prostate selected. During the course of the embolization, it became clear that collateral vessels from the lateral prostatic artery to the penis had opened up (Figure 1). This was treated with Gelfoam with further Gelfoam used at the end of the embolization procedure. A reasonable volume of embolic injected on this site, and hemostasis achieved without difficulty.

Immediately postembolization, Mr GM complained of perineal discomfort and urinary frequency. These symptoms are thought to be secondary to some off-target embolization to the tip of the penis as the arteries to the penis opened up during the course of embolization of the left-sided prostate artery. The patient developed a small area of punctate purple discoloration at the tip of the penis with sensitivity within the distal urethra and hypersensitivity and a painful glans penis. Since the patient was able to void, he was discharged home with simple analgesia.

However, the patient presented to the emergency department 5 days after embolization with a painful, dark glans penis consistent with an evolving PGN (Figure 2). He reports erectile dysfunction although he denied bowel issue, sensory change, or motor weakness to his gluteal or lower limb.

Following a discussion on his condition and various treatment options, he was referred to receive HBOT and completed 10 courses of therapy. At a follow-up visit 4 weeks following his last HBOT session, he reported resolution of his penile pain, glans discoloration, dysuria, and hematuria. The patient reported normal penile sensation, regained normal erection, and engaged in satisfactory sexual activity. Clinical examination showed almost complete resolution of his PGN.

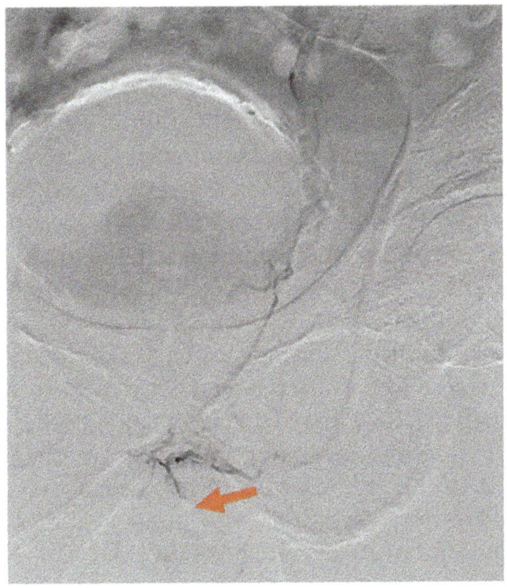

Figure 1: Presence of collateral vessels from the lateral prostatic artery to the penis and nontarget embolization of the penile artery (arrow).

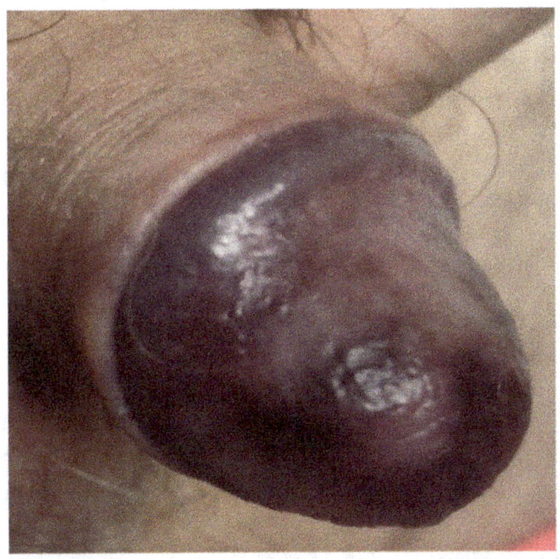

Figure 2: The appearance of penile glans necrosis at day 5 of postembolization.

3. Discussion

Preoperative workup includes CTA of the prostatic vessels to determine underlying prostatic vascular anatomy since multiple pelvic vessel anastomoses can present considerable technical challenges [4]. If significant vascular anastomoses are identified, the angiocatheter can be positioned distal to the vessel, or protective coil embolization is performed. Hence, PAE outcome can be variable and is highly operator-dependent; although there are concerted efforts to standardize and improve the reproducibility of PAE. Benign TRAE accounts for over 99% of all complications, and these include post-PAE syndrome, dysuria, urinary tract infection, hematuria, hematospermia, and urinary retention while serious complications due to nontarget embolization can result in ischemia of bladder, rectum, or penis [1–4]. However, the large variations in prostatic artery anatomy with collateral anastomoses can lead to nontarget embolization with subsequent ischemia, inflammation, and ulceration of affected organs such as PGN [6].

While the exact mechanism by which HBOT works is debatable, it is theorized that HBOT improves the oxygen concentration in a person's blood, thereby increasing the amount of oxygen reaching the areas that need to heal [7]. There are several beneficial properties of HBOT concomitant with the elevated oxygen distribution in tissue including anti-inflammation and promotion of neovascularization through vascular endothelial growth factor proliferation, augmented fibroblast, lymphocyte and macrophage activity, tissue, and wound repair as well as bactericidal activity. Furthermore, it is thought that HBOT may be able to support these mechanisms by increasing the amount of oxygen in the blood and directing it to the regions where it is needed most, thereby decreases the necessary time for wound healing as well as the induced rate of collagen deposition [7].

4. Conclusion

This unique but devastating case of PGN secondary to PAE illustrates the importance of discussing the risk of nontarget embolization with patients, and that HBOT can be an effective treatment option. As the practice of PAE takes off, education and mentoring are essential for its safe uptake worldwide. Clinicians must understand PAE's role with its strengths and weaknesses to enable optimal patient selection, ensure the best results, and minimize complications.

References

[1] S. M. Schreuder, A. E. Scholtens, J. A. Reekers, and S. Bipat, "The role of prostatic arterial embolization in patients with benign prostatic hyperplasia: a systematic review," *Cardiovascular and Interventional Radiology*, vol. 37, no. 5, pp. 1198–1219, 2014.

[2] S. Feng, Y. Tian, W. Liu et al., "Prostatic arterial embolization treating moderate-to-severe lower urinary tract symptoms related to benign prostate hyperplasia: a meta-analysis," *Cardiovascular and Interventional Radiology*, vol. 40, no. 1, pp. 22–32, 2017.

[3] F. C. Carnevale, A. M. Moreira, A. M. de Assis, and A. A. Antunes, "Prostatic artery embolization for the treatment of lower urinary tract symptoms due to benign prostatic hyperplasia: 10 years' experience," *Radiology*, vol. 296, no. 2, pp. 444–451, 2020.

[4] F. Sun, V. Crisóstomo, C. Báez-Díaz, and F. M. Sánchez, "Prostatic artery embolization (PAE) for symptomatic benign prostatic hyperplasia (BPH): part 2, insights into the technical rationale," *Cardiovascular and Interventional Radiology*, vol. 39, no. 2, pp. 161–169, 2016.

[5] A. M. Moreira, A. M. de Assis, F. C. Carnevale, A. A. Antunes, M. Srougi, and G. G. Cerri, "A review of adverse events related to prostatic artery embolization for treatment of bladder outlet obstruction due to BPH," *Cardiovascular and Interventional Radiology*, vol. 40, no. 10, pp. 1490–1500, 2017.

[6] N. Kisilevzky, C. Laudanna Neto, and A. Cividanes, "Ischemia of the glans penis following prostatic artery embolization," *Journal of Vascular and Interventional Radiology*, vol. 27, no. 11, pp. 1745–1747, 2016.

[7] J. Gandhi, O. Seyam, N. L. Smith, G. Joshi, S. Vatsia, and S. A. Khan, "Clinical utility of hyperbaric oxygen therapy in genitourinary medicine," *Medical Gas Research*, vol. 8, no. 1, pp. 29–33, 2018.

51

Brain Complete Response to Cabozantinib prior to Radiation Therapy in Metastatic Renal Cell Carcinoma

An Uche,[1] Chad Sila,[1] Tad Tanoura,[1] James Yeh,[1] Neil Bhowmick,[2] Edwin Posadas,[2] Robert Figlin,[2] and Jun Gong[3]

[1]*Division of Hematology/Oncology, Department of Medicine, Harbor-UCLA Medical Center, 1000 W Carson St, Torrance, CA 90509, USA*
[2]*Division of Hematology/Oncology, Department of Medicine, Cedars-Sinai Medical Center, 8700 Beverly Blvd, Los Angeles, CA 90048, USA*
[3]*Division of Hematology/Oncology, Department of Medicine, Cedars-Sinai Medical Center, 8700 Beverly Blvd, AC1042B, Los Angeles, CA 90048, USA*

Correspondence should be addressed to Jun Gong; jun.gong@cshs.org

Academic Editor: Apul Goel

Cabozantinib represents an established vascular endothelial growth factor- (VEGF-) tyrosine kinase inhibitor (TKI) in the treatment paradigm of metastatic renal cell carcinoma (mRCC). Its activity in mRCC patients with brain metastases (BMs) has been largely underreported in prospective clinical trials. We present the unique case of a heavily pretreated mRCC patient with BMs who achieved a brain complete response to cabozantinib prior to receiving radiation therapy. We end with a literature review and discussion of the biologic rationale and growing evidence supporting the intracranial activity of cabozantinib.

1. Introduction

Cabozantinib, a multitarget vascular endothelial growth factor- (VEGF-) tyrosine kinase inhibitor (TKI), is currently approved by the US Food and Drug Administration (FDA) for the first-line treatment of metastatic renal cell carcinoma (mRCC) based on a superior progression-free survival (PFS) benefit over sunitinib in the phase II CABOSUN trial [1] and the second-line and beyond treatment in mRCC based on a superior overall survival (OS), PFS, and overall response rate (ORR) benefit over everolimus in the phase III METEOR trial [2]. Despite the establishment of cabozantinib as a standard of care therapy in the treatment paradigm of mRCC, its activity in mRCC patients with brain metastases (BMs) remains largely unexplored. We present the case of a heavily pretreated mRCC patient with BMs who experienced an unusual brain complete response (CR) to cabozantinib.

2. Case Presentation

The patient is a 48-year-old male who presented with gross hematuria in February 2017. Computed tomography (CT) of the chest, abdomen, and pelvis (CAP) showed bilateral renal masses, numerous bilateral pulmonary nodules, and mediastinal and right hilar lymphadenopathy. Pathology from a transbronchial lymph node biopsy (station 11R) revealed metastatic renal cell carcinoma. He was started on sunitinib 50 mg daily for 14 days every 21 days cycle and experienced a partial response (PR) until April 2018 when he developed worsening flank pain. CT CAP showed progression of disease (PD) with an enlarging right renal mass and right hilar lymphadenopathy. He was started on nivolumab 3 mg/kg every 14 days. After 8 cycles of nivolumab, patient developed worsening headache and blurry vision of the left eye, which prompted a magnetic resonance imaging (MRI) of the brain that showed a 2.5 cm enhancing, right parietal mass associated with hemorrhage and edema as well as punctuate areas of enhancement in the left frontal lobe and left cerebellar peduncle. Of note, a baseline MRI brain obtained after his initial diagnosis was negative for metastatic disease. Repeat CT CAP also showed PD with an enlarging left renal mass and worsening mediastinal lymphadenopathy. Patient was started on third-line cabozantinib 60 mg daily

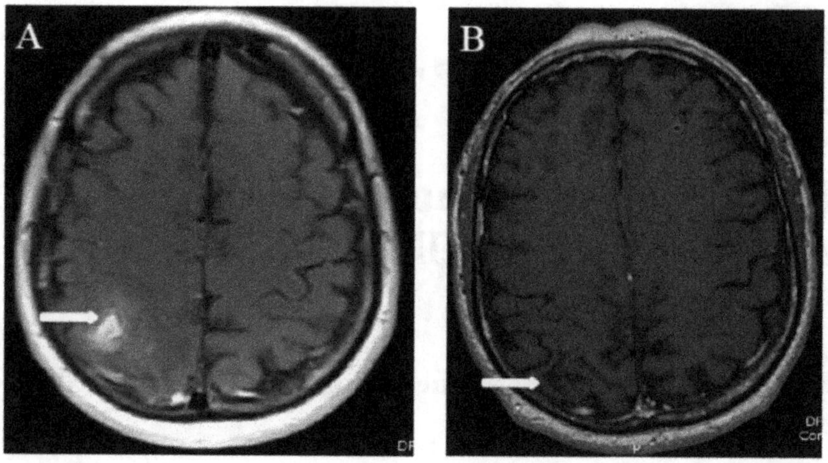

(a) (b)

Figure 1: *MRI brain.* (a) An axial, postcontrast-enhanced, fat-saturated T1-weighted image of the brain shows a 2.0 x 1.0 cm right parietal mass with ill-defined area of enhancement. (b) An axial, contrast enhanced, fat-saturated T1-weighted image of the brain, 3 weeks after therapy with cabozantinib, shows resolution of the prior mass and surrounding enhancement.

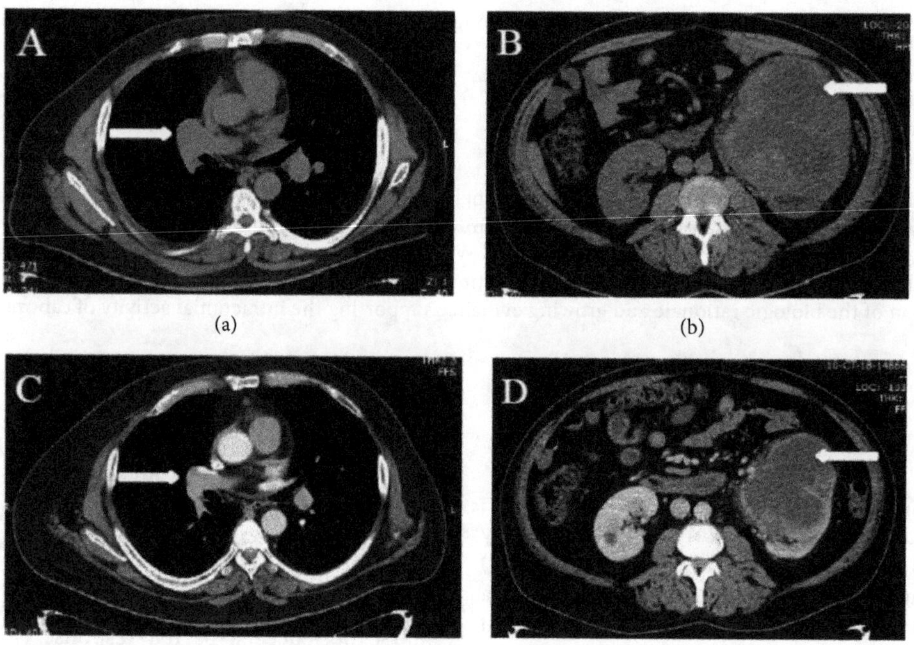

(a) (b) (c) (d)

Figure 2: *CT CAP.* (a) and (b) Axial images of CT CAP showed right sided hilar lymphadenopathy and a large left kidney mass. (c) and (d) Axial images of CT CAP showed improvement in right sided hilar lymphadenopathy and reduction in size of left kidney mass, after 8 weeks of therapy with cabozantinib.

and received a course of dexamethasone 4 mg twice daily with referral to radiation oncology for treatment of his brain metastases. Three weeks after starting cabozantinib, a repeat MRI brain was obtained for radiation planning and showed complete resolution of the right parietal mass with now encephalomalacia of the area (Figure 1). Patient also reported improvement of his headache and blurry vision. Due to resolution of the right parietal mass, radiation therapy was no longer deemed necessary and the patient remains on cabozantinib 60 mg daily. A CT CAP, obtained 8 weeks after initiation of cabozantinib therapy, showed partial response with reduction in size of mediastinal lymphadenopathy and bilateral renal masses (Figure 2).

3. Discussion

The median OS for mRCC has improved to approximately 30 months in the current decade from 13 months in the era of cytokine therapy nearly 3 decades ago [3, 4]. Although accounting for approximately 8% of all RCC metastatic sites [5], the survival of mRCC patients with BMs treated in the VEGF-TKI era remains poor with several retrospective series having shown that median OS ranges from 5.4-14.4 months [6–8]. In particular, patients with >4 BMs have a significantly worse OS (3.9 months) compared to those with ≤4 BMs (15.4 months; hazard ratio (HR) 3.02, 95% confidence interval (CI) 1.33-6.83, p=0.005) [6]. VEGF-TKI therapy has been shown to prolong time to BM development (median 28 months) compared to mRCC patients who did not receive TKI therapy (median 11.5 months) though preclinical investigations have demonstrated limited penetration of sorafenib or sunitinb across the blood-brain barrier [9].

Patients with BMs have historically been excluded from most prospective targeted therapy clinical trials in RCC; although the METEOR and CABOSUN trials allowed treatment of mRCC patients having BMs with cabozantinib, this subset was underrepresented (<1%) in METEOR and not reported in CABOSUN [1, 2]. Nevertheless, there exists biologic rationale for efficacy of cabozantinib in mRCC patients with BMs as expression of MET, a target of cabozantinib, was found to be in 35% of BMs compared to 0% of primary RCC tumors [10]. A separate series corroborated findings that cMET expression was significantly higher in metastatic sites compared to primary RCC tumor sites [11]. Furthermore, the ability of cabozantinib to penetrate the central nervous system (CNS) has recently been supported in several tumor types including glioblastoma, RCC metastatic to the brain, and non-small-cell lung cancer metastatic to the brain where cabozantinib demonstrated therapeutic efficacy [12–14].

Data on the efficacy of other commonly used VEGF-TKIs and systemic agents in treating RCC BMs are limited. Expanded access studies of sorafenib have shown a 12-week disease control rate (DCR) 60.7% and a median PFS of 7.4 months, while sunitinib has shown an ORR of 9% (clinical benefit rate or CBR of 42%) and median PFS of 5.3 months in RCC patients with BMs [15, 16]. In an expanded access study of nivolumab, an ORR of 18.8% or CBR of 53% was produced in RCC patients with BMs [17]. Data on the intracranial activity of nivolumab and ipilimumab in RCC BMs is limited, but in a melanoma BM cohort the combination showed an intracranial clinical benefit rate of 57% with a 26% CR rate and 30% PR rate [18]. In a triple-negative breast cancer preclinical study, the mTOR inhibitor temsirolimus had little activity in treating BMs at high concentrations of 100 nM [19]. In mouse models exploring the ability of pazopanib to penetrate the CNS, only 1.5% of the concentration in plasma was able to reach the brain implying severe restriction of this agent for brain penetration [20]. The variable ability of VEGF-TKIs to penetrate the CNS may be dependent on reliance on active uptake through drug transporters. For example, sorafenib and sunitinib showed low-moderate affinity for the ATP-binding cassette (ABC) transporter, ABCB1, where brain penetration was increased 1.9-fold and 2.9-fold for sorafenib and sunitinib, respectively, in knockout mice with the absence of ABCB1 when compared to controls [21].

Our case represents among the initial cases of a brain CR to cabozantinib in a heavily pretreated mRCC patient and adds to a growing body of evidence supporting its intracranial antitumor activity. Notably, nivolumab in combination with ipilimumab and nivolumab monotherapy comprise another FDA-approved standard of care therapy in the first-line and second-line treatment of mRCC, respectively; though patients with BMs were excluded in their registration trials [22, 23]. On this note, cabozantinib may represent a preferable option in mRCC patients with BMs given the current evidence at hand. Further investigation of the intracranial activity of cabozantinib in mRCC is warranted. Results of an ongoing BM-specific clinical trial (NCT02260531) are eagerly awaited in hope that the CNS penetrating ability and pharmacokinetics of cabozantinib will be better understood.

4. Conclusion

We have presented an unusual case of a patient with mRCC and BMs experiencing a brain CR to cabozantinib prior to radiation therapy. Our report contributes to the accumulating but overall limited evidence on the intracranial activity of cabozantinib. Further investigation is duly warranted to evaluate the ability of cabozantinib to penetrate the blood-brain barrier and elicit a clinical response. This is especially important in mRCC patients with BMs where this subset has been historically underrepresented in prospective VEGF-TKI clinical trials.

References

[1] T. K. Choueiri, S. Halabi, B. L. Sanford et al., "Cabozantinib versus sunitinib as initial targeted therapy for patients with metastatic renal cell carcinoma of poor or intermediate risk: the alliance A031203 CABOSUN trial," *Journal of Clinical Oncology: Official Journal of The American Society of Clinical Oncology*, vol. 35, no. 6, pp. 591–597, 2017.

[2] T. K. Choueiri, B. Escudier, T. Powles et al., "Cabozantinib versus everolimus in advanced renal cell carcinoma (METEOR): final results from a randomised, open-label, phase 3 trial," *The Lancet Oncology*, vol. 17, no. 7, pp. 917–927, 2016.

[3] J. J. Hsieh, M. P. Purdue, S. Signoretti et al., "Renal cell carcinoma," *Nature Reviews Disease Primers*, vol. 3, Article ID 17009, 2017.

[4] R. J. Motzer, J. Bacik, B. A. Murphy, P. Russo, and M. Mazumdar, "Interferon-alfa as a comparative treatment for clinical trials of new therapies against advanced renal cell carcinoma," *Journal of Clinical Oncology: Official Journal of The American Society of Clinical Oncology*, vol. 20, no. 1, pp. 289–296, 2002.

[5] M. Bianchi, M. Sun, C. Jeldres et al., "Distribution of metastatic sites in renal cell carcinoma: a population-based analysis," *Annals of Oncology: Official Journal of The European Society for Medical Oncology*, vol. 23, no. 4, pp. 973–980, 2012.

[6] M. M. Vickers, H. Al-Harbi, T. K. Choueiri et al., "Prognostic factors of survival for patients with metastatic renal cell carcinoma with brain metastases treated with targeted therapy: Results from the international metastatic renal cell carcinoma database consortium," *Clinical Genitourinary Cancer*, vol. 11, no. 3, pp. 311–315, 2013.

[7] J. Verma, E. Jonasch, P. K. Allen et al., "The impact of tyrosine kinase inhibitors on the multimodality treatment of brain

metastases from renal cell carcinoma," *American Journal of Clinical Oncology*, vol. 36, no. 6, pp. 620–624, 2013.

[8] I. Yildiz, A. Bilici, N. Karadurmuş et al., "Prognostic factors for survival in metastatic renal cell carcinoma patients with brain metastases receiving targeted therapy," *Tumori Journal*, vol. 104, no. 6, pp. 444–450, 2018.

[9] A. Z. Dudek, A. Raza, M. Chi et al., "Brain metastases from renal cell carcinoma in the era of tyrosine kinase inhibitors," *Clinical Genitourinary Cancer*, vol. 11, no. 2, pp. 155–160, 2013.

[10] L. Derosa, G. Le Teuff, M. Khordahi et al., "Inter and intra-tumor heterogeneity of PD-L1 and MET expression in metastatic renal cell carcinoma (mRCC)," *Journal of Clinical Oncology*, vol. 35, 15, p. 4569, 2017.

[11] A.-K. A. Lalani, K. P. Gray, L. Albiges et al., "Differential expression of c-Met between primary and metastatic sites in clear-cell renal cell carcinoma and its association with PD-L1 expression," *Oncotarget*, vol. 8, no. 61, pp. 103428–103436, 2017.

[12] S. J. Klempner, A. Borghei, B. Hakimian, S. M. Ali, and S.-H. I. Ou, "Intracranial activity of cabozantinib in MET exon 14–positive NSCLC with brain metastases," *Journal of Thoracic Oncology: Official Publication of the International Association for the Study of Lung Cancer*, vol. 12, no. 1, pp. 152–156, 2017.

[13] P. Y. Wen, J. Drappatz, J. De Groot et al., "Phase II study of cabozantinib in patients with progressive glioblastoma: subset analysis of patients naive to antiangiogenic therapy," *Neuro-Oncology*, vol. 20, no. 2, pp. 249–258, 2018.

[14] C. Ciccarese, R. Iacovelli, C. Mosillo, and G. Tortora, "Exceptional response to cabozantinib of rapidly evolving brain metastases of renal cell carcinoma: a case report and review of the literature," *Clinical Genitourinary Cancer*, vol. 16, no. 5, pp. e1069–e1071, 2018.

[15] J. Beck, G. Procopio, E. Bajetta et al., "Final results of the european advanced renal cell carcinoma sorafenib (EU-ARCCS) expanded-access study: a large open-label study in diverse community settings," *Annals of Oncology: Official Journal of The European Society for Medical Oncology*, vol. 22, no. 8, pp. 1812–1823, 2011.

[16] M. E. Gore, C. Szczylik, C. Porta et al., "Final results from the large sunitinib global expanded-access trial in metastatic renal cell carcinoma," *British Journal of Cancer*, vol. 113, no. 1, pp. 12–19, 2015.

[17] U. De Giorgi, G. Cartenì, D. Giannarelli et al., "Safety and efficacy of nivolumab for metastatic renal cell carcinoma: real-world results from an expanded access programme," *BJU International*, vol. 123, no. 1, pp. 98–105, 2019.

[18] H. A. Tawbi, P. A. Forsyth, A. Algazi et al., "Combined nivolumab and ipilimumab in melanoma metastatic to the brain," *The New England Journal of Medicine*, vol. 379, no. 8, pp. 722–730, 2018.

[19] H. Zhao, K. Cui, F. Nie et al., "The effect of mTOR inhibition alone or combined with MEK inhibitors on brain metastasis: an in vivo analysis in triple-negative breast cancer models," *Breast Cancer Research and Treatment*, vol. 131, no. 2, pp. 425–436, 2012.

[20] M. Minocha, V. Khurana, and A. K. Mitra, "Determination of pazopanib (GW-786034) in mouse plasma and brain tissue by liquid chromatography-tandem mass spectrometry (LC/MS-MS)," *Journal of Chromatography B, Analytical Technologies in The Biomedical and Life Sciences*, vol. 901, pp. 85–92, 2012.

[21] S. Hu, Z. Chen, R. Franke et al., "Interaction of the multikinase inhibitors sorafenib and sunitinib with solute carriers and ATP-binding cassette transporters," *Clinical Cancer Research: An Official Journal of The American Association for Cancer Research*, vol. 15, no. 19, pp. 6062–6069, 2009.

[22] R. J. Motzer, B. Escudier, D. F. McDermott et al., "Nivolumab versus everolimus in advanced renal-cell carcinoma," *The New England Journal of Medicine*, vol. 373, no. 19, pp. 1803–1813, 2015.

[23] R. J. Motzer, N. M. Tannir, D. F. McDermott et al., "Nivolumab plus ipilimumab versus sunitinib in advanced renal-cell carcinoma," *The New England Journal of Medicine*, vol. 378, no. 14, pp. 1277–1290, 2018.

52

Pyelolithotomy in a Patient with Complete Coraliform Calcification Induced by a Double-J Ureteral Stent

Miguel Bonfitto,[1] **Analaura de Oliveira Cury**,[2] **Victoria Caroline Pagelkopf**,[3] **Vinicius Ramos Bezerra de Morais**,[3] **and Carlos Abib Cury**[4]

[1] *São José do Rio Preto Base Hospital/Famerp, SP, Brazil*
[2] *Votuporanga School of Medicine, SP, Brazil*
[3] *São José do Rio Preto School of Medicine (Famerp), SP, Brazil*
[4] *Urology Sector, São José do Rio Preto School of Medicine (Famerp), SP, Brazil*

Correspondence should be addressed to Miguel Bonfitto; miguelbonfitto@gmail.com

Academic Editor: Mohamed A. Ghoneim

The placement of a double-J ureteral stent enables the treatment of upper urinary tract obstruction. Despite advances, forgetting the stent favors the occurrence of calcification, leading to increased morbidity rates, lawsuits, and a financial burden on the healthcare system. This paper describes a successful pyelolithotomy for the removal of a calcified double-J ureteral stent.

1. Introduction

The placement of a double-J ureteral stent enables the draining and relief of obstructive processes of the upper urinary tract [1]. Despite the benefits of this stent and its innovations, complications stemming from the implanted stent constitute an important cause of morbidity [1]. The main complications are occlusion, calcification, migration, fragmentation, the formation of calculus, and compromised kidney function, which can be caused by oversaturation or the long-term presence of the stent [1, 2]. The removal of a calcified stent can be a challenge to urologists and requires procedures ranging from noninvasive extracorporeal lithotripsy to open surgery [1–4].

We report the difficult treatment of a patient with complete coraliform calcification of a double-J stent, highlighting the importance of avoiding complications secondary to the presence of the ureteral stent, as such factors contribute to patient morbidity and mortality.

2. Presentation of Case

A 38-year-old male patient was sent to the urology clinic due to difficulty in removing a calcified double-J stent in the left ureter. The patient reported that he had sought a different medical center seven months earlier with the complaint of left-side renal colic associated with nausea and vomiting and was diagnosed with a ureteral stone. After referral to our service, the patient was asymptomatic and the physical examination revealed a good general health status with a flat, painless abdomen. Cystoscopy performed for the removal of the stent was unsuccessful. The patient was then submitted to computed tomography of the kidneys and urinary ducts (Figure 1), which revealed a stent on the left side with complete coraliform calcification extending to the ureteropelvic junction and obliteration of the adjacent fat. The patient was submitted to extracorporeal lithotripsy without success. Thirteen months after admission, extended pyelolithotomy was performed with complete dissection of the renal sinus, exposing the entire pelvis, followed by a U-shaped incision around the renal sinus, enabling access to all renal infundibula. The calcified double-J stent was then removed from the renal sinus toward the ureteropelvic junction. The patient demonstrated good postoperative evolution, with the absence of residual calculi in the follow-up abdominal X-ray (Figure 2), receiving discharge on the third day. The patient is currently in follow-up.

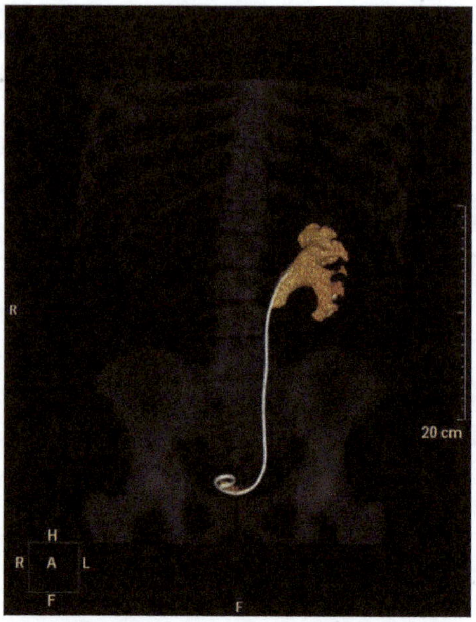

FIGURE 1: Abdominal computed tomography (coronal cut) showing complete coraliform calcification on double-J stent.

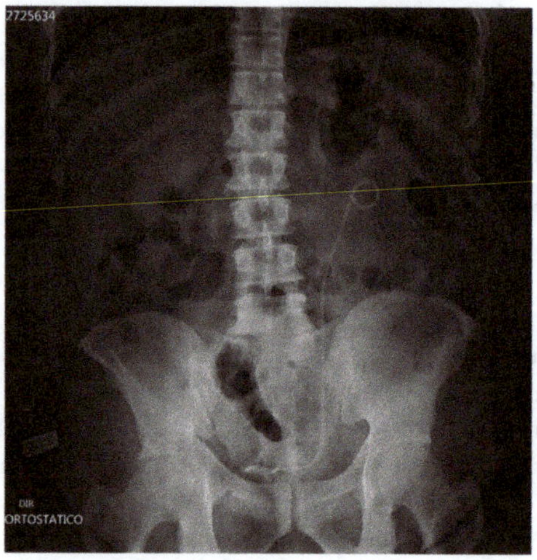

FIGURE 2: Abdominal X-ray showing absence of residual calculi in left pyelocalicial system.

3. Step by Step

(1) Left lumbar incision and opening of planes (superficial, muscular, pararenal, and perirenal), enabling retroperitoneal access to the kidney.

(2) Isolation of proximal ureter, with ascending dissection of the renal pelvis and left renal sinus, with ample exposure of the field to be operated.

(3) Inverted U-shaped incision in posterior portion of renal pelvis at its transition with the calyx infundibula, obtaining access to the double-J catheter completed encompassed by the pelvic calcified mass and its calyx branches.

(4) Anterograde removal of calcified double-J catheter from the renal sinus to the ureteropelvic junction.

4. Discussion

The double-J stent is a therapeutic option for different urological conditions [5, 6]. The main risk factors for the calcification of this stent are low schooling, time of use, sepsis, pyelonephritis, chronic kidney disease, recurring or residual kidney stones, congenital and metabolic abnormalities, and malignant ureteral obstruction due to chemotherapy with hyperuricosuria [5]. Physiological changes during pregnancy can also predispose the patient to calcification of the stent [6]. When removal by cystoscopy is not possible due to the calcification, another procedure is required [5, 6].

Treatment is generally performed using endourological (transurethral) procedures, with the rare need for open surgical techniques for patients in whom the stent remains for up to 30 months [7]. In such cases, percutaneous nephrolithotomy achieves good results. However, patients treated with this procedure for the resolution of complete calculi have residual calculi in up to 70% of times, which increases the risk of obstructive conditions in the postoperative period [8, 9]. The possible approaches to the removal of a calcified double-J stent are cystoscopy, extracorporeal lithotripsy, cystolithotripsy, ureterolithotripsy, percutaneous nephrolithotomy, or open surgery [9–13]. The video-assisted laparoscopic and robotic approaches can be indicated in select cases as methods for the treatment of coraliform calculi and pelvic calculi of a medium size and favorable anatomic access (extrarenal pelvis) [14–18]. Regarding the double-J catheter calcified in complete coraliform calculus, there is no report in the indexed literature on such techniques to date.

This study described a difficult case with three unsuccessful attempts at removing the calcified stent by cystoscopy and extracorporeal lithotripsy. We finally opted for extended pyelolithotomy due to the limitations of percutaneous nephrolithotomy for this case. The patient had no postoperative complications.

Calcification of the double-J stent is a common complication with a high rate of patient morbidity, requiring further surgical procedures and a consequent increase in financial expenses [19]. To avoid potential complications with the use of a double-J stent, the use of a spreadsheet available on the Internet is a viable control option that could be fundamental to the management of patients so that they are not forgotten, the consequences of which are possible lawsuits [19–22].

The double-J stent is part of the urological arsenal for the treatment of urinary tract infections. Despite advances in recent years, the complications due to its presence in the ureter can be challenging to urologists and patients alike, leading to an increase in the morbidity rate and a financial burden on the healthcare system. Greater control of patients with stents should be exercised, counseling them on the maximum time of stent use and the complications that can arise in cases of forgetfulness.

5. Conclusion

Patients with complete coraliform calcification induced by a double-J ureteral stent should be treated in an individualized manner and considering the limitation of percutaneous surgery regarding the removal of all fragments.

References

[1] G. Haleblian, K. Kijvikai, J. De La Rosette, and G. Preminger, "Ureteral stenting and urinary stone management: a systematic review," *The Journal of Urology*, vol. 179, no. 2, pp. 424–430, 2008.

[2] D. Gallego, J. B. Persiva, M. P. Mestre et al., "Double J catheter migrated to the bladder and encrusted. Case report and bibliographic review," *Archivos Españoles de Urología*, vol. 65, no. 2, pp. 251–255, 2012.

[3] V. M. Pais, B. Chew, O. Shaw et al., "Percutaneous nephrolithotomy for removal of encrusted ureteral stents: A multicenter study," *Journal of Endourology*, vol. 28, no. 10, pp. 1188–1191, 2014.

[4] C.-C. Tsai, J.-T. Shen, S.-P. Huang et al., "Use of a holmium laser to treat a forgotten double-j stent with whole stent encrustations: a case report," *Kaohsiung Journal of Medical Sciences*, vol. 25, no. 10, pp. 567–571, 2009.

[5] I. Singh, N. P. Gupta, A. K. Hemal, M. Aron, A. Seth, and P. N. Dogra, "Severely encrusted polyurethane ureteral stents: Management and analysis of potential risk factors," *Urology*, vol. 58, no. 4, pp. 526–531, 2001.

[6] B. A. Vanderbrink, A. R. Rastinehad, M. C. Ost, and A. D. Smith, "Encrusted urinary stents: Evaluation and endourologic management," *Journal of Endourology*, vol. 22, no. 5, pp. 905–912, 2008.

[7] H. Polat, M. Ö. Yücel, M. M. Utangaç et al., "Management of forgotten ureteral stents: relationship between indwelling time and required treatment approaches," *Balkan Medical Journal*, vol. 34, no. 4, pp. 301–307, 2017.

[8] M. S. Pearle, L. M. Watamull, and M. A. Mulligan, "Sensitivity of noncontrast helical computerized tomography and plain film radiography compared to flexible nephroscopy for detecting residual fragments after percutaneous nephrostolithotomy," *The Journal of Urology*, vol. 162, no. 1, pp. 23–26, 1999.

[9] F. Altunrende, A. Tefekli, R. J. Stein et al., "Clinically insignificant residual fragments after percutaneous nephrolithotomy: Medium-term follow-up," *Journal of Endourology*, vol. 25, no. 6, pp. 941–945, 2011.

[10] M. F. Bultitude, R. C. Tiptaft, J. M. Glass, and P. Dasgupta, "Management of encrusted ureteral stents impacted in upper tract," *Urology*, vol. 62, no. 4, pp. 622–626, 2003.

[11] R. Gupta, A. Gupta, A. Anand, and T. Azad, "Forgotten DJ stent a nagging problem -management and long term follow up," *JK Science*, vol. 19, no. 2, pp. 110–114, 2017.

[12] Y. Bostanci, E. Ozden, F. Atac, Y. K. Yakupoglu, A. F. Yilmaz, and S. Sarikaya, "Single session removal of forgotten encrusted ureteral stents: Combined endourological approach," *Urolithiasis*, vol. 40, no. 5, pp. 523–529, 2012.

[13] M. Robert, A.-M. Boularan, M. El Sandid, and D. Grasset, "Double-J ureteric stent encrustations: Clinical study on crystal formation on polyurethane stents," *Urologia Internationalis*, vol. 58, no. 2, pp. 100–104, 1997.

[14] A. K. Chow and L. A. Deane, "Robotic pyelolithotomy for the intact removal of a complete staghorn calculus: a feasible approach even after a previous open pyelolithotomy," *Urology*, 2019.

[15] M. H. Soltani, S. Hamedanchi, B. Shakiba, and H. Hoshyar, "Laparoscopic pyelolithotomy for management of complete staghorn stone of an ectopic pelvic kidney," *Urology Journal*, 2018.

[16] A. Nouralizadeh, N. Simforoosh, and M. H. Soltani, "Laparoscopic transperitoneal pyelolithotomy for management of staghorn renal calculi," *Journal of Laparoendoscopic & Advanced Surgical Techniques*, vol. 22, no. 1, 2012.

[17] Y. Xiao, Q. Li, C. Huang, P. Wang, J. Zhang, and W. Fu, "Perioperative and long term results of retroperitoneal laparoscopic pyelolithotomy versus percutaneous nephrolithotomy for staghorn calculi?: a single center randomized controlled trial," *World Journal of Urology*, 2018.

[18] M. Mujeeburahiman and C. Vipin, "Laparoscopic pyelolithotomy as a monotherapy for the management of intermediate," *Sized Renal Pelvic Stones*, pp. 189–192, 2018.

[19] P. Paulo Polotto, J. Paulo Pretti Fantin, T. Litaiff Padilha et al., "Computerized system for online control of ureteral catheters hosted on google drive: an alert tool," *International Journal of Sciences*, vol. 3, no. 09, pp. 79–81, 2017.

[20] S. Agarwal, R. Sarpal, P. Pathak et al., "Tricks and tacks in the management of the forgotten double J stent," *International Surgery Journal*, vol. 5, no. 3, pp. 792–795, 2018.

[21] A. A. Sancaktutar, A. Tepeler, H. Söylemez et al., "A solution for medical and legal problems arising from forgotten ureteral stents: Initial results from a reminder short message service (SMS)," *Urolithiasis*, vol. 40, no. 3, pp. 253–258, 2012.

[22] J. S. Lam and M. Gupta, "Tips and tricks for the management of retained ureteral stents," *Journal of Endourology*, vol. 16, no. 10, pp. 733–741, 2002.

Normotensive, Oversized Pheochromocytoma in Twin-Pregnancy: Analysis of Therapeutic Challenges in a Rare Case

Bora Özveren,[1] **Halim Ulugöl**,[2] **and Levent Türkeri**[1]

[1]*Acibadem Mehmet Ali Aydinlar University, School of Medicine, Department of Urology, Turkey*
[2]*Acibadem Mehmet Ali Aydinlar University, School of Medicine, Department of Anesthesiology & Reanimation, Turkey*

Correspondence should be addressed to Bora Özveren; ozverenb@yahoo.com

Academic Editor: David Duchene

An asymptomatic, normotensive 36-year-old woman in the second trimester of a twin-gestation was diagnosed with a 11 cm adrenal pheochromocytoma. Considering the hemodynamic stability of the patient, tumor size, and gestational age, the therapeutic decision of a multidisciplinary team ensued open surgical excision without any preoperative antihypertensive preparation. Following successful removal of pheochromocytoma, the patient had a normal subsequent course of pregnancy and cesarean section delivery of healthy twins at term. This unique case of a normotensive, incidental, large-sized pheochromocytoma in a twin-pregnancy illustrates that the decisions of management in such a rare occurrence should be based on individual features of the patient. Our experience supports that α-adrenergic blockade may not be essential in normotensive pheochromocytoma in pregnancy and open-surgery remains as a safe approach in the management of large adrenal tumors in twin-pregnant patients following a multidisciplinary consultation.

1. Introduction

Pheochromocytoma (PC) in pregnancy is extremely rare, with an estimated incidence of 1 in 50,000 patients [1]. Historically, PC in pregnancy carried significant risks with mortality rates for both mother and fetus of up to 58% [2]. Maternal and fetal survival greatly depend on a timely diagnosis, an appropriate medical management, and a correct timing of delivery and surgery. When diagnosed antenatally, PC is associated with more successful outcomes, with a maternal mortality rate of 0-2% but still significant risk of fetal loss at a rate of 11-15% [3].

Current report presents the management of a unique case of a twin-pregnancy with an incidentally discovered, asymptomatic large adrenal PC.

2. Case Presentation

A 36-year-old woman (G4,P2), at the 15th gestational week of twin-pregnancy following IVF-embryo transfer, was found to have a solid adrenal mass on a regular checkup. MRI revealed a 11×7.5 cm right suprarenal hypervascular mass with mixed signal intensity in T2-weighted images (Figure 1). The diagnosis of PC was confirmed by laboratory analysis (Table 1). The patient had no genetic testing and her family history was not indicative of any hereditary disease. She had two previous vaginal deliveries (14 and 11 years ago) and a history of one abortus at 10-week gestation two years earlier. The patient confirmed that she had no symptoms relating to PC in her previous deliveries. She had no genetic testing and her family history was not indicative of hereditary disease. She was asymptomatic and normotensive and had no hemodynamic instability during pregnancy. She was asymptomatic and normotensive and had no hemodynamic instability during pregnancy. Perinatological ultrasonography revealed normal morphology of dichorionic and diamniotic male and female fetuses.

A multidisciplinary team consisting of urologists, anesthesiologists, endocrinologist, and obstetricians focused on the therapeutic approach. The patient did not receive any

TABLE 1: Pre- and postoperative catecholamines.

	Preoperative	Postoperative	
24-hour urinary			
† Vanillyl mandelic acid	--	6.6 mg/day	(<8.0)
† Metanephrines	699.4 μg/day	78.0 μg/day	(<180)
† Normetanephrines	16510 μg/day	265.9 μg/day	(<419)
Plasma			
† Epinephrine	157 pg/ml	8.3 pg/ml	(<85)
† Norepinephrine	9577 pg/ml	108.7 pg/ml	(<420)
† Dopamine	--	3.5 pg/ml	(<50)

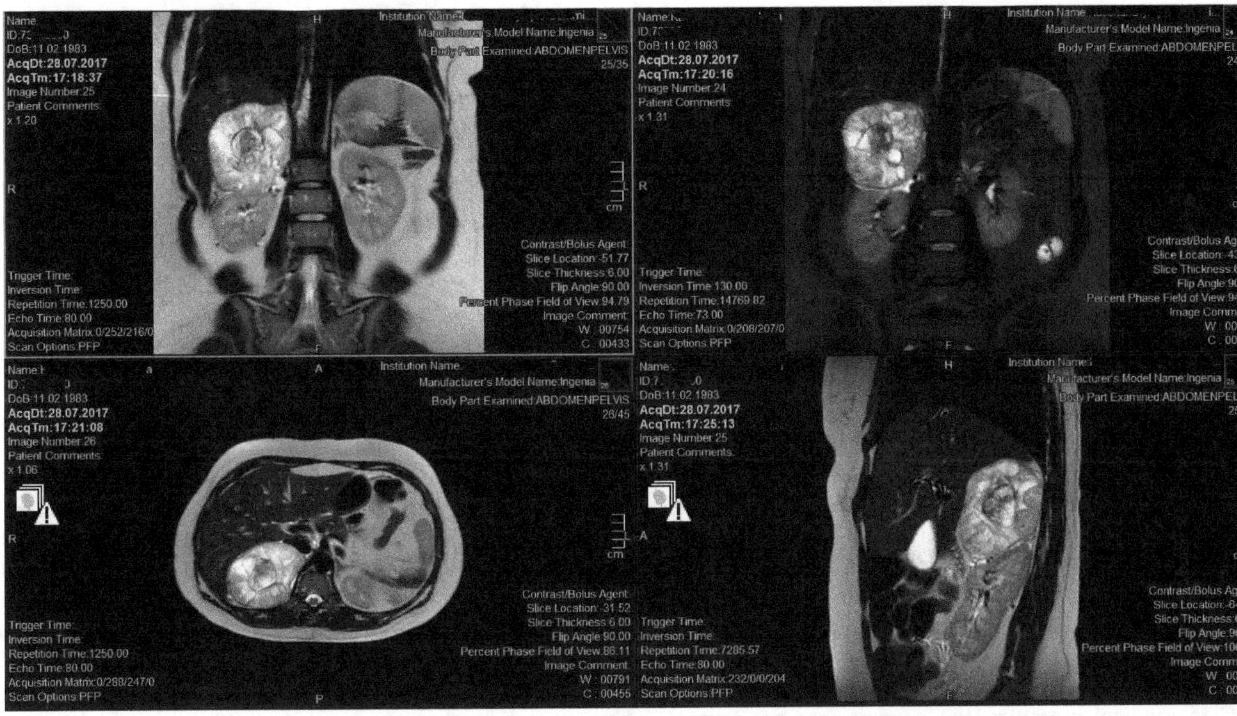

FIGURE 1: MRI examination showing a 11×7.5 cm right suprarenal hypervascular mass with mixed signal intensity in T2-weighted images.

medical treatment for alpha or beta blockade preoperatively. She underwent laparotomy with a subcostal incision and transperitoneal tumor resection at 17 weeks of gestation (Figure 2). During surgery blood pressure (BP) was stabilized with phentolamine and esmolol, with occasional bouts of brief hypertensive periods up to 240 mm Hg systolic pressure. A hypervascular mass with fragile large veins was dissected free of the upper pole of the right kidney, between the vena cava and the lower border of the liver. The estimated blood loss was 1100 ml. The patient was transfused with 3 units of erythrocyte suspensions. The postoperative period was uneventful and she remained hemodynamically stable. Histopathological examinations were in accordance with a PC.

She had a normal subsequent course of pregnancy and cesarean section delivery of healthy twins at term. Nine months after delivery, follow-up ultrasonography revealed no recurrent mass. Urinary and plasma catecholamine levels were in normal range.

3. Discussion

Hypertension is the most common presenting feature of pheochromocytoma in pregnancy, reported in 87% [4]. Establishing the diagnosis can be challenging considering the varied modes of presentation, which may mimic other common disorders of pregnancy such as gestational hypertension, atypical preeclampsia, or gestational diabetes.

The medical management primarily aims to prevent hypertensive crisis and usually includes alpha and beta blockers or calcium channel blockers. Surgery is the definitive treatment of PC, but the timing remains a challenging and controversial issue, depending on the gestational age, clinical response to medical treatment, the accessibility of the tumor, and the presence of fetal distress [5].

There are only 2 previous cases of twin-pregnancy complicated by PC. The first patient was a primigravid presenting with high BP, a 7 cm adrenal mass found on ultrasonography, and elevated urinary and plasma catecholamines. Despite

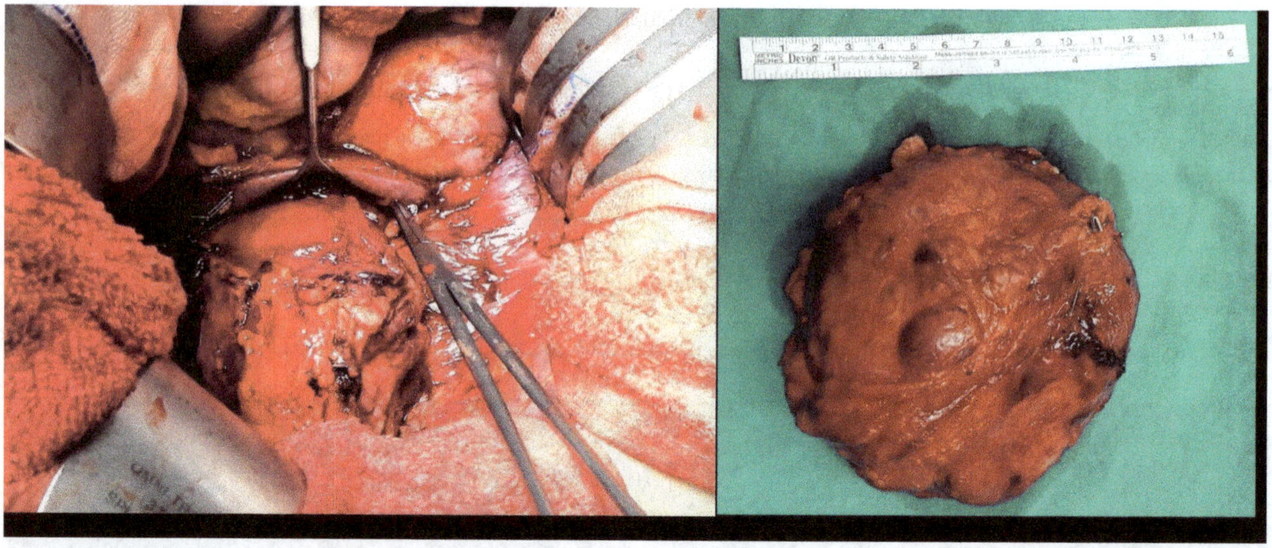

FIGURE 2: Transperitoneal resection of the hypervascular tumor located above the upper pole of the right kidney, between the vena cava and the lower border of the liver.

an add-on therapy of beta blockers to a high dose of phenoxybenzamine, the pregnancy was complicated with the demise of one of the twins at 29 weeks of gestation and resulting in an emergency cesarean section for the surviving twin shortly after [6]. The second case was a chronic, severely hypertensive woman with 13 weeks of twin-gestation. Evaluation for secondary hypertension disclosed high levels of urinary (nor)metanephrines and a 2.9 cm adrenal mass on MRI. She underwent laparoscopic left adrenalectomy for PC without complications. She had normal BP for the remainder of pregnancy and delivered healthy twins via cesarean section [7].

In addition to being the third report on a twin-gestation with PC in medical literature, the current case has several distinctive features. To the best of our knowledge, we report the largest PC complicating a pregnancy in literature to date, which is treated by open surgical excision in the second trimester with successful maternofetal outcome. Analysis of contemporary series of PC in pregnancy showed that average tumor size is about 3-4 cms (min: 2 cm, max:10 cm) [3, 5, 8, 9]. Adrenal PCs above 7 cm are considered large-sized, and laparoscopic surgery is contraindicated. Moreover, large (5 cm or greater) size is one of the high risk factors predictive of malignant pheochromocytoma [10]. The timing and the method of surgical intervention depend on the size/location of the tumor as well as the gestational age and maternal/fetal response to medical pretreatment. If diagnosed early in pregnancy, it is generally suggested to remove the tumor in the second trimester, following the appropriate medical management of BP and heart rate. In the third trimester, when medical pretreatment is sufficient, it is usually recommended to postpone adrenalectomy until the time of or after delivery. In our case, the considerable size and hypervascularity of the tumor as well as the dimensions of the uterus bearing twin-fetuses substantiated prompt intervention with open surgical approach for safety concerns.

Another foremost difference of our case remains the unusual presentation as an incidental discovery of normotensive PC during twin-pregnancy. The typical clinical manifestation of PC is paroxysmal or sustained hypertension. In the nonpregnant population, absence of hypertension or hemodynamic manifestations are reported in 10 to 40% of incidental PC cases [11]. Despite the frequency of this hemodynamically silent presentation, little is known about the characteristics of normotensive incidentally discovered PCs. Furthermore, there is a paucity of information concerning epidemiology and specific clinical features of normotensive incidental PC in pregnancy due to its extremely rare occurrence. Clinically overt PC in pregnancy may be triggered by several mechanisms such as intra-abdominal pressure, fetal movement, uterine contraction, process of delivery, an abdominal intervention, and general anesthesia. Lafont et al. suggested that normotensive incidental PCs (in nonpregnant patients) are roughly comparable to hypertensive PCs in terms of hemodynamic instability during surgical resection [12]. Furthermore, in their retrospective cohort, they identified no differences in hemodynamic instability in terms of presence or absence of preoperative use of antihypertensive agents.

For nonpregnant patients, the current standard of care consists of a medical pretreatment with α-adrenergic receptor blockade for at least 10–14 days before surgery in order to lower the risks of perioperative and postoperative hemodynamic complications. However, in pregnant patients, optimal medical therapy for PC is not clearly defined and target BP is not known, since the published literature largely comprises case reports. While effective control of maternal hypertension is crucial to avoid complications owing to the effects of raised catecholamine levels, medical management requires a balance of maintaining sufficient uteroplacental circulation to prevent fetal growth impairment or demise. The drug of choice, phenoxybenzamine, is a *pregnancy class C* medication that crosses the placenta. Neonates born to mothers receiving phenoxybenzamine should be monitored closely in an intensive care unit, with particular observation for hypotension and respiratory distress [13]. The risk of neonatal cardiac failure may be associated to the large proportion of α-receptors in the neonatal heart. However, the relation between phenoxybenzamine and respiratory distress is not clear.

In our case, the hemodynamic stability of the asymptomatic pregnant patient and the probability of adverse effects of antihypertensive medications in the perioperative period warranted a shared-decision of omitting antihypertensive preparation prior to surgery. The current case demonstrates that, in normotensive incidental PC patients, intraoperative hemodynamic stability can successfully be maintained without the requirement of preoperative α1-adrenoceptor antagonist therapy.

4. Conclusion

We report a patient with 17 weeks of twin-gestation and a diagnosis of asymptomatic normotensive pheochromocytoma who was successfully treated with open-surgery without any preoperative antihypertensive preparation. Multidisciplinary approach and judicious anesthetic management resulted in a successful outcome without compromising the fetal well-being of the twins in this extraordinarily rare case. Considering the lack of treatment guidelines of this rare condition, further evidence is needed to define the best management of pheochromocytoma in pregnant patients.

References

[1] J. L. Harrington, D. R. Farley, J. A. Van Heerden, and K. D. Ramin, "Adrenal tumors and pregnancy," *World Journal of Surgery*, vol. 23, no. 2, pp. 182–186, 1999.

[2] M. Mannelli and D. Bemporad, "Diagnosis and management of phaeochromocytoma during pregnancy," *Journal of Endocrinological Investigation*, vol. 25, p. 567, 2002.

[3] M. A. Biggar and T. W. J. Lennard, "Systematic review of phaeochromocytoma in pregnancy," *British Journal of Surgery*, vol. 100, no. 2, pp. 182–190, 2013.

[4] K. Van Der Weerd, C. Van Noord, M. Loeve et al., "Pheochromocytoma in pregnancy: Case series and review of literature," *European Journal of Endocrinology*, vol. 177, no. 2, pp. R49–R58, 2017.

[5] R. Oliva, P. Angelos, E. Kaplan, and G. Bakris, "Pheochromocytoma in pregnancy: a case series and review," *Hypertension*, vol. 55, no. 3, pp. 600–606, 2010.

[6] M. M. Kennelly, S. G. Ball, V. Robson, and M. J. Blott, "Difficult alpha-adrenergic blockade of a phaeochromocytoma in a twin pregnancy," *Journal of Obstetrics & Gynaecology*, vol. 27, no. 7, pp. 729-730, 2007.

[7] M. A. Miller, P. J. Mazzaglia, L. Larson, G. M. Ankner, G. R. Bourjeily, and P. Curran, "Laparoscopic adrenalectomy for phaeochromocytoma in a twin gestation," *Journal of Obstetrics & Gynaecology*, vol. 32, no. 2, pp. 186-187, 2012.

[8] G. Donatini, J. L. Kraimps, C. Caillard et al., "Pheochromocytoma diagnosed during pregnancy: lessons learned from a series of ten patients," *Surgical Endoscopy*, vol. 32, no. 9, pp. 3890–3900, 2018.

[9] A. Yulia, I. W. Seetho, A. Ramineni, and R. A. K. Jaiyesimi, "Pheochromocytoma in pregnancy: a review of the literature," *Obstetrics and Gynaecology Cases-Reviews*, vol. 3, p. 096, 2016.

[10] F. Feng, Y. Zhu, X. Wang et al., "Predictive factors for malignant pheochromocytoma: analysis of 136 patients," *The Journal of Urology*, vol. 185, no. 5, pp. 1583–1589, 2011.

[11] M. Haissaguerre, M. Courel, P. Caron et al., "Normotensive incidentally discovered pheochromocytomas display specific biochemical, cellular, and molecular characteristics," *The Journal of Clinical Endocrinology & Metabolism*, vol. 98, no. 11, pp. 4346–4354, 2013.

[12] M. Lafont, C. Fagour, M. Haissaguerre et al., "Per-operative hemodynamic instability in normotensive patients with incidentally discovered pheochromocytomas," *The Journal of Clinical Endocrinology & Metabolism*, vol. 100, no. 2, pp. 417–421, 2015.

[13] S. C. Aplin, K. F. Yee, and M. J. Cole, "Neonatal effects of long-term maternal phenoxybenzamine therapy," *Anesthesiology*, vol. 100, no. 6, pp. 1608–1610, 2004.

54

Giant Primary Scrotal Lipoma: A Rare Entity with Diagnostic Pitfalls

Louis Vignot, Elie Saad, Michael Peyromaure, and Nicolas Barry Delongchamps

Department of Urology, Cochin Hospital, University of Paris Descartes, Paris, France

Correspondence should be addressed to Louis Vignot; vignot.l@chu-nice.fr

Academic Editor: Apul Goel

Primary scrotal lipomas are rare. We describe the case of a 47-year-old male with a giant scrotal lipoma who underwent a surgical excision. We report the clinical and radiological approach as well as the treatment of this atypical benign tumor.

1. Introduction

In urological practice, intrascrotal lesions are frequent, and the major challenge is to distinguish a benign lesion from a malignant one. Lipomas represent a small proportion of scrotal swellings, but it is necessary to have knowledge of this benign entity as a differential diagnosis.

2. Case Presentation

The patient was a 46-year-old man with no relevant medical history who presented in our institution with a large left scrotal mass. He first noticed a swelling ten years ago and reported a very progressive growth of this lump that became discomfortable and dysesthetic. No other symptoms were reported in anamnesis. Physical examination revealed a large, nonreductible, soft, and painless left scrotal mass with well-defined margins. Both testicles were not palpable due to the large size of the mass.

The patient underwent scrotal ultrasonography (Figure 1(a)) to confirm the prima facie clinical diagnosis of hydrocele. The scrotal ultrasound revealed a large heterogeneous solid mass of 16 × 12 × 8 cm, showing weak vascularization on Doppler imaging, pushing both testicles upwards and to the right. The testicles, epididymis, and spermatic cords were intact.

Magnetic resonance imaging (MRI) showed a large extratesticular and extraepididymal mass with smooth margins and no intra-abdominal extension through the inguinal canal (Figures 1(b) and 1(c)). T2-weighted sequences revealed an encapsulated fat-containing mass, and T1-contrast enhanced sequences showed a very slight enhancement. This initial workup did not show any evidence of invasiveness of adjacent structures and did not support the diagnosis of malignant tumor. The most likely diagnosis was a lipoma. However, the radiologist could not formally rule out a diagnosis of liposarcoma because of the tumor's size.

An ultrasound guided biopsy was performed and confirmed the diagnosis of lipoma.

Surgical removal of the left scrotal mass was planned under general anesthesia, and a scrotal incision was performed. The lump appeared to be composed of fat, looked encapsulated, and was easily removed (Figure 1(d)). The testicles were not examined intraoperatively, because the tunica vaginalis testis was not opened and stayed intact during the whole procedure.

Immediate postoperative course was uneventful, and the patient was discharged on postoperative day one. Unfortunately, postoperative period was marked by the occurrence of a voluminous scrotal hematoma on day four, which required reintervention for drainage.

On gross examination, the specimen weighted 480 g, measured 17 × 11 × 6 cm and was roughly oval. It was multi-

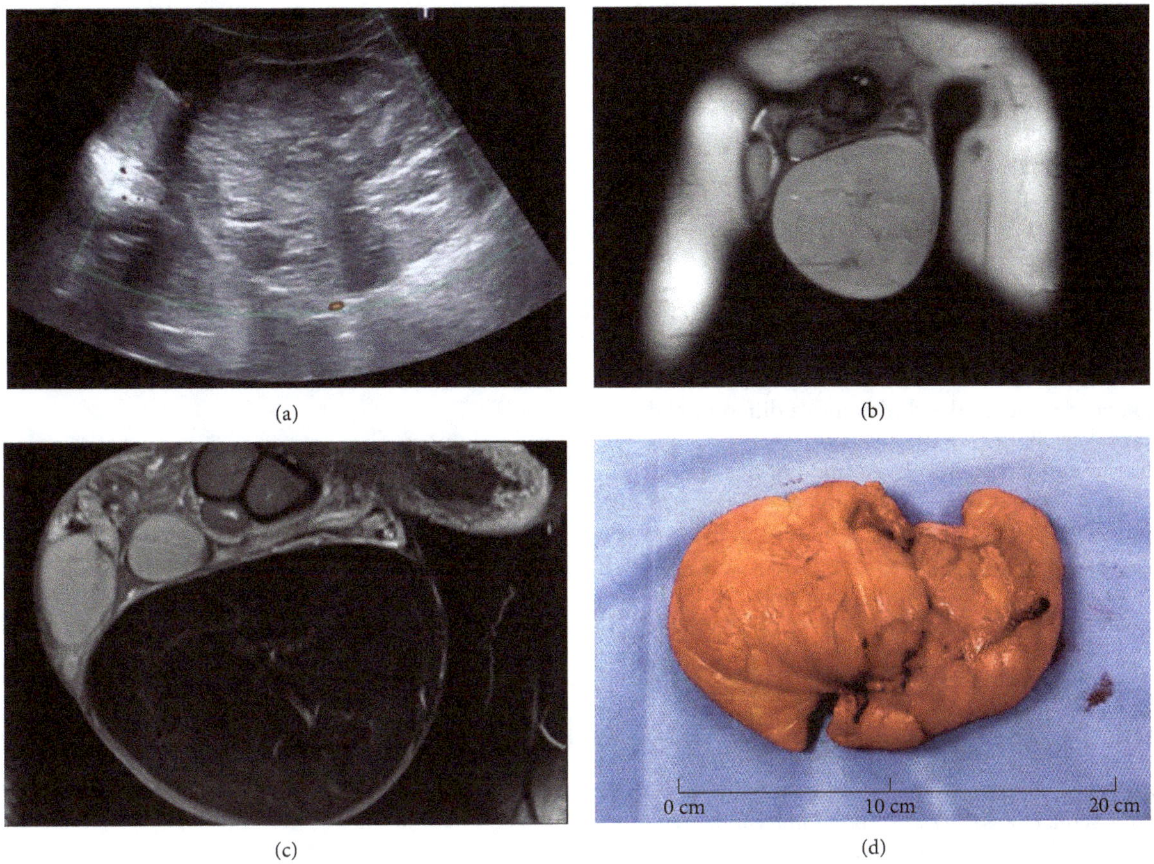

FIGURE 1: Imaging and gross pathologic features of primary scrotal lipoma. (a) On a color Doppler image, the lesion lacks internal flow. (b) Coronal T2-weighted image of the scrotum shows a lesion with homogeneous high signal intensity. (c) Coronal contrast-enhanced T1-weighted MRI shows very low enhancement of the tumor. (d) Gross examination of the surgical specimen.

lobulated, yellowish with soft to firm consistency. Histopathological examination showed a proliferation of well-differentiated and mature adipocytes of various sizes in all samples.

3. Discussion

Intrascrotal lesions are a heterogeneous entity. Although benign in most cases, clinical examination alone may not exclude malignancy. Many diagnostic pitfalls exist, and multiple anatomical structures in a confined space with all their own pathologies do not make the clinician's task any easier [1].

Scrotal lipomas can originate from three different regions: (a) from the adipose tissue posterior to the spermatic cord, (b) from the spermatic cord, and (c) from the scrotal wall [2]. The last entity is called "primary scrotal lipoma" and is rarely seen. In most cases, it is not easy to identify the precise origin of the lesion.

Intratesticular masses are 95% malignant while nonepididymal extratesticular tumors, including those originating from the scrotum and spermatic cord, are most commonly mesenchymal benign tumors (97%) [3]. However, a diagnosis of extratesticular malignancy such as liposarcoma, leiomyosarcoma, lymphoma, or mesothelioma should not be missed. Although lipomas are the most common benign neoplasms in the scrotum, they remain a rare entity [4].

To our knowledge, there are very few cases of primary scrotal lipoma described in the scientific literature. Symptoms and patient discomfort vary according to the size of the lipoma: their weight varies from 225 g to 9 kg [5]. Clinically, it can mimic an inguinal hernia or a scrotal hematoma, hence the essential contribution of imaging. Ultrasonography is the first-line imaging and helps to specify the solid or cystic nature of the lesion as well as its location. While most of the extratesticular solid tumors are benign like the one reported, there may be some doubt especially concerning very large tumors. Magnetic resonance imaging (MRI) is then a valuable tool in such cases because it is the most precise resource in distinguishing a malignant tumor from a benign one. A homogeneous, encapsulated, and well-limited fat mass would be strongly in favor of a benign lipoma. But a huge tumor, although benign, may have a small proportion of muscle vessels or fibers, mimicking a well-differentiated liposarcoma. Moreover, O'Donnell et al. showed that experienced observers could differentiate well-differentiated liposarcoma from benign lipoma in only 69% of cases using only MRI [6]. Lipoma can be differentiated from liposarcoma by the lack of any enhancing soft tissue within a lipoma and more heterogeneous content of liposarcomas [3].

The biopsy performed in this context does not exclude a malignant focus because of the size of the lesion and its possible heterogeneity. Being an encapsulated and noninfiltrative mass helped us differentiate it from lipomatosis and the absence of abnormal mitosis and cellular atypia to differentiate from liposarcoma. Some very rare cases of malignant degeneration of giant scrotal lipomas have been described in scientific literature [7].

4. Conclusion

Primary scrotal lipomas are rare and benign tumors but should be kept in mind by the clinician as a differential diagnosis of scrotal swelling.

First line imaging remains ultrasound but does not allow differentiating a lipoma from a liposarcoma with certainty and must therefore be complemented by scrotal MRI, especially in the case of a large tumor.

The treatment of choice is surgical excision, and the histological analysis of the specimen allows a diagnosis of certainty.

References

[1] J. S. Montgomery and D. A. Bloom, "The diagnosis and management of scrotal masses," *The Medical Clinics of North America*, vol. 95, no. 1, pp. 235–244, 2011.

[2] N. Fujimura and K. Kurokawa, "Primary lipoma of the scrotum," *European Urology*, vol. 5, pp. 182-183, 2017.

[3] D. J. Deccia, R. J. Krane, and C. A. Olsson, "Clinical management of non-testicular intrascrotal tumors," *The Journal of Urology*, vol. 116, pp. 476–479, 1976.

[4] D. J. Wolfman, J. Marko, C. F. Gould, I. A. Sesterhenn, and G. E. Lattin Jr., "Mesenchymal extratesticular tumors and tumorlike conditions: from the radiologic pathology archives," *Radiographics*, vol. 35, no. 7, pp. 1943–1954, 2015.

[5] J. F. J. Leyson, L. W. Doroshow, and M. A. Robbins, "Extratesticular lipoma: report of 2 cases and a new classification," *The Journal of Urology*, vol. 116, no. 3, pp. 324–326, 1976.

[6] P. W. O'Donnell, A. M. Griffin, W. C. Eward et al., "Can experienced observers differentiate between lipoma and well-differentiated liposarcoma using only MRI?," *Sarcoma*, vol. 2013, Article ID 982784, 6 pages, 2013.

[7] M. Ongari, C. Bazzoni, M. Serini, M. Alleva, C. Sguazzini, and C. Lombardi, "Sarcomatous degeneration of a giant scrotal lipoma," *Minerva Urologica e Nefrologica*, vol. 45, pp. 72–75, 1993.

Dorsal Onlay Oral Mucosa Graft Urethroplasty: A Case Report and Review of Literature

Kwaku Addai Arhin Appiah,[1,2,3] Christian Kofi Gyasi-Sarpong,[1,2] Edwin M. T. Yenli,[4] Patrick Opoku Manu Maison,[5] Charles Kwame Adofo,[6] George Amoah,[1] Roland Azorliade,[1] Dominic Annor Mintah,[1] and Augustina Badu-Peprah[7,8]

[1]*Department of Surgery, Komfo Anokye Teaching Hospital, Kumasi, Ghana*
[2]*Department of Surgery, KSMD, College of Health Sciences, KNUST, Kumasi, Ghana*
[3]*Kings Medical Consult (Specialist Urology Clinic), Kumasi, Ghana*
[4]*University for Development Studies-SMHS, Department of Surgery, Urology Unit, Tamale, Ghana*
[5]*Department of Surgery, School of Medical Sciences, UCC, Cape Coast, Ghana*
[6]*Seventh Day Adventist Hospital, Dominase, Ghana*
[7]*Department of Radiology, Komfo Anokye Teaching Hospital, Kumasi, Ghana*
[8]*Department of Radiology, KSMD, College of Health Sciences, KNUST, Kumasi, Ghana*

Correspondence should be addressed to Kwaku Addai Arhin Appiah; addaiarhin@yahoo.com

Academic Editor: Giorgio Carmignani

The use of buccal mucosa grafts in urethral reconstruction for complex anterior urethral strictures has gained popularity over the years with very good outcomes reported in literature. We report on the successful repair of a complex anterior urethral stricture in a 14-year-old boy following catheterization using this method at the Komfo Anokye Teaching Hospital. The aim is to describe the method of dorsal onlay oral mucosa graft urethroplasty and to review the literature.

1. Introduction

Urethral strictures in children are uncommon. They may present as lower urinary tract symptoms or acute urine retention [1]. The causes could be congenital, iatrogenic, posthypospadias repair, or traumatic [2, 3]. The diagnosis involves a detailed history, physical examination, and appropriate radiological and endoscopic investigations [4].

Retrograde urethrography (RUG) with or without micturating cystourethrogram (MCUG) is the gold standard confirmatory test. In some situations, urethroscopy may be required for confirmation and treatment. Penile and long bulbar urethral strictures are generally regarded as complex strictures. This is because they do not lend themselves to simple excision and primary anastomosis [5].

They require tissue transfer in the form of grafts, flaps, or staged repair. Since the 1990s, the use of the buccal mucosal grafts to repair such complex anterior strictures has gained enormous popularity and acceptance due to its reproducibility and durable long term success rates of 85% and beyond [6–8].

Of significant debate is whether to place the graft ventrally or dorsally on the urethra. The dorsal approach seems cumbersome but the outcome is definitely better due to the mechanical support offered to the graft by the ventral aspect of the corporeal bodies [9–11].

We report on the successful application of the use of the oral mucosa graft dorsal onlay urethroplasty technique as described by Guido Barbagli [12] in a 14-year-old boy with a 7 cm Peno-bulbar urethral stricture at the Komfo Anokye

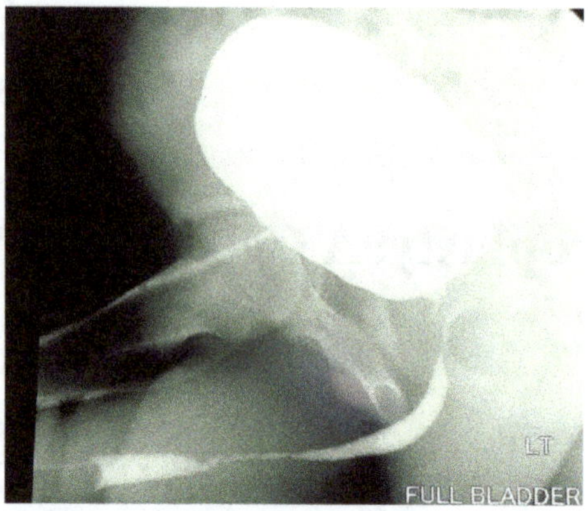

Figure 1: RUG in the left oblique view showing a 7 cm long partial occlusion of the penile and bulbar urethra.

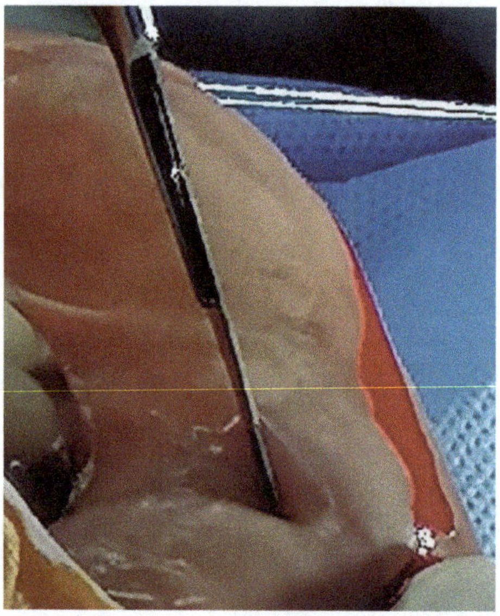

Figure 2: Harvesting oral mucosa graft from the lower lip, and a wheal raised with epinephrine solution.

Teaching Hospital (KATH). The objective is to highlight the technique of dorsal onlay oral mucosa graft urethroplasty and to review the literature.

2. Case Report

A 14-year-old boy had laparotomy for a mesenteric cyst 7 years ago during which he had a transurethral bladder catheter passed. Few weeks after discharge from the hospital, he began to experience difficulty in passing urine. It started as straining at urination with a poor stream which worsened over time. Over the cause of the past 7 years, he has had multiple dilatations which did not resolve the problem until a suprapubic catheter was passed for him a year ago and referred to see the urologist at KATH.

On examination, he had normal growth for his age. He had a two-way suprapubic catheter in situ with indurations along the penile and bulbar urethra.

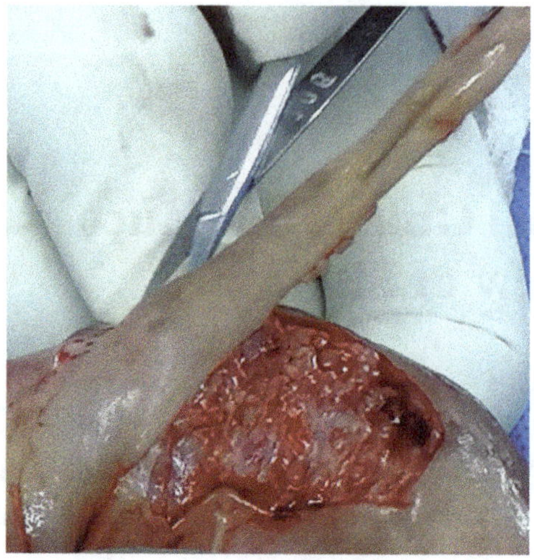

Figure 3: Oral mucosa graft being harvested from the lower lip.

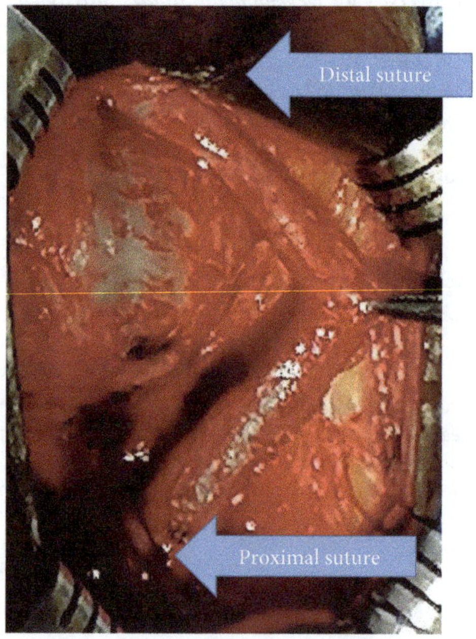

Figure 4: Urethra mobilized completely off the ventral surface of the corporeal bodies and rotated 180° with the aid of distal and proximal sutures (arrows).

A retrograde urethrogram demonstrated a partial narrowing of the penile and bulbar urethra (Figure 1).

2.1. Preoperative Preparation. A routine urine examination was done which revealed leukocytosis for which reason a urine culture was requested that isolated Klebsiella species sensitive to only amikacin.

A one-week course of parenteral amikacin was given after which a repeat urine culture was negative.

Other tests done included a full blood count and kidney function tests which were all within normal ranges. Thus, patient was scheduled for urethroplasty.

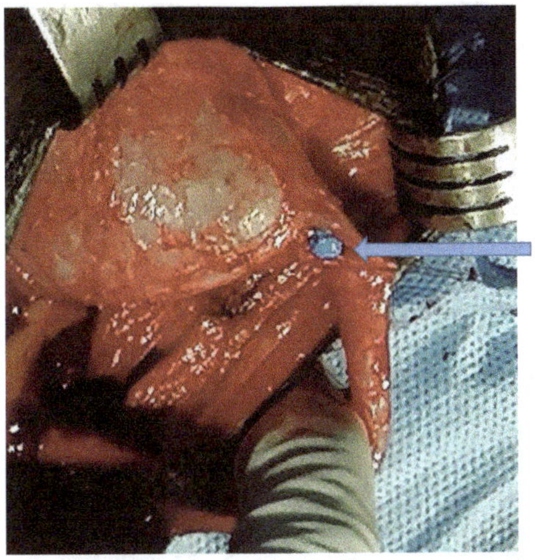

FIGURE 5: Initial dorsal incision on the catheter tip (arrow) to expose a healthy urethral lumen.

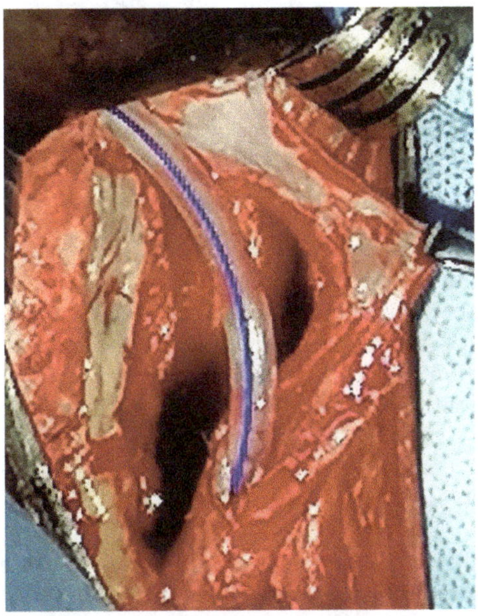

FIGURE 6: The narrowed urethral segment has been opened up under direct vision, and the oral mucosa graft has been quilted to the underside of the corporeal bodies.

Patient positioning was the standard lithotomy with padding of the pressure points with administration of general anaesthesia with oropharyngeal intubation.

2.2. Description of the Surgical Procedure

2.2.1. Step 1. Harvesting the Graft. A 7 cm × 2 cm lower lip oral mucosa graft starting from the right lateral angle of the mouth extending to the left cheek (Figures 2 and 3) was harvested. The submucosa was injected with lidocaine mixed with epinephrine (1 : 200,000) to raise a wheal which helped with easy harvesting of the graft while ensuring adequate haemostasis. A gauze was placed appropriately in the pharynx to prevent blood from entering the trachea or oesophagus. The mucosal defect at the donor site was left to heal by secondary intention. The graft was defatted removing all

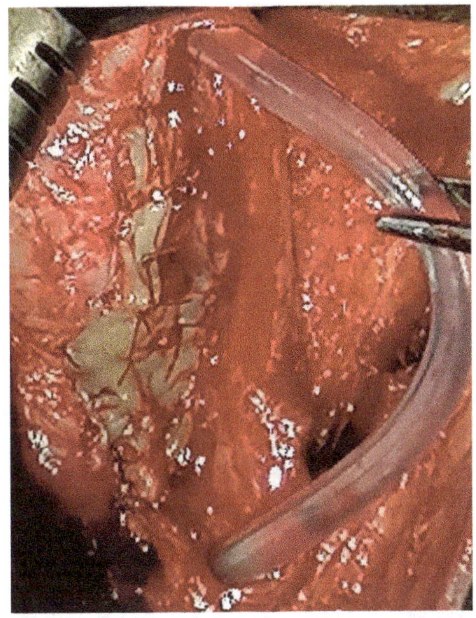

FIGURE 7: Suturing the left edge to the urethral plate to the left lateral aspect of the graft.

muscle fibers to retain only mucosa and lamina propria. Tiny fenestrations were made into it and then kept in saline until needed.

2.2.2. Step 2. Preparation of the Recipient Site. A midline perineal incision was made through the skin, subcutaneous tissues, and fascia. The perineal muscles were divided in the midline and carefully dissected away from the urethra. The urethra was then circumferentially mobilized off the corporeal bodies from the bulbar to the penile urethra going beyond the strictured segments as defined by a catheter passed per the urethral meatus and a bougie dilator proximally from the cystostomy wound by sharp dissection with fine scissors.

The urethra was then rotated 180° bringing the dorsal aspect ventrally with the aid of sutures placed proximally and distally on the dorsal aspect of the urethra (Figure 4). A dorsal stricturotomy was made over the strictured segment starting distally from the immediately adjacent patent urethral segment over the catheter tip (Figures 5 and 6). This was to ensure that the urethral mucosa was visible throughout the stricturotomy.

The oral mucosa graft was quilted to the ventral aspect of the corporeal bodies, and the left edge of the urethral plate was sutured to the left lateral aspect of the graft in interrupted fashion using vicryl 4/0 (Figures 6 and 7).

A size of 16Fr urethral catheter was advanced into the bladder, and the contralateral edge of the urethral plate was then sutured to the right edge of the oral mucosa graft over it (Figure 8).

2.3. Postoperative Management. Postoperatively, a size of 16Fr catheter wound drain was left in situ and closed wound dressing done (Figure 9). A spigot was applied to the urethral catheter which was then plastered loosely to the thigh to

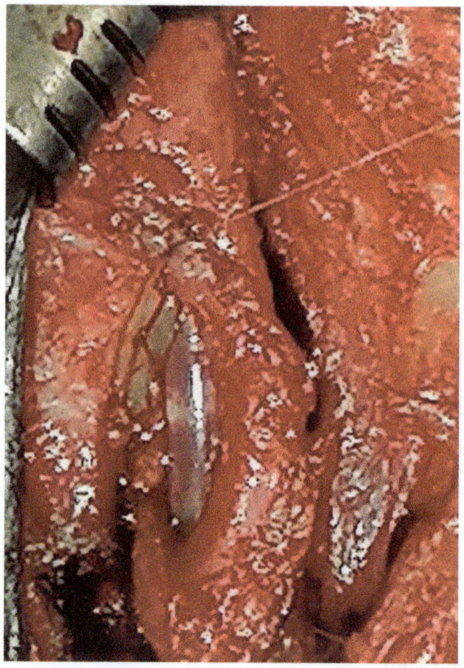

Figure 8: Suturing the right edge of the graft to the right aspect of the urethral plate over the size 16Fr catheter.

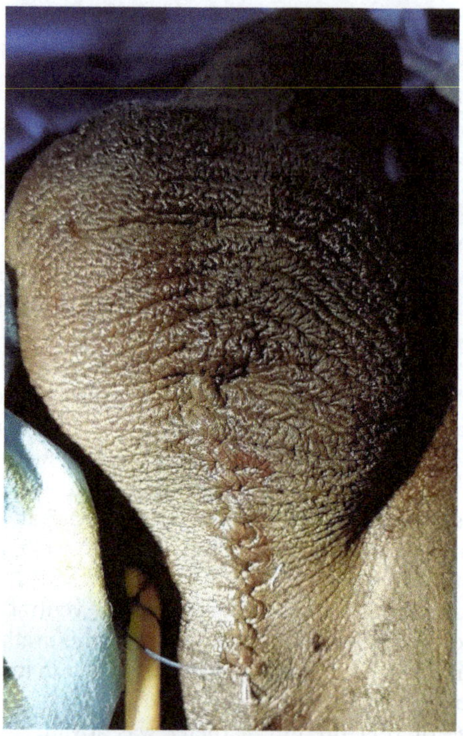

Figure 9: Final wound closure with a catheter drain left in situ.

prevent excessive movement within the urethra. A urine bag was connected to the suprapubic catheter for continuous drainage of urine. Patient was continued on parenteral cefuroxime for one more week. The wound drain was removed on day 2 when it was found not to drain any longer.

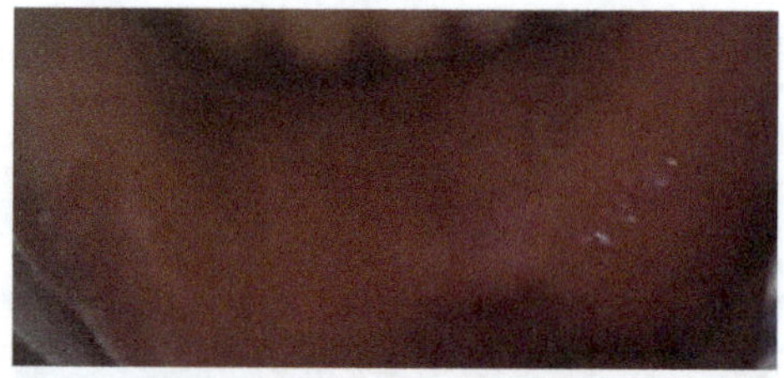

Figure 10: Healed donor site.

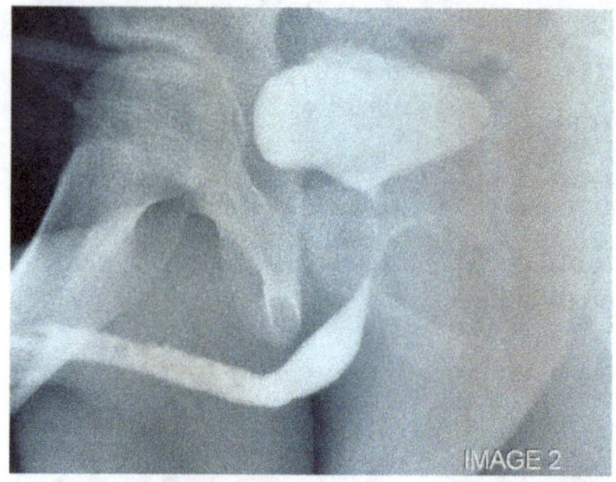

Figure 11: RUG in the left oblique view 4 weeks posturethroplasty showing normal caliber anterior urethra with no contrast extravasation.

The donor site healed within 7 days without any complications with no special dressing (Figure 10).

Both the suprapubic and urethral catheters were removed 4 weeks postoperatively when RUG showed no urinary extravasation (Figure 11). Patient has been reviewed at 3, 6, and 12 months postoperatively with no urinary concerns.

3. Discussion

Poor quality latex catheters are known to cause extensive anterior urethral strictures mainly from allergic reactions and urethritis [13–15].

Repeated minimally invasive treatment options like dilatation and direct vision internal urethrotomy (DVIU) have not been found useful in the management of complex anterior strictures [16] as happened in this patient.

The management of such complex strictures relies on tissue transfer techniques or staged urethroplasty [17, 18].

Staged urethroplasty beyond the high revision rates has the tendency to increase morbidity and financial burden and has challenges with psychosocial adjustment [17, 19]. In a boy of school going age, a prompt solution in a single stage is a welcome relief as it allows him to return to normalcy without the need for regular hospital attendance.

The use of genital fasciocutaneous flaps is a viable option for managing such complex anterior urethral strictures in a single stage [9]. It also has a durable long-term success rate of about 79% [20]. However, it may be complicated by flap and proximal penile skin necrosis, penile oedema, wound haematoma, infection, etc. There is also the risk of penile shortening and chordee beyond issues of cosmesis [21–23].

Buccal mucosa has become the graft material of choice in the management of complex anterior urethral strictures. This is because it is readily available and easily harvested from the cheek or lip, allowing for the scar to be hidden with low oral morbidity. It is also hairless, with a thick elastin-rich epithelium, which makes it tough yet easy to handle and a thin and highly vascular lamina propria, which facilitates graft take and survival [24]. We chose the lower lip mucosa for ease of harvest and avoidance of injury to Stenson's duct.

The use of skin, bladder, lingual, and rectal mucosa for onlay urethroplasty has also been reported in literature when certain conditions preclude the use of buccal mucosa [25].

Buccal mucosa grafts for dorsal onlay urethroplasty as first described by Barbagli is a versatile technique as it obviates a lot of the challenges associated with the ventral onlay approach such as sacculations, diverticulum formation, and troublesome postvoid dribbling due to inadequacy of the graft support [26]. This is because the ventral aspect of the corporeal bodies provide a much more solid mechanical support for the graft compared with the corpus spongiosum [10].

However, the abundant corpus spongiosum of the proximal bulbar urethra lends adequate support to a ventrally placed graft as opposed to strictures involving the distal bulbar and penile urethra, in which the dorsal approach is preferable due to the paucity of the corpus spongiosum [27, 28].

The success rate of buccal mucosa graft urethroplasty has been estimated in literature to range from 80 to 95% with the dorsal onlay approach having a slight advantage over the ventral approach [29–31].

We chose the oral mucosa graft dorsal onlay urethroplasty technique for this patient because it is fairly simple to harvest the graft with little morbidity at the donor site and has excellent cosmesis with durable long-term success rate.

This patient had no major complications following the surgery and has a good stream of urine with a peak flow rate of 24mls/s after one year of follow-up.

4. Conclusion

The oral mucosa graft dorsal onlay urethroplasty for complex anterior urethral strictures is applicable to complex anterior urethral strictures in children. The technique is simple to perform with minimal morbidities and has good outcomes.

Authors' Contributions

Kwaku Addai Arhin Appiah and Charles Kwame Adofo were the surgeons who performed the surgery. The first three authors conceived and designed the study. All authors have made significant contributions in drafting the paper in terms of relevant literature search, critical analysis and interpretation of data, and final approval of the paper for submission.

References

[1] M. F. Campbell, "Stricture of the urethra in children," *The Journal Pediatrics*, vol. 35, no. 2, pp. 169–179, 1949.

[2] M. W. Vetterlein, L. Weisbach, S. Riechardt, and M. Fisch, "Anterior urethral strictures in children: disease etiology and comparative effectiveness of endoscopic treatment vs. open surgical reconstruction," *Frontiers in Pediatrics*, vol. 7, 2019.

[3] A. S. Fenton, A. F. Morey, R. Aviles, and C. R. Garcia, "Anterior urethral strictures: etiology and characteristics," *Urology*, vol. 65, no. 6, pp. 1055–1058, 2005.

[4] G. W. Kaplan and W. A. Brock, "Urethral strictures in children," *The Journal of Urology*, vol. 129, no. 6, pp. 1200–1203, 1983.

[5] A. Srivastava, S. Vashishtha, U. P. Singh et al., "Preputial/penile skin flap, as a dorsal onlay or tubularized flap: a versatile substitute for complex anterior urethral stricture," *BJU International*, vol. 110, no. 11c, pp. E1101–E1108, 2012.

[6] H. Wessells and J. W. McAninch, "Current controversies in anterior urethral stricture repair: free-graft versus pedicled skin-flap reconstruction," *World Journal of Urology*, vol. 16, no. 3, pp. 175–180, 1998.

[7] G. Barbagli, S. Sansalone, R. Djinovic, G. Romano, and M. Lazzeri, "Current controversies in reconstructive surgery of the anterior urethra: a clinical overview," *International Brazilian Journal of Urology*, vol. 38, no. 3, pp. 307–316, 2012.

[8] G. Barbagli and M. Lazzeri, "Surgical treatment of anterior urethral stricture diseases: brief overview," *International Braz J Urol*, vol. 33, no. 4, pp. 461–469, 2007.

[9] D. Dubey, V. Vijjan, R. Kapoor et al., "Dorsal onlay buccal mucosa versus penile skin flap urethroplasty for anterior urethral strictures: results from a randomized prospective trial," *The Journal of Urology*, vol. 178, no. 6, pp. 2466–2469, 2007.

[10] M. Bhandari, D. Dubey, and B. S. Verma, "Dorsal or ventral placement of the preputial/penile skin onlay flap for anterior urethral strictures:does it make a difference?," *BJU International*, vol. 88, no. 1, pp. 39–43, 2001.

[11] C. E. Iselin and G. D. Webster, "Dorsal onlay urethroplasty for urethral stricture repair," *World Journal of Urology*, vol. 16, no. 3, pp. 181–185, 1998.

[12] G. Barbagli, C. Selli, A. Tosto, and E. Palminteri, "Dorsal free graft urethroplasty," *The Journal of Urology*, vol. 155, no. 1, pp. 123–126, 1996.

[13] M. Ruutu, O. Alfthan, M. Talja, and L. C. Andersson, "Cytotoxicity of latex urinary catheters," *British Journal of Urology*, vol. 57, no. 1, pp. 82–87, 1985.

[14] J. N. Nacey, A. G. S. Tulloch, and A. F. Ferguson, "Catheter-induced urethritis: a comparison between latex and silicone catheters in a prospective clinical trial," *British Journal of Urology*, vol. 57, no. 3, pp. 325–328, 1985.

[15] N. Lumen, P. Hoebeke, P. Willemsen, B. De Troyer, R. Pieters, and W. Oosterlinck, "Etiology of urethral stricture disease in the 21st century," *The Journal of Urology*, vol. 182, no. 3, pp. 983–987, 2009.

[16] S. W. Waxman and A. F. Morey, "Management of urethral strictures," *The Lancet*, vol. 367, no. 9520, pp. 1379-1380, 2006.

[17] S. Kulkarni, J. Kulkarni, S. Surana, and P. M. Joshi, "Management of panurethral stricture," *Urologic Clinics of North America*, vol. 44, no. 1, pp. 67–75, 2017.

[18] K. J. Carney and J. W. McAninch, "Penile circular fasciocutaneous flaps to reconstruct complex anterior urethral strictures," *The Urologic Clinics of North America*, vol. 29, no. 2, pp. 397–409, 2002.

[19] D. E. Andrich, T. J. Greenwell, and A. R. Mundy, "The problems of penile urethroplasty with particular reference to 2-

stage reconstructions," *The Journal of Urology*, vol. 170, no. 1, pp. 87–89, 2003.

[20] J. M. Whitson, J. W. McAninch, S. P. Elliott, and N. F. Alsikafi, "Long-term efficacy of distal penile circular fasciocutaneous flaps for single stage reconstruction of complex anterior urethral stricture disease," *The Journal of Urology*, vol. 179, no. 6, pp. 2259–2264, 2008.

[21] H. A. Aldaqadossi, H. Shaker, Y. Kotb, H. Youssof, and S. Elgamal, "Penile fasciocutaneous flap urethroplasty for the reconstruction of pediatric long anterior urethral stricture," *Journal of Pediatric Urology*, vol. 14, no. 6, pp. 555.e1–555.e6, 2018.

[22] A. F. Morey, L. K. Tran, and L. M. Zinman, "Q-flap reconstruction of panurethral strictures," *BJU International*, vol. 86, no. 9, pp. 1039–1042, 2000.

[23] L. Boccon-Gibod and B. Le Portz, "One-stage urethroplasty for urethral stricture. Free full thickness skin graft versus cutaneous island flap urethroplasty," *European Urology*, vol. 10, no. 1, pp. 32–35, 1984.

[24] G. Barbagli, E. Palminteri, S. D. Stefani, and M. Lazzeri, "Harvesting buccal mucosal grafts: the authors present a simple, safe, and reliable technique for harvesting buccal mucosa that is based on sound anatomic principles and is reproducible in the hands of any surgeon," *Contemporary Urology*, vol. 18, pp. 16–27, 2006.

[25] B. M. Browne and A. J. Vanni, "Use of alternative techniques and grafts in urethroplasty," *The Urologic Clinics of North America*, vol. 44, no. 1, pp. 127–140, 2017.

[26] Y. J. Lee and S. W. Kim, "Current management of urethral stricture," *Korean Journal of Urology*, vol. 54, no. 9, pp. 561–569, 2013.

[27] S. Kulkarni, G. Barbagli, S. Sansalone, and M. Lazzeri, "One-sided anterior urethroplasty: a new dorsal onlay graft technique," *BJU International*, vol. 104, no. 8, pp. 1150–1155, 2009.

[28] G. Barbagli, S. Sansalone, G. Romano, and M. Lazzeri, "Ventral onlay oral mucosal graft bulbar urethroplasty," *BJU International*, vol. 108, no. 7, pp. 1218–1231, 2011.

[29] A. Meneghini, A. Cacciola, L. Cavarretta, G. Abatangelo, P. Ferrarrese, and A. Tasca, "Bulbar urethral stricture repair with buccal mucosa graft urethroplasty," *European Urology*, vol. 39, no. 3, pp. 264–267, 2001.

[30] D. E. Andrich, C. J. Leach, and A. R. Mundy, "The Barbagli procedure gives the best results for patch urethroplasty of the bulbar urethra," *BJU International*, vol. 88, no. 4, pp. 385–389, 2001.

[31] A. W. El-Kasaby, M. Fath-Alla, A. M. Noweir, M. R. El-Halaby, W. Zakaria, and M. H. El-Beialy, "The use of buccal mucosa patch graft in the management of anterior urethral strictures," *Journal of Urology*, vol. 149, no. 2, pp. 276–278, 1993.

56

Scrotal Skin Metastases Revealing a Prostatic Adenocarcinoma

Idriss Ziani,[1] Zayd El Boukili El Makhoukh,[1] Ahmed Ibrahimi,[1] Omar Bellouki,[1] Jihane Benahmed,[2] Yasmine Laraqui,[3] Fouad Zouidia,[3] Hachem El Sayegh,[1] Lounis Benslimane,[1] and Yassine Nouini[1]

[1]*Department of urological surgery "A"-Ibn Sina University Hospital RABAT-Faculty of Medicine of RABAT, Mohammed V University, Rabat, Morocco*
[2]*Department of dermatology and venereology-Ibn Sina University Hospital RABAT-Faculty of Medicine of RABAT, Mohammed V University, Rabat, Morocco*
[3]*Department of Anatomopathology and Cytology-Ibn Sina University Hospital RABAT-Faculty of Medicine of RABAT, Mohammed V University, Rabat, Morocco*

Correspondence should be addressed to Idriss Ziani; idrissziani20@gmail.com

Academic Editor: Apul Goel

Introduction. Prostate cancer is the most common cancer in men. Cutaneous metastasis from prostate cancer is an unusual clinical finding. Scrotal skin metastasis revealing a prostate adenocarcinoma is even rarer. *Case Report.* We report the case of a 78-year-old patient, who initially consulted for nonspecific scrotal skin lesions evolving for 4 months. Patient's past history revealed urinary disorders. Physical examination and PSA levels led to perform a prostate biopsy, and the diagnosis of prostate adenocarcinoma was made. Bone scintigraphy showed that the cancer has spread to the bones. Imaging studies showed that the cutaneous lesions were limited to the scrotal wall. Cutaneous metastasis was suspected and was proven on skin biopsy. The patient received second-generation hormone therapy with good clinical and biological outcomes. *Discussion.* Based on literature review of nearly 2,500 skin metastases, we found that only 436 were spreading from the genitourinary tract. Skin metastasis from prostate adenocarcinoma is a rare entity with a low incidence rate (0.36%). *Conclusion.* Skin metastases, and especially in the scrotum, are exceptional in prostate cancer. However, in any patient with a prostate adenocarcinoma, nonspecific cutaneous lesions should lead to perform skin biopsy in order to identify and initiate treatment of cutaneous metastases.

1. Introduction

According "Cancer Statistics" from 2019 [1], around 174,650 new cases of prostate adenocarcinoma have been reported in men (20%), with very variable mortality rates [2]. In 2018, the highest death rates were recorded in Central America (10.7 per 100,000 inhabitants), followed by Australia and New Zealand (10.2) and Western Europe (10.1) [2]. The 5-year relative survival rate for localized and regional prostate adenocarcinomas is 100%, compared to 30.5% for metastatic ones [3].

The most common metastatic sites are the pelvic lymph nodes, bones, and lungs. Other abdominal and thoracic sites are very rarely reported [4].

Skin metastases are a rare entity with a recorded frequency of 0.7 to 9% of all metastatic malignancies [5].

Despite the fact that prostate cancer is the most common in men, it is exceptionally presented with skin metastases with a published incidence rate of 0.36% [6].

We illustrate through this case report of a rare occurrence of scrotal metastasis revealing prostate adenocarcinoma.

To our knowledge, this is the first observation of scrotal metastases from a prostate adenocarcinoma published in the literature.

2. Case Report

A 78-year-old man, with no notable medical history, consults for painless scrotal lesions evolving for 4 months, without any other signs.

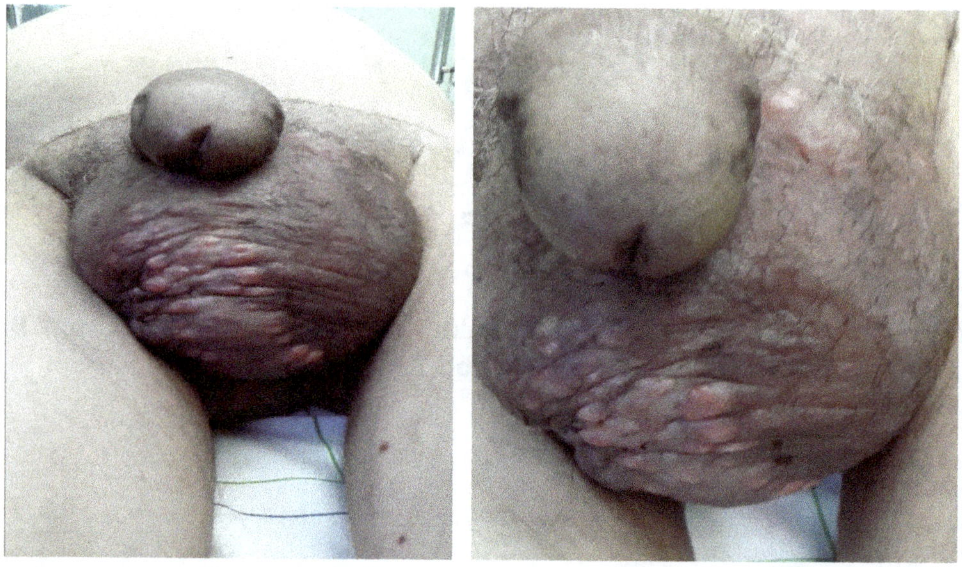

Figure 1: Clinical image of scrotal lesions palpable, firm, soft, and mobile subcutaneous nodules.

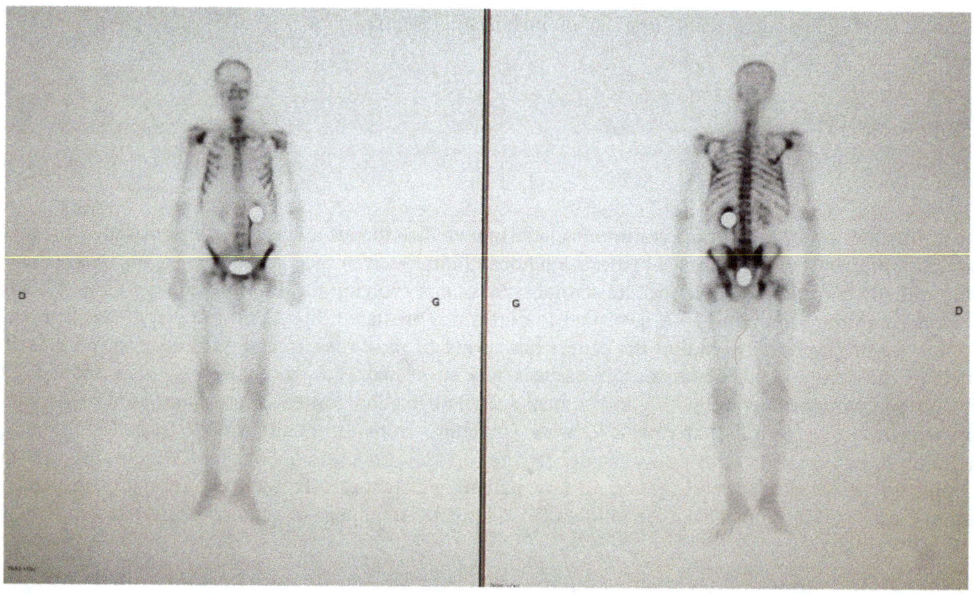

Figure 2: Bone scintigraphy showing several metastatic lesions, including in the lumbar spine.

The patient reported lower urinary tract symptoms that started 8 months ago, associated to rapidly progressive bones pain, especially in the pelvis, a 10 kg weight loss in 2 months, and deterioration of general condition. Physical examination showed soft, mobile, subcutaneous nodules, and erythematous papules of different sizes (0.5 to 1.5 cm in diameter) in the scrotum (Figure 1).

Abnormal digital rectal examination of the prostate with high PSA levels (321 ng/mL) led to perform a prostate biopsy and the diagnosis of prostate adenocarcinoma was made with a Gleason score of 10 (5 + 5) with perineural invasion. Bone scintigraphy revealed bone metastases, which were also identified on the MRI, a lumbar epiduritis was also noted (Figures 2 and 3). Chest and abdominopelvic CT-scan showed no other metastases. At this point of the investigation, scrotal skin metastasis was suspected. The skin biopsy revealed carcinoma cells proliferation organized in a thin stroma. The cells had an abundant cytoplasm with a monomorphic nucleus, some with a nucleolus. This description was compatible with a metastasic scrotal location of a prostate adenocarcinoma. PSA immunohistochemistry (IHC) was positive which confirms the prostatic origin (Figures 4 and 5).

Radiotherapy was urgently performed to treat spinal cord compression. Androgen suppression therapy has been indicated combining an LH-RH analog with second-generation hormone therapy. Abiraterone acetate was used given the high metastatic volume of the cancer. After 3 months, PSA levels dropped to 45 ng/mL

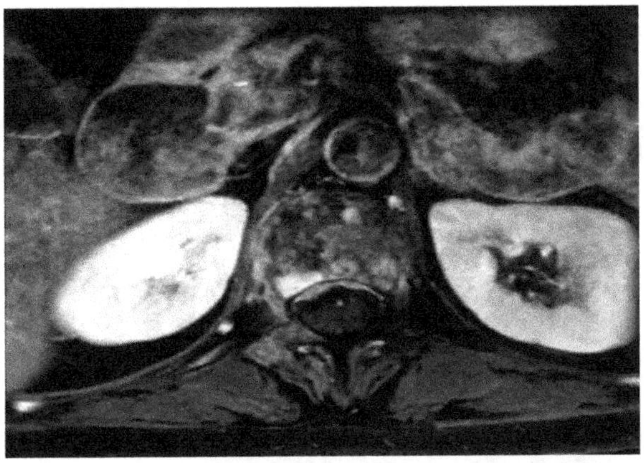

FIGURE 3: Axial section of an MRI in weighted sequence T1 with gadolinium injection showing irregular contrast uptake of epidural space with heterogeneity of the bone structure vertebral.

and a considerable regression of scrotal skin lesions was noted (Figure 6).

3. Discussion

Most common metastatic sites of prostate adenocarcinoma are bones, lungs, liver, and adrenal glands. Skin metastases are rare and usually appear as nodular lesions involving the suprapubic area and the anterior aspect of the thighs [7]. Skin metastases are considered a marker of advanced disease and are correlated with a poor prognosis with an average survival of 6 months [8].

In 2004, Mueller reviewed all the literature on skin metastases of genitourinary origin. Of nearly 2,500 skin metastases, only 436 were from the urogenital tract. He established the incidence rate of skin metastases from prostate cancer at 0.36% [6].

Based on our literature review, we found 59 articles documenting 71 cases of skin metastases. The average age was 67, with extremes of 50 to 81. In 63% of cases, the diagnosis was already known, but it was not specified in 21%. In only 15% of cases, the skin lesions led to the diagnosis of primary prostate cancer [9, 10], which is the case for our patient.

Small cell carcinoma, a very undifferentiated histological form of prostate cancer, is known to have a high metastatic potential with various reported cases of cutaneous metastatic tumors [11, 12].

Four mechanisms of metastasis in prostate adenocarcinoma were identified: local extension from an underlying tumor, implantation in a surgical scar, lymphatic spread, and hematogenous spread.

Skin metastasis is a complex process. Theoretically, the metastatic cells will circulate in the blood or lymphatic vessels and extravasate into dermis in order to proliferate to form the metastatic mass [13].

The clinical presentation can be variable; usually, it appears as erythematous subcutaneous nodules [14, 15]. The unusual, painful erysipelas-like appearance of extensive metastatic lesions was noted [16]. Less often, it may be associated to telangiectasias [17].

Cutaneous metastases are a diagnostic challenge to the pathologists. In prostate adenocarcinoma, skin lesions are reported to be similar to the primary tumor, including dermal invasion with undifferentiated carcinoma cells, often with a clearly visible Grenz area and nuclear atypia characterized by hyperchromasia and prominent eosinophilic nucleoli; connective tissue can also be infiltrated by malignant cells [9, 18]. In addition, immunohistochemistry has been useful to confirm the prostatic origin of atypical metastatic sites. The PSA, a protein normally produced by prostate cells, has been widely used as an immunohistochemical marker, as almost 97% of prostatic metastases can express it [19]. Human Ki-67 protein and CD10 can also be useful as they are often associated with cell proliferation, aggressive migration, and advanced diseases [20, 21].

A particular entity of metastatic skin lesion, described in 1949, is Sister Mary Joseph's nodule. A separate entity defined by nodular metastasis located under the umbilical subcutaneous skin. The nodule is often described as erythematous, firm, elastic, painful, and irregular. It can also appear as an eroded and bloody vascular mass. In 40% of cases, it is a primary malignant tumor. It can also be found in endometriosis (30%) and metastatic skin lesions (20%) [22]. The most common origins of this very rare entity are gastrointestinal and genitourinary tracts.

Therapeutically, many options are reported to manage prostate adenocarcinoma with skin metastases. Mainly, it is a palliative treatment based on tumor excision, radiotherapy, intralesional chemotherapy and treatment of primary neoplasia (i.e., chemotherapy, hormonal, or surgical treatments) [9–22].

In our observation, our patient was treated by second-generation hormone therapy without local treatment of scrotal metastases with good clinical and biological outcomes.

Our case presents the peculiarity of the scrotal localization from a metastatic prostate adenocarcinoma. To the best of our knowledge, it is the first case report in the literature for this particular metastatic site. On the other hand, the fact that skin metastases have appeared before the initial diagnosis of prostate cancer means that dermatologists may be the first to discover the disease. This form of revelation were reported in only 15% of published case reports. Another particular aspect of our case is the regression of the scrotal skin lesions after administration of systemic treatment with second-generation hormone therapy which raises the possibility of systemic preservative treatment for this type of metastasis.

4. Conclusion

Skin metastases in prostate cancer are exceptional. The incidence prostate adenocarcinoma with skin metastases is 0.36% of all skin metastases of genitourinary origin.

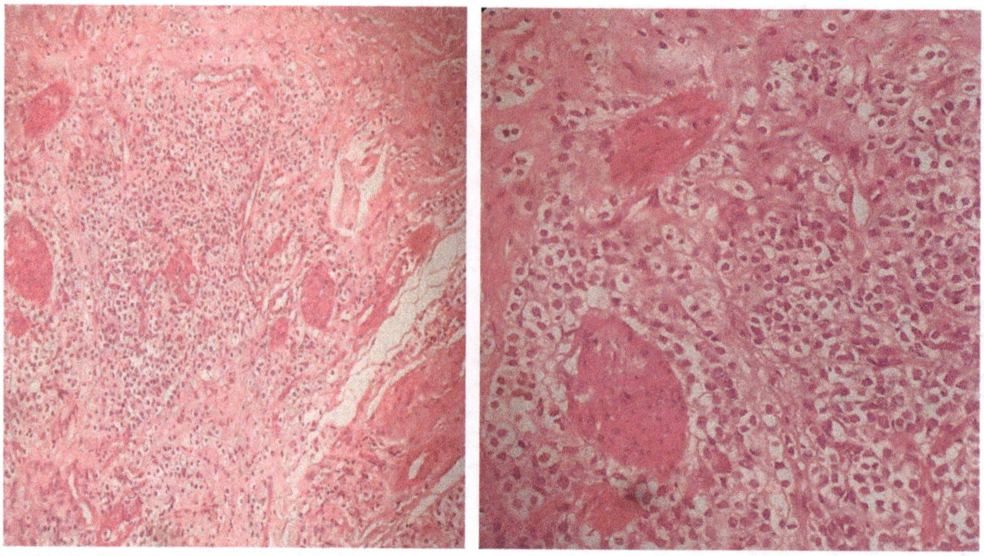

FIGURE 4: A carcinomatous tumor proliferation located in a small cell stroma, a cytoplasmic shelter, and a monomorphic nucleus sometimes nucleated in the scrotal skin tissue.

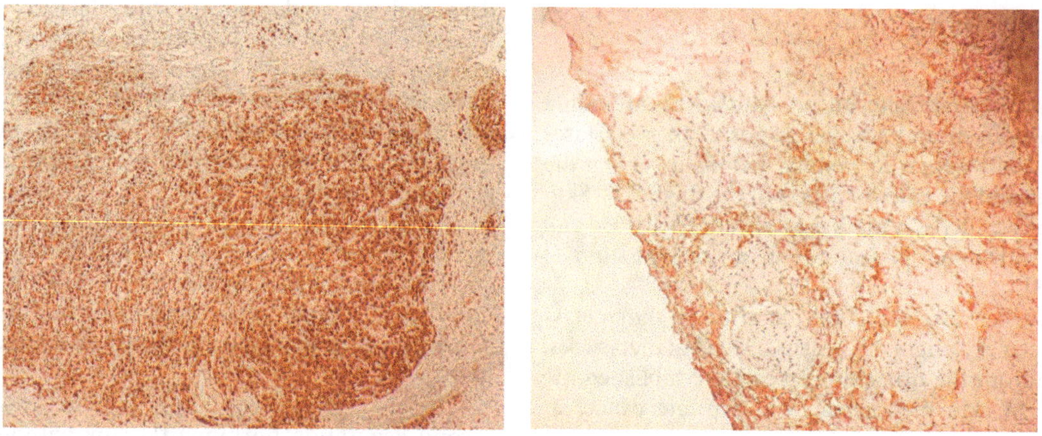

(a) (b)

FIGURE 5: (a) Immunohistochemistry (G ×100): positive labeling with anti-PSA antibody. (b) Immunohistochemistry (×40): positive labeling with anti-PSA antibody with image of perineural neoplastic invasion.

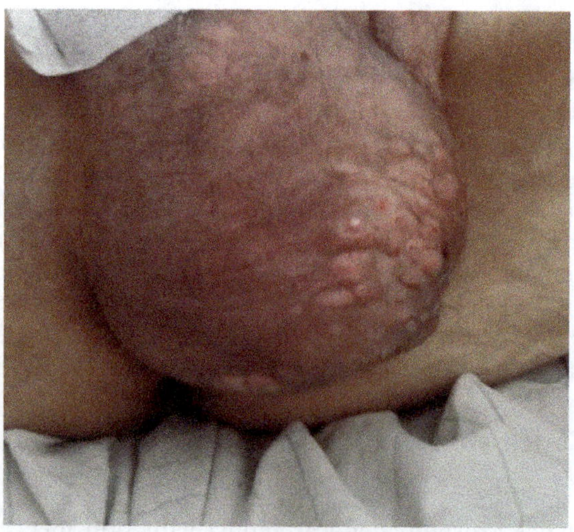

FIGURE 6: Regression of skin nodules after hormone therapy.

Of those, a scrotal localization is even more exceptional. However, in any patient with a prostate adenocarcinoma, nonspecific cutaneous lesions should lead to perform skin biopsy in order to identify and initiate treatment of cutaneous metastases. Given their rarity in the literature, their management has not yet been codified.

References

[1] R. L. Siegel, K. D. Miller, and A. Jemal, "Cancer Statistics, 2019," *CA: A Cancer Journal for Clinicians*, vol. 69, no. 1, pp. 7–34, 2018.

[2] J. Ferlay, M. Ervik, F. Lam et al., "Global cancer observatory: cancer today. Lyon, France: International Agency for Research on Cancer," February 2019, https://gco.iarc.fr/today.

[3] Cancer Stat Facts, *Prostate cancer*, National Cancer Institute, 2009–2015, https://seer.cancer.gov/statfacts/html/prost.html.

[4] L. Bubendorf, A. Schöpfer, U. Wagner et al., "Metastatic patterns of prostate cancer: an autopsy study of 1,589 patients," *Human Pathology*, vol. 31, no. 5, pp. 578–583, 2000.

[5] U. Gül, A. Kiliç, M. Gönül, S. KülcüCakmak, and C. Erinçkan, "Spectrum of Cutaneous metastases in 1287 cases of internal Malignancies: a study from Turkey," *Acta Dermato-Venereologica*, vol. 87, no. 2, pp. 160–162, 2007.

[6] T. J. Mueller, H. Wu, R. E. Greenberg et al., "Skin metastases of genitourinary malignancies," *Urology*, vol. 63, pp. 1021–1026, 2004.

[7] C. Jones and T. Rosen, "Multiple red nodules on lower abdomen," *Archives of Dermatology*, vol. 128, no. 11, pp. 1538–1538, 1992.

[8] S. Q. Wang, P. S. Mecca, P. L. Myskowski, and S. F. Slovin, "Scrotal and penile papules and plaques as the initial manifestation of a cutaneous metastasis of adenocarcinoma of the prostate: case report and review of the literature," *Journal of Cutaneous Pathology*, vol. 35, no. 7, pp. 681–684, 2008.

[9] N. Abrol, A. Seth, and P. Chattergee, "Cutaneous metastasis of prostate carcinoma to neck and upper chest," *Indian Journal of Pathology and Microbiology*, vol. 54, no. 2, pp. 394-395, 2011.

[10] J. Thivolet, C. Molinie, G. Moulin, and J. Proust, "Les métastases de la verge au cours du cancer prostatique," *Dermatology*, vol. 130, no. 4, pp. 221–230, 1965.

[11] Y. Yildirim, Y. Akcay, O. Ozyilkan, and B. Celasun, "Prostate small cell carcinoma and skin metastases: a rare entity," *Medical Principles and Practice*, vol. 17, no. 3, pp. 250–252, 2008.

[12] M. Kaplan, I. H. Atakan, S. Bilgi, and O. Inci, "Case report: subcutaneous metastasis from small cell carcinoma of the prostate," *International Urology and Nephrology*, vol. 39, no. 1, pp. 157–160, 2007.

[13] D. P. Lookingbill, N. Spangler, and F. M. Sexton, "Skin involvement as the presenting sign of internal carcinoma," *Journal of the American Academy of Dermatology*, vol. 22, no. 1, pp. 19–26, 1990.

[14] N. Ali, M. Ali, I. Sabir, R. Azhar, and S. Mansoor, "Skin metastasis from prostate adenocarcinoma," *Journal of the College of Physicians and Surgeons–Pakistan: Jcpsp*, vol. 13, no. 1, pp. 53-54, 2003.

[15] E. P. Duran, A. Paradela, M. C. Fariña et al., "Cutaneous metastases from prostatic carcinoma," *Journal of Surgical Oncology*, vol. 62, no. 2, pp. 144–147, 1996.

[16] C. S. Ng, "Carcinoma erysipeloides from prostate cancer presenting as cellulitis," *Cutis*, vol. 65, no. 4, pp. 215-216, 2000.

[17] S. Reddy, R. H. Bang, and M. E. Contreras, "Telangiectatic cutaneous metastasis from carcinoma of the prostate," *The British Journal of Dermatology*, vol. 156, no. 3, pp. 598–600, 2007.

[18] G. Brown, D. Kurtzman, F. Lian, and J. Sligh, "Eruptive nodules of the head and neck: a case report of metastatic prostate cancer," *Dermatology Online Journal*, vol. 20, no. 2, 2014.

[19] T. Sheridan, M. Herawi, J. I. Epstein, and P. B. Illei, "The role of P501S and PSA in the diagnosis of metastatic adenocarcinoma of the prostate," *The American Journal of Surgical Pathology*, vol. 31, no. 9, pp. 1351–1355, 2007.

[20] M. A. Dall'Era, L. D. True, A. F. Siegel, M. P. Porter, T. M. Sherertz, and A. Y. Liu, "Differential expression of CD10 in prostate cancer and its clinical implication," *BMC Urology*, vol. 7, no. 1, 2007.

[21] R. Li, K. Heydon, M. E. Hammond et al., "Ki-67 staining index predicts distant metastasis and survival in locally advanced prostate cancer treated with radiotherapy: an analysis of Patients in radiation therapy Oncology Group Protocol 86-10," *Clinical Cancer Research*, vol. 10, no. 12, pp. 4118–4124, 2004.

[22] R. Gabriele, M. Conte, F. Egidi, and M. Borghese, "Umbilical metastases: current viewpoint," *World Journal of Surgical Oncology*, vol. 3, no. 1, p. 13, 2005.

Primary Paratesticular Leiomyosarcoma: A Case Report and Literature Review

Zeineb Naimi,[1,2] **Semia Zarraa**,[2] **Salma Kammoun**,[3] **Safia Yahyaoui**,[2] **Maha Driss**,[3] **and Chiraz Nasr**[2]

[1] *University of Tunis El Manar, Faculty of Medicine of Tunis, 1007 Tunis, Tunisia*
[2] *Department of Radiation Oncology, Salah Azaiez Institute, 1006 Tunis, Tunisia*
[3] *Department of Pathology, Salah Azaiez Institute, 1006 Tunis, Tunisia*

Correspondence should be addressed to Zeineb Naimi; zeinebnaimi89@gmail.com

Academic Editor: Fumitaka Koga

Paratesticular soft tissue sarcomas are very rare malignant mesenchymal tumors. With only few cases reported in the literature, data regarding diagnostic and management of these tumors are limited. We reported a case of primary paratesticular leiomyosarcoma in a 72-year-old man complaining of a progressively growing painless right scrotal mass. The patient underwent radical inguinal right orchiectomy and adjuvant 3D conformal radiotherapy to the tumor bed including the surgical scar. The prescription dose was 54 Gy, and no pelvic irradiation was performed. He remained free of recurrence for the last 16 months.

1. Introduction

Soft tissue sarcomas of the genitourinary tract are rare malignant tumors accounting for less than 2% of all urological tumors [1, 2]. More specifically, primary sarcomas of the paratesticular tissue are very uncommon with only around 500 cases described in the literature [3, 4]. Due to their low prevalence, medical research remains difficult, and prospective trials are unfeasible. Literature data only consist of few individual case-reports and very small heterogeneous series. The most commonly reported histological subtypes are liposarcoma, followed by leiomyosarcoma, and rhabdomyosarcoma [4]. Here, we report a case of primary paratesticular leiomyosarcoma in a 72-year-old man who underwent radical right orchiectomy and adjuvant radiotherapy.

2. Case Presentation

A 72-year-old man with past medical history of hypertension and atrial fibrillation presented to the hospital with a progressively growing painless swelling in his right hemiscrotum as a chief complaint. No lower urinary tract symptoms were reported. Physical examination revealed a 3 cm firm-to-hard mass, isolated from the epididymis. Right epididymis and testis were normal. Scrotal ultrasound revealed a 4×3 right extra testicular heterogeneous lesion with peripheral vascularity. The patient underwent radical right inguinal orchiectomy. Grossly, the resected specimen measured 9 cm, showing a 3 cm testis covered by intact tunicae and a distant white surface mass measuring 2 cm. Four satellite nodules were associated, ranging from 2 to 5 mm. Combined histological examination and immunohistochemical study revealed a primary paratesticular grade 1 (score3) leiomyosarcoma arising from the spermatic cord (Figures 1–2). Resection margins were negative. Metastatic workup included a thoracic-abdominal-pelvic computed tomography and showed no distant metastases. The patient was planned for adjuvant 3D conformal radiotherapy to the primary tumor bed (Figure 3). He was clearly informed about the risk of radiation induced infertility and did not wish for sperm banking. Planning CT scan was performed in supine position, with both arms on the chest and legs separated with a diamond-shaped device. CT images were not contrast enhanced and were acquired with a 3 mm slice thickness. Treatment planning was performed using the Varian Eclipse® treatment planning system version 13.7. Clinical

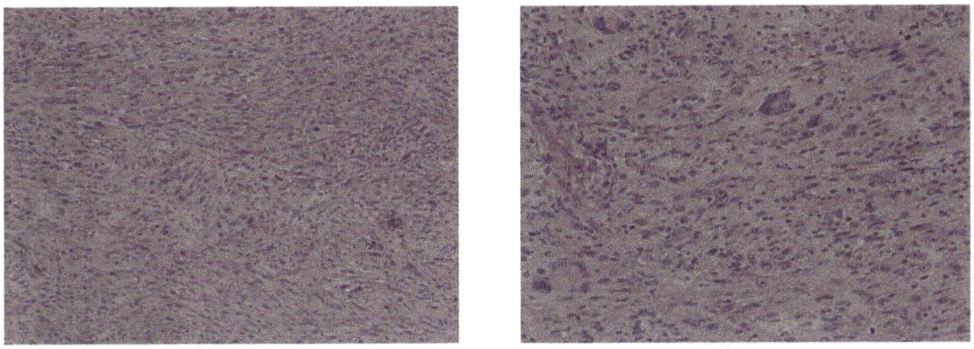

(a) (b)

Figure 1: Spindle cell proliferation arranged in interlacing fascicles (×100) (a), with marked cytonuclear atypia at high magnification (×200) (b).

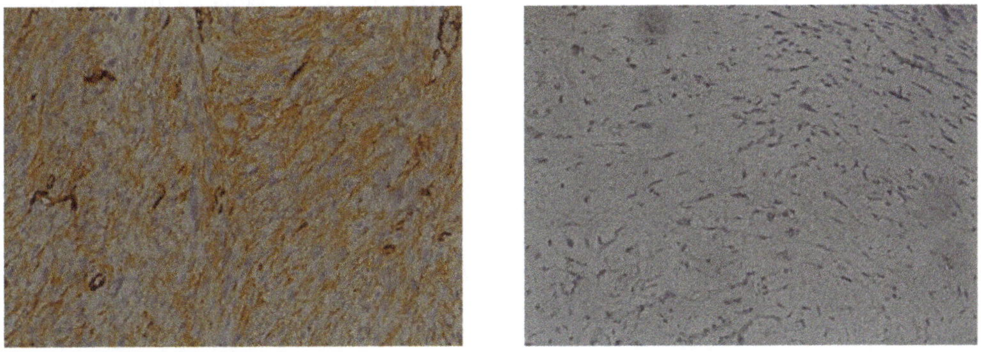

(a) (b)

Figure 2: Immunohistochemistry findings showing positive staining for caldesmon (a) and myogenin (b) negativity. Original magnification ×200.

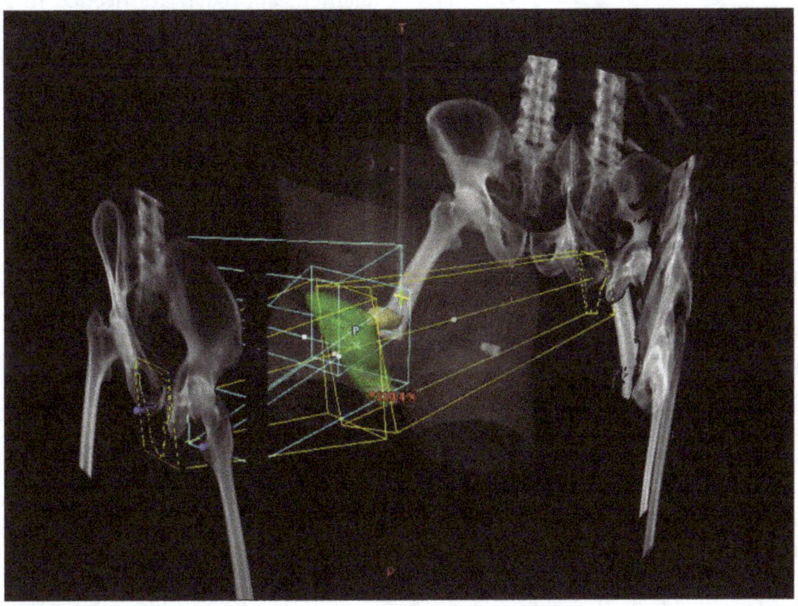

Figure 3: 3D reconstruction of radiotherapy beams.

target volume (CTV) was defined by the right scrotal and inguinal regions and included the surgical scar. Planning target volume (PTV) was defined by a 10 mm CTV expansion. No pelvic irradiation was performed. The prescription dose was 54 Gy delivered in 2 Gy single daily fraction, 5 fractions per week. Radiotherapy was delivered with 6 and 18 MV photon beams generated by the Clinac iX® Varian linear accelerator. The treatment plan was optimized using beam modifiers such as wedges, angles, collimator angles, multileaf collimators (MLC), and field-in-field technique in order to respect the organ at risk (bladder, rectum, femoral heads, penile bulb, and contralateral testis) dosimetric constraints. Radiotherapy was well tolerated, and no radiation dermatitis was reported. The patient was regularly followed-up for 16 months, with physical examination and scrotal ultrasound every 3 months and annual chest CT. He remained free of local recurrence and distant metastases for the last 16 months.

3. Discussion

Paratesticular leiomyosarcoma are unfrequently encountered malignant soft tissue tumors that may arise either from the epididymis, the scrotum, or the spermatic cord [5, 6]. Few cases have been reported in the literature with peak incidence in the 6th and 7th decades and survival rates ranging from 50% to 80% [7, 8]. Nazemi et al. have recently published a large population-based analysis of genitourinary sarcomas [4]. Authors reported a median overall survival of 130 months for paratesticular sarcomas with rhabdomysarcomas showing the best survival. Although little is known about the clinicopathologic features of these neoplasms, tumor grade seems to be the most important prognostic factor and has been related to both local recurrence and distant metastases [9, 10].

Typically, paratesticular leiomyosarcoma presents as a firm nontender scrotal painless mass, independent from the testis on physical examination. Scrotal ultrasound is the primary imaging modality for the evaluation of a scrotal mass, differentiating extratesticular from intratesticular lesions and dismissing several differential diagnoses such as epididymitis, cysts, and hydrocele [11]. However, with no specific imaging features, preoperative diagnosis remains difficult, and histological examination of the resected specimen is required for definitive diagnosis [12].

Due to the rarity of these malignancies, literature data regarding the optimal therapeutic management are inconclusive. However, most of the authors recommend radical orchiectomy with high ligation of the spermatic cord as the standard surgery [13]. Adjunctive prophylactic nodal dissection is rarely performed. With reported nodal involvement rate of up to 29% [14], Banowsky et al. investigated the role of extensive retroperitoneal nodal dissection in a series of 101 patients. No survival benefit was reported [15].

Adjuvant management of paratesticular leiomyosarcoma remains controversial. The Memorial Sloan-Kettering Cancer Center released one of the largest retrospective studies on urologic sarcomas, including 131 patients, of whom 57 presenting with paratesticular localisation [1]. However, data regarding adjuvant treatment were insufficient and therefore not included in analysis. Earlier reports showed high rates of local failure with surgery alone, suggesting the potential benefit of adjuvant radiotherapy in local control improvement [16, 17]. In a series of 18 patients from Massachusetts General Hospital, five of nine patients treated with orchiectomy alone developed locoregional failure, whereas no relapse was reported for the irradiated group [16]. Nonetheless, the median follow-up was shorter for the irradiated group (63 versus 123 months). Similar findings were reported by a retrospective analysis of 21 adult paratesticular sarcomas, showing significantly higher 5-year disease-free survival rate for patients receiving adjuvant radiotherapy (100% versus 56%; $p < 0.01$) [17]. Data regarding the optimal dose are lacking and reported radiotherapy modalities are inconsistent. The prescription dose ranged from 48 to 64 Gy, and pelvic irradiation was not systematically performed [10, 17]. By analogy with the efficacy of radiation in the management of soft tissue sarcomas in general, adjuvant radiotherapy should be considered for paratesticular leiomyosarcoma, especially for patients with high grade tumors and positive margins. Except for pediatric rhabdomyosarcoma, systemic therapy has not shown any strong evidence of benefit in the management of soft tissue sarcoma [18]. Therefore, adjuvant chemotherapy has been rarely considered for paratesticular sarcomas.

4. Conclusion

With limited available data, the diagnostic and treatment of paratesticular leiomyosarcoma remains challenging. Although radical inguinal orchiectomy is the mainstay of treatment, adjuvant radiotherapy may improve recurrence-free survival and should be considered, particularly for high-grade tumors. Multi-institutional collaboration and a centralized case management approach are needed to gain experience and better define the optimal management of these tumors.

Consent

The consent to publish this information was obtained from study participant. We confirm that written proof of consent to publish study participant's data is available when requested and at any time.

References

[1] Z. A. Dotan, R. Tal, D. Golijanin et al., "Adult genitourinary sarcoma: the 25-year Memorial Sloan-Kettering experience," *The Journal of Urology*, vol. 176, no. 5, pp. 2033–2039, 2006, discussion 8-9.

[2] P. Russo, M. S. Brady, K. Conlon et al., "Adult urological sarcoma," *The Journal of Urology*, vol. 147, no. 4, pp. 1032–1036, 1992, discussion 6-7.

[3] R. Kamitani, K. Matsumoto, T. Takeda, R. Mizuno, and M. Oya, "Optimal treatment strategy for paratesticular liposarcoma: retrospective analysis of 265 reported cases," *International Journal of Clinical Oncology*, 2020.

[4] A. Nazemi and S. Daneshmand, "Adult genitourinary sarcoma: a population-based analysis of clinical characteristics

and survival," *Urologic Oncology: Seminars and Original Investigations*, vol. 38, no. 5, pp. 334–343, 2020.

[5] A. B. Galosi, M. Scarpelli, R. Mazzucchelli et al., "Adult primary paratesticular mesenchymal tumors with emphasis on a case presentation and discussion of spermatic cord leiomyosarcoma," *Diagnostic Pathology*, vol. 9, no. 1, p. 90, 2014.

[6] J. Alfarelos, G. Gomes, F. Campos, M. Matias, A. Canelas, and M. Gonçalves, "Paratesticular leiomyosarcoma: a case report and review of the literature," *Urology Case Reports*, vol. 11, pp. 30–32, 2017.

[7] J. Moloney, J. Drumm, and D. M. Fanning, "A rare case of paratesticular leiomyosarcoma," *Clinics and practice*, vol. 2, no. 1, p. 29, 2012.

[8] L. Gatto, M. Del Gaudio, M. Ravaioli et al., "Paratesticular Mesenchymal Malignancies: A Single-Center Case Series, Clinical Management, and Review of Literature," *Integrative Cancer Therapies*, vol. 19, 2020.

[9] C. Fisher, J. R. Goldblum, J. I. Epstein, and E. Montgomery, "Leiomyosarcoma of the paratesticular region: a clinicopathologic study," *The American Journal of Surgical Pathology*, vol. 25, no. 9, pp. 1143–1149, 2001.

[10] P. H. Blitzer, D. E. Dosoretz, K. H. Proppe, and W. U. Shipley, "Treatment of malignant tumors of the spermatic cord: a study of 10 cases and a review of the literature," *The Journal of Urology*, vol. 126, no. 5, pp. 611–614, 1981.

[11] S. Haran, V. Balakrishan, and G. Neerhut, "A rare case of paratesticular leiomyosarcoma," *Case reports in urology*, vol. 2014, Article ID 715395, 4 pages, 2014.

[12] M. Secil, M. Bertolotto, L. Rocher et al., "Imaging features of paratesticular masses," *Journal of Ultrasound in Medicine*, vol. 36, no. 7, pp. 1487–1509, 2017.

[13] D. Rodríguez and A. F. Olumi, "Management of spermatic cord tumors: a rare urologic malignancy," *Therapeutic Advances in Urology*, vol. 4, no. 6, pp. 325–334, 2012.

[14] C. Catton, M. Jewett, B. O'Sullivan, and R. Kandel, "Paratesticular sarcoma: failure patterns after definitive local therapy," *The Journal of Urology*, vol. 161, no. 6, pp. 1844–1847, 1999.

[15] L. H. Banowsky and G. N. Shultz, "Sarcoma of the spermatic cord and tunics: review of the literature, case report and discussion of the role of retroperitoneal lymph node dissection," *The Journal of Urology*, vol. 103, no. 5, pp. 628–631, 1970.

[16] M. A. Fagundes, A. L. Zietman, A. F. Althausen, J. J. Coen, and W. U. Shipley, "The management of spermatic cord sarcoma," *Cancer*, vol. 77, no. 9, pp. 1873–1876, 1996.

[17] C. N. Catton, B. J. Cummings, V. Fornasier, B. O'Sullivan, I. Quirt, and D. Warr, "Adult paratesticular sarcomas: a review of 21 cases," *The Journal of Urology*, vol. 146, pp. 342–345, 1991.

[18] P. J. Woll, M. van Glabbeke, P. Hohenberger et al., "Adjuvant chemotherapy (CT) with doxorubicin and ifosfamide in resected soft tissue sarcoma (STS): Interim analysis of a randomised phase III trial," *Journal of Clinical Oncology*, vol. 25, 18_suppl, p. 10008, 2007.

Permissions

All chapters in this book were first published by Hindawi Publishing Corporation; hereby published with permission under the Creative Commons Attribution License or equivalent. Every chapter published in this book has been scrutinized by our experts. Their significance has been extensively debated. The topics covered herein carry significant findings which will fuel the growth of the discipline. They may even be implemented as practical applications or may be referred to as a beginning point for another development.

The contributors of this book come from diverse backgrounds, making this book a truly international effort. This book will bring forth new frontiers with its revolutionizing research information and detailed analysis of the nascent developments around the world.

We would like to thank all the contributing authors for lending their expertise to make the book truly unique. They have played a crucial role in the development of this book. Without their invaluable contributions this book wouldn't have been possible. They have made vital efforts to compile up to date information on the varied aspects of this subject to make this book a valuable addition to the collection of many professionals and students.

This book was conceptualized with the vision of imparting up-to-date information and advanced data in this field. To ensure the same, a matchless editorial board was set up. Every individual on the board went through rigorous rounds of assessment to prove their worth. After which they invested a large part of their time researching and compiling the most relevant data for our readers.

The editorial board has been involved in producing this book since its inception. They have spent rigorous hours researching and exploring the diverse topics which have resulted in the successful publishing of this book. They have passed on their knowledge of decades through this book. To expedite this challenging task, the publisher supported the team at every step. A small team of assistant editors was also appointed to further simplify the editing procedure and attain best results for the readers.

Apart from the editorial board, the designing team has also invested a significant amount of their time in understanding the subject and creating the most relevant covers. They scrutinized every image to scout for the most suitable representation of the subject and create an appropriate cover for the book.

The publishing team has been an ardent support to the editorial, designing and production team. Their endless efforts to recruit the best for this project, has resulted in the accomplishment of this book. They are a veteran in the field of academics and their pool of knowledge is as vast as their experience in printing. Their expertise and guidance has proved useful at every step. Their uncompromising quality standards have made this book an exceptional effort. Their encouragement from time to time has been an inspiration for everyone.

The publisher and the editorial board hope that this book will prove to be a valuable piece of knowledge for researchers, students, practitioners and scholars across the globe.

List of Contributors

Katharina Mitchell
West Virginia University School of Medicine, Morgantown, WV, USA
West Virginia University Department of Urology, USA

John Barnard
West Virginia University School of Medicine, Morgantown, WV 26506, USA
Department of Urology, West Virginia University School of Medicine, Morgantown, WV 26506, USA
West Virginia University, Department of Urology, Morgantown, WV, USA
West Virginia University Department of Urology, USA

Julian Fazi, David Adkins, Jennifer Knight and Adam Luchey
Department of Urology, West Virginia University, Morgantown, WV 26505, USA

Nassib Abou Heidar
Department of Surgery, Division of Urology, American University of Beirut Medical Center, Beirut, Lebanon

Hussein Elsemesmani, Ahmad Elamine and Mustafa Natout
Department of Radiology, American University of Beirut Medical Center, Beirut, Lebanon

Mishal AlArifi
College of Medicine, Imam Abdulrahman Bin Faisal University, Dammam, Saudi Arabia

Magdi Al-Gahwary and Mohamed Gomha
Department of Urology, King Fahad Specialist Hospital, Dammam, Saudi Arabia

Adama Ouattara, Abdoul Karim Paré, Gnimdou Botcho, Abdoul Aziz Ouédraogo, Amidou Bako, Rigobert Kiba and Timothée Kambou
Division of Urology, Souro Sanou University Teaching Hospital, Bobo-Dioulasso, Burkina Faso

Aristide F. Kaboré, Clotaire Yaméogo and Désiré Ky
Division of Urology, Yalgado Ouedraogo University Teaching Hospital, Ouagadougou, Burkina Faso

Zakari Nikiéma
Division of Radiology and Imaging, Souro Sanou University Teaching Hospital, Bobo-Dioulasso, Burkina Faso

Bashir Yunusa, Kalamon Wullie, Soeghen E. Willie, Solomane Konneh, Swaliho Sherriff and Edit Ikpi
Department of Surgery, Liberia College of Physicians and Surgeons, Monrovia, Liberia

Ayun Cassell
Département d'Urologie et d'Andrologie, Hôpital Général de Grand Yo, Dakar, Senegal

Faten Gargouri
Department of Pathology, Military Hospital of First Instruction of Tunis, Tunisia
Faculty of Medicine of Tunis, University Tunis El Manar, Department of Pathology, Military Hospital of First Instruction of Tunis, Tunisia

Prodromos Philippou, Christos Kitsios and Maria Miliatou
St George's Medical School, University of Nicosia, Nicosia, Cyprus
Apollonion Hospital, Nicosia, Cyprus

Christiana Poullou and Pavlos Konstantinou
Histopathology and Cytology Laboratory Services, Nicosia, Cyprus
School of Medicine, European University of Cyprus, Cyprus

Edward Assaf and Imad Ghantous
Urology Department, St George Hospital University Medical Center, University of Balamand, Beirut, Lebanon

Rawad Abou Zahr
Urology Department, St George Hospital University Medical Center, University of Balamand, Beirut, Lebanon
Urology Department, Erasme Hospital, Université Libre de Bruxelles, Brussels, Belgium

Elie Ghabi
Faculty of Medicine and Medical Sciences, St George Hospital University Medical Center, University of Balamand, Beirut, Lebanon

Amanda E. Kahn and David D. Thiel
Department of Urology, Mayo Clinic, Jacksonville, FL, USA

Kevin J. Wu
Department of Pathology, Mayo Clinic, Jacksonville, FL, USA

Chrysovalantis Gkekas, Vasileios Kalyvas, Evangelos N. Symeonidis, Apostolos Malioris and Michail Papathanasiou
Department of Urology, 424 General Military Hospital of Thessaloniki, Thessaloniki, Greece

Nikolaos Kalinderis, KyriakosMoisidis and Konstantinos Hatzimouratidis
2nd Department of Urology, Aristotle University ofThessaloniki, Thessaloniki, Greece

Ali Tavoosian, Sana Ahmadi and Seyed Mohammad Kazem Aghamir
Urology Research Center, Tehran University of Medical Sciences, Tehran, Iran

Ankur Choksi, Benjamin Press, Cayce Nawaf and Thomas V. Martin
Department of Urology, Yale University School of Medicine, New Haven, CT, USA

Shannon Longyear and Marc Ferrante
Department of Radiology and Biomedical Imaging, Yale University School of Medicine, New Haven, CT, USA

Mohamed Ali Nouioui, Tarek Taktak, Seif Mokadem and Houssem Mediouni
Department of Urology, Military Hospital of First Instruction of Tunis, University of Tunis El Manar, Tunisia

Cale E. Leeson
Division of Urology, Department of Surgery, University of Ottawa, Ottawa, Ontario, Canada

Brianna-Lee Beaudry
Faculty of Medicine, Northern Ontario School of Medicine, Thunder Bay, Ontario, Canada

Geoffrey R. Wignall
Division of Urology, Grey Bruce Health Services, Owen Sound, ON, Canada

Spyridon Paparidis, Antonios Katsimantas and Nikolaos Ferakis
Urology Department, Korgialenio-Benakio Hellenic Red Cross Hospital, Athanasaki 1, 11526 Athens, Greece

Dimitrios Oikonomidis
Second Cardiology Department, Korgialenio-Benakio Hellenic Red Cross Hospital, Athanasaki 1, 11526 Athens, Greece

Sabrina L. Noyes
Spectrum Health, Grand Rapids, MI, USA

Jacob W. Bruinius
Spectrum Health, Grand Rapids, MI, USA
Helix Scribes Solutions, Grand Rapids, MI, USA

Karl J. Dykema
Van Andel Research Institute, Grand Rapids, MI, USA

Bin Tean Teh
National Cancer Centre Singapore, Singapore

Brian R. Lane
Spectrum Health, Grand Rapids, MI, USA
Michigan State University College of Human Medicine, Grand Rapids, MI, USA

Jaisukh Kalathia, Kaushal Patel and Santosh Agrawal
Department of Urology and Kidney Transplantation, Fortune Urology Clinic, India

Mizuki Kasahara, Tomo Shimizu, Hiroshi Aoki, Mizuho Okawa, Fumito Yamabe, Hideyuki Kobayashi, Koichi Nagao, Koichi Nakajima and Yozo Mitsui
Department of Urology, Toho University Faculty of Medicine, 143-8540 Tokyo, Japan

Jamil S. Syed, Cayce B. Nawaf, Ghazal Khajir, Darryl T. Martin, Michael S. Leapman, Preston C. Sprenkle and Kamyar Ghabili
Department of Urology, Yale University School of Medicine, New Haven, CT, USA

Nathan Paulson, Angelique Levi and Peter A. Humphrey
Department of Pathology, Yale University School of Medicine, New Haven, CT, USA

John Onofrey and Jeffrey C. Weinreb
Department of Radiology and Biomedical Imaging, Yale University School of Medicine, New Haven, CT, USA

Kazuya Kashiyama, Motoi Nakano, Akihito Higashi and Shoko Ashizuka
Department of Plastic and Reconstructive Surgery, Nagasaki Harbor Medical Center, Nagasaki, Japan
Department of Plastic and Reconstructive Surgery, Nagasaki University Hospital, Nagasaki, Japan

Yuki Moriuchi, Atsuhiko Iwao and Katsumi Tanaka
Department of Plastic and Reconstructive Surgery, Nagasaki University Hospital, Nagasaki, Japan

Charalampos Mavridis, George Georgiadis, Iordanis Skamagkas, Ioannis Heretis and Charalampos Mamoulakis
Department of Urology, University General Hospital of Heraklion, University of Crete, Medical School, Heraklion, Crete, Greece

Eleni D. Lagoudaki, Anastasios V. Koutsopoulos
Department of Pathology, University General Hospital of Heraklion, University of Crete, Medical School, Heraklion, Crete, Greece

John Michael Nesemann
University of California Los Angeles, David Geffen School of Medicine, Los Angeles, USA

Kathy Huen
Department of Urology, University of California Los Angeles David Geffen School of Medicine, Los Angeles, USA

Jonathan Bergman
Olive-View UCLA Medical Center, Veterans Association Greater Los Angeles, David Geffen School of Medicine, Los Angeles, USA

Agustín Fraile Poblador, Manuel Hevia Palacios, Alberto Artiles Medina, Enrique Sanz Mayayo, Silvia García Barreras, Guillermo Fernández Conejo, Rafael Rodríguez Patrón and Javier Burgos Revilla
Urology Department, IRYCIS (Institute of Biosanitary Research of the Ramon y Cajal Hospital), Crta Colmenar Viejo, Km 9, 100,28034 Madrid, Spain

Manuel Rodríguez Vegas
Plastic Surgery Department, IRYCIS (Institute of Biosanitary Research of the Ramon y Cajal Hospital), Crta Colmenar Viejo, Km 9,100, 28034 Madrid, Spain

Varona Crespo Constatino and Ana Saiz González
Anatomic Pathology Department, IRYCIS (Institute of Biosanitary Research of the Ramon y Cajal Hospital), Crta Colmenar Viejo, Km 9, 100, 28034 Madrid, Spain

Amine Hermi, Hamza Ichaoui, Aziz Kacem, Houcem Hedhli, Ramzi Khiari and Samir Ghozzi
Faculty of Medicine of Tunis, University Tunis El Manar, Department of Urology, Military Hospital of First Instruction of Tunis, Tunisia

Tariq Hameed, Sudhir Kumar Jain, Faiz Manzar Ansari and Amrita Dua
Department of Surgery, Maulana Azad Medical College, Delhi, India

Pansy Uberoi and Forrest Jellison
San Antonio Uniformed Services Health Education Consortium, USA

Rojan Adhikari, Hari Prasad Baral, Utsav Bhattarai, Ravi Kiran Gautam, Kiran Jung Kunwar, Dipesh Shrestha and Bijay Mansingh Katwal
Department of Urology and Kidney Transplant, Shahid Dharmabhakta National Transplant Centre, Bhaktapur, Nepal

Tateki Yoshino, Ayako Itakura, Shinnosuke Fujikawa, Tomoyuki Sugitani, Kazuo Kawakami and Shota Oshima
Department of Urology, Shimane Prefectural Central Hospital, Shimane, Japan

Emi Ishibashi and Koji Kodama
Department of Radiology, Shimane Prefectural Central Hospital, Shimane, Japan

Manolis Pratsinis, Olivia Köhle, Hans-Peter Schmid and Patrick Betschart
Department of Urology, Cantonal Hospital St. Gallen, St. Gallen, Switzerland

Charlotte Düwel
Department of Urology, Klinikum Rechts der Isar, Technical University of Munich, Munich, Germany

Annette Enzler-Tschud
Department of Pathology, Cantonal Hospital St. Gallen, St. Gallen, Switzerland

Lennert Eismann, Christian G. Stief and Frank Strittmatter
Department of Urology, Ludwig-Maximilians-University, Munich, Germany

Sabine Kess
Department of Gynecology and Obstetrics, University Hospital of Heidelberg, Heidelberg, Germany

Nastaran Mahmoudnejad
Assistant Professor of Urology, Fellowship of Female Urology, Labbafinejad Hospital, Urology and Nephrology Research Center, Shahid Beheshti University of Medical Sciences (SBMU), Tehran, Iran

Alireza Zadmehr
Resident of Urology, Labbafinejad Hospital, Urology and Nephrology Research Center, Shahid Beheshti University of Medical Science (SBMU), Tehran, Iran

Mohammad Hamidi Madani
Department of Urology, Labbafinejad Hospital, Shahid Beheshti University of Medical Science (SBMU), Tehran, Iran

Masayuki Tomioka, Makoto Kawase, Daiki Kato, Manabu Takai, Koji Iinuma, Kengo Horie, Keita Nakane and Takuya Koie
Department of Urology, Gifu University Graduate School of Medicine, Gifu, Japan

Natsuko Suzui and Tatsuhiko Miyazaki
Department of Pathology, Gifu University Graduate School of Medicine, Gifu, Japan

Tatsuya Umemoto and Hidenori Zakoji
Department of Urology, Tokai University Hachioji Hospital, 1838 Ishikawa-machi, Hachioji, Tokyo 192-0032, Japan

Jun Naruse and Hideshi Miyakita
Department of Urology, Tokai University Oiso Hospital, 21-1, Gakkyo, Oiso-machi, Naka-gun, Kanagawa 259-0198, Japan

Yukio Usui
Department of Urology, Shizuoka City Shimizu Hospital, Miyakami 1231, Shimizu Ward Shizuoka City, Shizuoka 424-8636, Japan

Akira Miyajima
Department of Urology, Tokai University School of Medicine, 143 Shimokasuya, Isehara, Kanagawa 259-1193, Japan

Catti Massimo, Nappo Gerocarni Simona, Tadini Barbara, Cerchia Elisa, Ferrero Luisa and Elisabetta Teruzzi
Paediatric Urology, Città Della Salute e Della Scienza Torino, Italy

Gambella Alessandro
Pathology Unit, Department of Medical Sciences, Città Della Salute e Della Scienza Torino, Italy

Pacchioni Donatella
Pathology Unit, Città Della Salute e Della Scienza Torino, Italy

Marco Falcone, Sedigh Omidreza and Gontero Paolo
Urology Department, Città Della Salute e Della Scienza Torino, Italy

Kazuhiro Watanabe, Noboru Hara and Tsutomu Nishiyama
Department of Urology, Uonuma Institute of Community Medicine, Niigata University Medical and Dental Hospital, Urasa 4132, Minamiuonumashi, Niigata 949-7302, Japan

Go Hasegawa
Department of Pathology, Uonuma Institute of Community Medicine, Niigata University Medical and Dental Hospital, Minamiuonumashi, Niigata 949-7302, Japan

Yohei Ikeda
Department of Diagnostic Radiology, Uonuma Institute of Community Medicine, Niigata University Medical and Dental Hospital, Minamiuonuma, Niigata, Japan

Yasuhiro Hashimoto and Yuichiro Suzuki
Department of Urology, Hirosaki University Graduate School of Medicine, Aomori, Japan

Yoshiomi Hatayama
Department of Radiation Oncology, Hirosaki University Graduate School of Medicine, Aomori, Japan

Futoshi Kimura
Department of Anesthesiology, Hirosaki University Graduate School of Medicine, Aomori, Japan

Tyler L. Overholt and Robert J. Evans
Department of Urology, Wake Forest Baptist Health, USA

Christina Ross
Wake Forest Institute for Regenerative Medicine, USA

Stephen J. Walker
Department of Urology, Wake Forest Baptist Health, USA
Wake Forest Institute for Regenerative Medicine, USA

Chad Crigger and Chad Morley
West Virginia University Department of Urology, USA

Vidas Dumasius
Marietta Memorial Hospital Department of Cosmetic, Plastic and Reconstructive Surgery, USA

Masaki Murata, Kohei Inui, Moto Hasegawa and Yuki Nakagawa
Department of Urology, Uonuma Institute of Community Medicine, Niigata University Medical and Dental Hospital, Niigata, Japan

Salman Soltani
Kidney Transplantation Complications Research Center, Mashhad University of Medical Sciences, Mashhad, Iran

Mahdi Mottaghi
Students Research Committee, Faculty of Medicine, Mashhad University of Medical Sciences, Mashhad, Iran

Amir Jafarpisheh
Department of Urology, Faculty of Medicine, Mashhad University of Medical Sciences, Mashhad, Iran

Mahmoud Tavakkoli
Kidney Transplantation Complications Research Center, Mashhad University of Medical Sciences, Mashhad, Iran

George Khludenev, Akshay Reddy, Sinan Akosman and Michael J. Whalen
George Washington University School of Medicine, 2300 I St NW, Washington, DC 20052, USA

Madison Caja and Michaela Lamonde
West Virginia University School of Medicine, Morgantown, WV 26506, USA
Department of Obstetrics & Gynecology,West Virginia University School of Medicine, Morgantown, WV 26506, USA

Stanley Zaslau and Robert E. Shapiro
West Virginia University School of Medicine, Morgantown, WV 26506, USA
Department of Obstetrics & Gynecology,West Virginia University School of Medicine, Morgantown, WV 26506, USA
Department of Urology,West Virginia University School of Medicine, Morgantown, WV 26506, USA

Goran Benko and Marin Plantak
Department of Urology, Varaždin General Hospital, I. Meštrovića 1, Varaždin, Croatia

Andrina Kopjar
Department of Pathology, Varaždin General Hospital, I. Meštrovića 1, Varaždin, Croatia

Danijel Cvetko
Department of Radiology, Dubrava Clinical Hospital, Av. Gojka Šuška 6, Zagreb, Croatia

Manish Swarnkar
Department of Surgery, LN Medical College, Madhya Pradesh, 462042, Bhopal, India

Vicko Glunčić
Department of Anesthesia, Advocate Illinois Masonic Medical Center, 836 W Wellington Ave, Chicago, IL 60657, USA

Anita Lukić
Department of Anaesthesiology, Reanimatology, and Intensive Care, Varaždin General Hospital, I. Meštrovića 1, Varaždin, Croatia

Ezra Shoen, Benjamin Zollinger, Tripp Gresham, Katayoon M. Rezaei and Michael Whalen
School of Medicine and Health Sciences, The George Washington University, Washington, D.C., 20037, USA

Ahmed Osama Mohamed, Bala Eradi, Anthony Owen and Ashok Rajimwale
Department of Paediatric Surgery, Leicester Royal Infirmary, Infirmary Square, leicester, LE1 5WW, UK

Mehdi Chennoufi, Ibrahim Boukhannous, Mohamed Mokhtari, Anouar El Moudane, Mohamed Irzi, Abdelghani Ouraghi, Issam Jandou and Ali Barki
Department of Urology, Mohamed VI University Hospital Center, Mohamed I University, Oujda, Morocco

Achraf Miry
Department of Pathology, Mohamed VI University Hospital Center, Mohamed I University, Oujda, Morocco

Pathan Tanveer Khan
Department of General Surgery, JNMC, Maharashtra, 442001, Wardha, India

Mehdi Idrissi-Kaitouni and Thierry Roumeguere
Urology Department, Erasme Hospital, Université Libre de Bruxelles, Brussels, Belgium

Eric Chung
AndroUrology Centre, Brisbane QLD, Australia
University of Queensland, Princess Alexandra Hospital, Brisbane, QLD, Australia
Macquarie University Hospital, Sydney, NSW, Australia

An Uche, Chad Sila, Tad Tanoura and James Yeh
Division of Hematology/Oncology, Department of Medicine, Harbor-UCLA Medical Center, 1000WCarson St, Torrance, CA 90509, USA

Neil Bhowmick, Edwin Posadas and Robert Figlin
Division of Hematology/Oncology, Department of Medicine, Cedars-Sinai Medical Center, 8700 Beverly Blvd, Los Angeles, CA 90048, USA

Jun Gong
Division of Hematology/Oncology, Department of Medicine, Cedars-Sinai Medical Center, 8700 Beverly Blvd, AC1042B, Los Angeles, CA 90048, USA

Miguel Bonfitto
São José do Rio Preto Base Hospital/Famerp, SP, Brazil

Analaura de Oliveira Cury
Votuporanga School of Medicine, SP, Brazil

Victoria Caroline Pagelkopf and Vinicius Ramos Bezerra de Morais
São José do Rio Preto School of Medicine (Famerp), SP, Brazil

Carlos Abib Cury
Urology Sector, São José do Rio Preto School of Medicine (Famerp), SP, Brazil

Bora Özveren and Levent Türkeri
Acibadem Mehmet Ali Aydinlar University, School of Medicine, Department of Urology, Turkey

Halim Ulugöl
Acibadem Mehmet Ali Aydinlar University, School of Medicine, Department of Anesthesiology & Reanimation, Turkey

Louis Vignot, Elie Saad, Michael Peyromaure and Nicolas Barry Delongchamps
Department of Urology, Cochin Hospital, University of Paris Descartes, Paris, France

George Amoah, Roland Azorliade and Dominic Annor Mintah
Department of Surgery, Komfo Anokye Teaching Hospital, Kumasi, Ghana

Edwin M. T. Yenli
University for Development Studies-SMHS, Department of Surgery, Urology Unit, Tamale, Ghana

Patrick Opoku Manu Maison
Department of Surgery, School of Medical Sciences, UCC, Cape Coast, Ghana

Charles Kwame Adofo
Seventh Day Adventist Hospital, Dominase, Ghana

Augustina Badu-Peprah
Department of Radiology, Komfo Anokye Teaching Hospital, Kumasi, Ghana
Department of Radiology, KSMD, College of Health Sciences, KNUST, Kumasi, Ghana

Kwaku Addai Arhin Appiah
Department of Surgery, Komfo Anokye Teaching Hospital, Kumasi, Ghana
Department of Surgery, KSMD, College of Health Sciences, KNUST, Kumasi, Ghana
Kings Medical Consult (Specialist Urology Clinic), Kumasi, Ghana

Christian Kofi Gyasi-Sarpong
Department of Surgery, Komfo Anokye Teaching Hospital, Kumasi, Ghana
Department of Surgery, KSMD, College of Health Sciences, KNUST, Kumasi, Ghana

Idriss Ziani, Zayd El Boukili El Makhoukh, Ahmed Ibrahimi, Omar Bellouki, Hachem El Sayegh, Lounis Benslimane and Yassine Nouini
Department of urological surgery "A"-Ibn Sina University Hospital RABAT-Faculty of Medicine of RABAT, Mohammed V University, Rabat, Morocco

Jihane Benahmed
Department of dermatology and venereology-Ibn Sina University Hospital RABAT-Faculty of Medicine of RABAT, Mohammed V University, Rabat, Morocco

Yasmine Laraqui and Fouad Zouidia
Department of Anatomopathology and Cytology-Ibn Sina University Hospital RABAT-Faculty of Medicine of RABAT, Mohammed V University, Rabat, Morocco

Zeineb Naimi
University of Tunis El Manar, Faculty of Medicine of Tunis, 1007 Tunis, Tunisia
Department of Radiation Oncology, Salah Azaiez Institute, 1006 Tunis, Tunisia

Semia Zarraa, Safia Yahyaoui and Chiraz Nasr
Department of Radiation Oncology, Salah Azaiez Institute, 1006 Tunis, Tunisia

Salma Kammoun and Maha Driss
Department of Pathology, Salah Azaiez Institute, 1006 Tunis, Tunisia

Index

A

Abdominal Pain, 4-5, 45, 104-105, 107-108, 185

Abdominoscrotal Hydrocele, 191-193

Adenocarcinoma, 12, 68-72, 74, 115-117, 130, 141-143, 145-146, 163-168, 221-225

Antigen, 68, 72, 101, 103, 115-117, 145, 189

Antituberculosis Drugs, 131-135

B

Bacteriuria, 52-54, 110-111

Bladder Stones, 49, 51, 105, 107, 109, 156

C

Cancer Cells, 69-70, 127-129, 142, 146

Chemotherapy, 2, 23, 57, 68, 95-96, 99, 127-130, 137, 139, 141-142, 145-147, 164-165, 167-168, 178-179, 188, 196-197, 206, 223, 228-229

Collagen, 151, 196, 198, 200

Colon Cancer, 35, 68-71, 168

Colostomy, 28, 95, 152, 154, 169, 181, 183

Cutaneous Metastases, 221, 223-225

Cystectomy, 97-98, 100, 127, 130, 149, 163-165, 167-168, 194, 196-197

Cystolithotomy, 49-50, 107-109

Cystoscopy, 2, 15-16, 30, 44-46, 48-49, 51-53, 84, 98, 100-104, 108-109, 115-116, 127, 137, 141, 158, 163-164, 177, 181-182, 205-206

D

Diaphragmatic Crus, 110-114

Diaphragmatic Hernia, 4-5, 7, 110-114

E

Edema, 41, 152, 162, 192-193, 201

Embolization, 25-26, 56, 69, 198-200

Enucleation, 178-180

Epididymitis, 10, 52-53, 76

Epididymo-orchitis, 40-42, 133

Escherichia Coli, 89, 107-108, 110-111

F

Fasciocutaneous Flap, 94-95, 220

Flank Pain, 25-27, 87, 110-111, 113, 115-116, 201

G

Genomic Score, 72, 75

H

Hematuria, 1-5, 8, 14-15, 26, 44-45, 50, 52-53, 56, 82, 84, 97-98, 101, 105, 107-108, 111, 115, 131, 133, 135, 139, 141, 156, 158, 163-164, 166, 177, 194, 198-199, 201

Hepatic Atrophy, 110-112, 114

Hydronephrosis, 1, 4-6, 101, 107-108, 110-112, 115, 174, 177, 181-182

Hypertension, 4, 21, 26, 52, 87, 97, 100, 135, 169, 174, 199, 209-211, 226

I

Immune Response, 34, 131, 135

Ischemia, 30-31, 151, 160, 198-200

Ischiopubic Branch, 93, 95

K

Keratinization, 94-95

Kidney Disease, 94, 177, 206

L

Leiomyosarcoma, 196, 226, 228-229

Lesions, 13, 19-20, 22-23, 32-38, 40, 68-69, 83, 111, 116, 123-125, 127-128, 135, 164, 173-175, 185, 187, 189, 195, 212-213, 221-224, 228

Leydig Cells, 42, 76

Liposarcoma, 18-20, 173-175, 212-214

Lymph Node, 1-2, 60, 74, 92-93, 95-96, 127-128, 145, 163-164, 201, 229

Lymphadenopathy, 7, 97, 114, 128, 164, 178, 186, 194, 201-202

M

Malignant Cells, 127-128, 130-131, 223

Malignant Tumors, 77, 83, 92, 99, 229

Methylprednisolone, 131-135

O

Orchiectomy, 1, 18, 40-42, 68-70, 152, 154, 226, 228

P

Palpation, 13-14, 21, 41, 68, 87, 94, 107-108

Papilloma, 22, 137, 139

Penile Glans Necrosis, 198-199

Perforator Flap, 76-77, 81

Perineal Carcinoma, 92-93, 96

Plasmacytoma, 185, 187-190

Posterior Urethral Valves, 181, 183-184

Prostatic Artery, 198-200

Pulse Therapy, 131-136

Pyelography, 110-114

Q

Quinolones, 132-133

R

Recurrent Dysuria, 107-108

Renal Dysfunction, 111, 114, 169

S

Scrotum, 18-20, 28, 41, 67-69, 76-80, 117, 152, 154-155, 191-192, 213-214, 221-222, 228

Skin Flaps, 76-79

Skin Metastases, 221, 223, 225

Soft Tissue, 19-20, 32-33, 67, 85, 94, 151-152, 179, 185, 189, 196, 213, 226, 228-229

Spermatogenesis, 76, 192

Surgical Debridement, 151

Surgical Excision, 10, 36, 38, 65-66, 120-121, 124-125, 158, 173, 193, 208, 210, 212, 214

Surgical Repair, 4-6, 110-113

T

Testicular Tumor, 68-71

Testis, 2, 8, 18-20, 40-43, 68-71, 76-78, 191, 212, 226, 228

U

Ultrasonography, 12, 19, 48-49, 56-57, 65, 68-69, 89, 91, 102, 107-108, 174, 191, 208-209, 212-213

Ureteral Hernias, 4, 111, 114

Ureteral Loops, 111-112

Urethral Stricture, 89, 92-93, 95, 122, 134-135,

137, 215, 219-220

Urethroplasty, 92, 95, 137-140, 215-216, 218-220

Urinalysis, 4, 37, 48, 50, 86-87, 109-111

Urinary Bladder, 3, 48-49, 51, 54, 84-85, 97-98, 100-103, 107-109, 127-128, 130, 141, 145-146, 164, 167-168, 182, 193-195, 197

Urinary Retention, 2, 52, 87, 90, 107, 198

Urinary Symptoms, 48-49, 84, 115, 139, 198

Urinary Tract, 3, 8, 11, 29, 40, 43, 48-49, 51-56, 86-90, 101, 103, 106-109, 111-112, 114, 135, 141-143, 156, 158-159, 161, 166, 169, 174, 180, 182, 198, 200, 205-206, 215, 222, 226

Urothelial Carcinoma, 127, 139, 141-144, 58-159, 165, 167, 177-180

www.ingramcontent.com/pod-product-compliance
Lightning Source LLC
LaVergne TN
LVHW082134200926
848484LV00008B/2053